THE NEW TESTOSTERONE TREATMENT

THE NEW TESTOSTERONE TREATMENT

HOW YOU AND YOUR DOCTOR CAN FIGHT BREAST CANCER PROSTATE CANCER AND ALZHEIMER'S

DR. EDWARD FRIEDMAN

WITH WILLIAM CANE

FOREWORD BY PAUL SAVAGE, MD

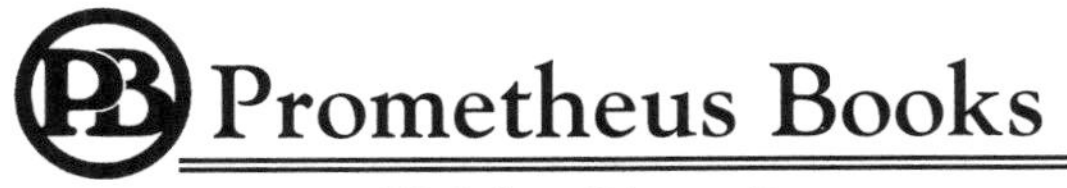

Prometheus Books
59 John Glenn Drive
Amherst, New York 14228–2119

Published 2013 by Prometheus Books

Cover design by Grace M. Conti-Zilsberger

Inquiries should be addressed to
Prometheus Books
59 John Glenn Drive
Amherst, New York 14228–2119
VOICE: 716–691–0133 • FAX: 716–691–0137
WWW.PROMETHEUSBOOKS.COM

17 16 15 14 13   5 4 3 2 1

Library of Congress Cataloging-in-Publication Data

Friedman, Edward, 1949-
The new testosterone treatment : how you and your doctor can fight breast cancer, prostate cancer, and Alzheimer's / by Edward Friedman, Ph.D. with William Cane.
p. cm.
Includes bibliographical references and index.
ISBN 978-1-61614-723-5 (pbk. : alk. paper)
ISBN 978-1-61614-724-2 (ebook)
1. Testosterone—Therapeutic use. 2. Testosterone—Physiological effect. 3. Chronic diseases—Chemotherapy. I. Cane, William. II. Title.

RM296.5.T47F75 2013
615.5--dc23

2013003789

Printed in the United States of America on acid-free paper

DISCLAIMER

The ideas, opinions, and suggestions expressed in *The New Testosterone Treatment* are intended to be used only for educational purposes. This book is sold with the understanding that the authors and publisher are not rendering medical advice of any kind, nor is this book intended to replace medical advice, nor to diagnose, prescribe, or treat any disease, condition, illness, or injury.

It is important that, before beginning any supplement or hormone replacement program, including any aspect of the program or protocols outlined herein, you receive full medical clearance from a licensed physician.

Author and publisher claim no responsibility to any person or entity for any liability, loss, or damage caused or alleged to be caused directly or indirectly as a result of the use, application, or interpretation of the material in this book.

PART 4. NEW TREATMENT PROTOCOLS: USING HORMONES TO FIGHT DISEASE

FOREWORD

I'm honored that I've been asked by my colleague Dr. Edward Friedman to introduce you to him and his work. The reason for my reaction will become clear as you read this foreword.

I began my professional career in mathematics. And while I went on to become a physician and a nationally acknowledged expert in anti-aging medicine, Ed went on to do the kind of research that turns heads, not only in biology departments, but also in departments of urology and oncology.

Because of Ed's research into the origins and treatment of prostate cancer and breast cancer, I recently invited him to speak at an Ageology conference, a consortium of experts in bioidentical hormone therapy. I must confess that I'm rather outgoing and like to walk around and mingle at these events. Ed is much quieter, maybe even a little reserved.

I feared the lecture might be a problem for the audience, especially because Ed never tells jokes. Since I had worked with him, discussing his research which I knew so well, I wished I could get up on the stage and give the lecture for him. Glad to say, my concerns were groundless. Once he began talking, his compelling concepts built one upon the other to a stunning conclusion in which he demonstrated that current theories of breast cancer are incomplete. His explanation of how hormones interact with their receptors revealed an effective new way to treat this cancer nonsurgically. A few doctors even came up to him after the presentation to tell him that for the first time in their lives they felt they truly understood breast cancer.

That same bold logic applies to Alzheimer's and leads to an exciting new hormonal protocol that promises new hope for preventing and possibly even treating this disease as well.

As a physician now for over twenty-five years, I have seen only a handful of discoveries that have ushered in a new day in medicine. Ultrasound and MRIs changed the way we image. Laparoscopic surgeries changed the way we operate. New-generation antibiotics and antivirals changed the way we treat infections. Believe me when I tell you that Ed's work belongs in this category. The book you're reading is going to change the way people look at breast cancer and prostate cancer. In fact, his model is so close to the bull's-eye that we're not going to find very much that needs to be added to it, if anything. Dr. Friedman's Hormone Receptor Model *answers* all the tough questions.

Yes, I blush when I say this because I feel I've been asked by a giant to talk about his work. My sincere hope is that this book is picked up by universities, cancer research centers, and urologists who are interested in prostate cancer and, most importantly, patients who have prostate cancer, breast cancer, or Alzheimer's and the people who love them.

It would not be a great surprise to me if at some point Dr. Friedman gets nominated for a Nobel Prize for his research. It has been a pleasure to have worked with Ed in the last five years and to have discussed exciting new ideas with him as he developed a theory that will surely bring us all into a new state of vibrant health.

Paul Savage, MD
CEO, Ageology
www.ageology.com

INTRODUCTION

I am a theoretical biologist and I've devoted my life to conducting research and publishing in professional journals that are read primarily by scientists. But in the summer of 2005 I made an unexpected discovery about prostate cancer that had far-reaching implications for preventing and treating the disease, and doctors and laypeople have been clamoring for additional information ever since.

In the years following my discovery, I uncovered other surprising facts about breast cancer and Alzheimer's that were all tied to my initial findings. I published additional articles about my discoveries in professional journals, and I have spoken at medical conferences to explain to physicians and researchers how prostate cancer and breast cancer can be prevented and how Alzheimer's can be halted and in some cases cured. I've also detailed for these medical professionals exactly how to treat patients who have these diseases—nonsurgically.

Other than posting on forums for prostate cancer patients, this book represents the first time I've addressed my remarks to laypeople, and I'm pleased to have finally written an easy-to-understand explanation of my work for a general audience. It is my sincere hope that the information contained in the following chapters will increase your chance of living a long, happy life, free from prostate cancer, breast cancer, and Alzheimer's.

You don't have to be a scientist to understand this book, although it is aimed at doctors as well as laypeople. You don't even need to have done well in high school biology or chemistry. In fact, I've done all the work for you, and I'll explain my findings in language that anyone can understand. More than this, I'm confident that the explanation of my discoveries will be as exciting for you as a reader as they were for me as a researcher—because the promise I hold out is one that is truly miraculous; indeed, I still sometimes have to stop and ask myself, Is it really true? Have we really found the cause of these three scourges of humankind? And is this treatment plan really going to save lives?

But all I have to do is mentally review the steps I took to arrive at my discoveries, and I can sit back and confidently predict that the answer to all three questions is a resounding *Yes*.

I have been trained to do one thing and do it well: cull through scientific studies and understand the implications of the results. My background usually allows me to draw conclusions that go beyond what the authors of individual articles have found. Keep in mind that there are twenty-two million articles in medical databases like PubMed®, and five hundred thousand new articles added each year. No one can read them all, and even if they could it is doubtful that anyone would understand all that information. The science is often difficult, and the citations in each article present a staggering mountain of information and cross-references. Luckily, I've been trained to find patterns in such mountains of data, and my ability to do so was given a thunderous jolt in 2004 when some of these diseases touched members of my family. Suddenly I started reading these articles as if my life depended on it. Within a matter of a few years, I had discerned a pattern that no one else had seen, a pattern that explained how prostate cancer starts from high local levels of estradiol (an estrogen). More than this, my understanding of how hormone receptors worked enabled me to see that this explained some previously inexplicable behavior of the disease, namely, why prostate cancer reacts in seemingly contradictory ways to testosterone.

Hormone receptors, I should add, are one of the key players in the story that follows. Before we go any further, allow me to introduce you to the major players so that you can become familiar with their names before we jump into the story.

Hormone receptors are proteins that bind to testosterone and estrogen. Hormone receptors are found in your cells.

Testosterone and **estrogen** are hormones. In essence, hormones are chemical messengers that travel through the blood and tell cells what to do. Hormones tell cells to produce proteins, divide and multiply, and die a noble death, among other things.

Apoptosis is the process of a cell self-destructing and dying a noble and honorable death to make way for new cells. If apoptosis occurs, then cancer cannot thrive since the cancer cells die. But, as we will see, cancer cells have ways of stopping apoptosis. The good news is that we have ways of starting it up again.

Prostate cancer is the number one cancer in men, after skin cancer.

Breast cancer is the number one cancer in women, after skin cancer.

Alzheimer's disease is a cognitive impairment that affects the elderly.

These are the characters in a drama unfolding in your body even as you read this book. The fact is that these players are doing things to either make you healthy or to disrupt your happy world. The more you know about these subjects, the more prepared you can be to take action to prevent disease in the first place and to fight it successfully if it occurs.

Because clinicians usually work on one little piece of the puzzle at a time, they rarely have an opportunity to see how their findings fit into the wider picture. Luckily, I wasn't hampered by such limitations. In fact, I used a technique called meta-analysis, which involves combing through hundreds of scientific studies, and in doing so I stumbled across the answer to one of the most vexing puzzles of modern medicine. The puzzle had stymied researchers for decades. But before I tell you what this puzzle is, and the answer I found, I need to explain something even more important, namely, why hormones have gotten a bad name.

Mention hormones to the average person and they get fearful. They think of baseball players and Olympic athletes who used steroids and the trouble they got into. People also think of studies that have linked hormones to cancer. For heaven's sake, even doctors suffer from the common misconception that hormones are bad.

For heaven's sake, even doctors suffer from the common misconception that hormones are bad.

But when you think about it logically, this attitude makes no sense. How can hormones be bad? Our body produces them. They're necessary for life. Instead of being bad, just the opposite is true. Hormones are good, so good that they can even make us feel wonderful. If you're male and you have lots of testosterone flowing through your veins, you're likely to feel calm and confident. You're fearless, you have motivation and youthful energy. If you're a woman the same great feeling happens when you have adequate amounts of estrogen in your body. You're energized and feel on top of the world.

This book is all about how to use hormones to fight disease with unprecedented efficacy. The treatment plan requires absolutely no surgery or radiation. But it gets even better. Because in addition I'm going to promise that the treatments I recommend will also make you feel younger, too.

So how did hormones get such a bad reputation? I'll go into that in more detail in chapter 1, but for now let's leave it at this: There was a colossal misunderstanding in the medical community and a flood of bad information. It all started when a small percentage of people began getting sick while using *synthetic* hormones. This book doesn't recommend the use of synthetic hormones, only bioidentical hormones. Later I'll talk about the significant differences between the two, but it needs to be emphasized that the treatment plans I'll recommend in this book are all based on hormones that have a safety profile identical to the hormones already in a person's body.

And now we're ready to talk about the puzzle that baffled doctors for decades. It can be stated quite simply: How is it that testosterone can sometimes protect against prostate cancer (as it clearly does in teenage males who almost never get the disease) and can sometimes cause cancer to grow (as it does in a small percentage of men who have advanced prostate cancer)? In other words, how can one hormone, testosterone, have diametrically opposite effects?

The answer to this puzzle (thoroughly explained in chapter 7) led me to discover that prostate cancer and breast cancer are similar diseases. In fact, they're the identical disease manifesting itself in different genders. The key to fighting both these cancers is to understand what causes them, and I explain their cause in chapter 4 (prostate cancer) and chapter 5 (breast cancer). The cause of Alzheimer's is outlined in chapter 6.

Prostate cancer is caused by high local levels of estradiol, the same hormone that causes breast cancer.

One of the most important things that I'll explain in this book is that prostate cancer is caused by high local levels of estradiol, the same hormone that causes breast cancer. I will also explain why surgery can sometimes cure prostate cancer, and why it does so at a high cost. Because much of the prostate's job is to produce semen and contribute to sexual pleasure, its removal during surgery can lead to a loss of sexual functioning.

The solution I talk about in this book is much more elegant and ultimately safer since no surgery is involved. It is a way to fight prostate cancer, reduce its aggressiveness, and make it die. *I would like to note here that the treatment protocol for fighting prostate cancer with testosterone is being used with a terrific success rate by a number of forward-thinking physicians worldwide, including a well-known California doctor, and it's also the technique being used in two contemporary clinical trials. But my protocol even promises to improve upon their extraordinary results.*

I think it's important to note that my treatment plan is based on the first theoretical model of prostate cancer that accounts for all the known important facts about the disease, including the fact that testosterone sometimes causes cancer and sometimes cures it. My research also reveals a method of treating breast cancer that is more promising than current protocols. And my work on hormone receptors also demonstrates how Alzheimer's can be cured in its early stages and halted in its later stages, primarily using testosterone. In summary, then, this book will address the following questions:

1. What causes prostate cancer? (chapter 4)
2. What can prevent it? (chapter 11)
3. What can treat it better than surgery? (chapter 12)
4. What causes breast cancer? (chapter 5)
5. What can prevent it? (chapter 11)

6. What can fight it better than surgery? (chapter 13)
7. What causes Alzheimer's? (chapter 6)
8. Is it true that early-stage Alzheimer's can be cured? (chapter 14)
9. What can prevent it? (chapter 11)
10. Why has one California doctor had such phenomenal success treating prostate cancer with testosterone? And how can his results be improved? (chapter 12)
11. Why are most theories about prostate cancer unconvincing? (chapter 4)
12. Why is eating broccoli no guarantee that I won't get prostate cancer? (chapter 15)
13. What should I eat and do to prevent prostate cancer, breast cancer, and Alzheimer's? (chapter 11)

The rest of this book will take you on a journey of discovery similar to the one I embarked on when I started studying hundreds of scientific articles in 2004. I begin by telling you about the safety and efficacy of bioidentical hormones. I then take you into the interior of the cell and explain how hormones work. In my opinion, this should be one of the most enjoyable parts of the book because, like the characters in Isaac Asimov's *Fantastic Voyage*, you'll shrink down in size and enter the cell itself. When you discover what's happening inside the cell, I think you'll be as happy as I was at the discoveries I made.

Finally, I tell you how to prevent and treat prostate cancer, breast cancer, and Alzheimer's based on the properties of hormones and hormone receptors. Just so you know, the treatment plans I present in the book can all be used today, with existing hormones and FDA-approved drugs. My treatment plans are also relatively inexpensive. And, best of all, the treatment doesn't hurt, like surgery does. Just the opposite: the use of hormones will make you feel young again, with a new vitality, energy, and zest for life.

PART 1

HORMONE HEALTH: A TWENTY-FIRST-CENTURY PROMISE

CHAPTER 1

WHY HORMONES HAVE GOTTEN A BAD RAP: BUT WHY THEY SHOULDN'T FRIGHTEN *YOU*

The story you're about to read is so shocking you may not believe it. But that only goes to show that truth is indeed stranger than fiction.

It was 1991, the final year of the Cold War, and the Soviet Union had collapsed. Erwin Neher and Bert Sakmann won the Nobel Prize in Medicine for discoveries about the inner workings of the cell. And one of the world's foremost medical research centers, the National Institutes of Health (NIH), launched an unprecedented investigation aimed at helping women age gracefully. Optimism about humankind's ability to fix political and medical problems soared to an all-time high. In the wake of this near-universal confidence, no one—least of all the hundreds of scientists involved in the Women's Health Initiative, as the study was called—could have predicted that their well-meaning investigation would ultimately cause an enormous setback to medical science.

How had it happened? What had gone so terribly wrong? In those early days, when scientists had high hopes for the study, none of them could have guessed that their work would have a major adverse effect on the health of untold numbers of women. One of the most unfortunate results of this study was that hormones got a black eye and were painted in such a negative light that people—especially people who needed them most, the elderly and infirm—began to *fear* hormones and consider them the equivalent of poison.

Before I launch into the core of this book and the lifesaving information it offers to men and women of all ages, let me correct the common misperception about hormones promulgated by the Women's Health Initiative (WHI). Errors in thinking about hormones are so widespread in our society that hardly a day goes by without some news outlet foisting stories on us about the sinister dangers of hormones. So how did it happen that a study intending to *help* women turned out to harm them instead? The saddest part is that this study is still, to this day, continuing to spread misinformation about hormones, misinformation your doctor probably subscribes to right now.

Well, sometimes even umpires get it wrong. Everybody knows that. After all, they're only human and they, too, can make mistakes. The purpose of the initiative, of course, was to investigate how hormones impact women's health. More specifically, the scientists were hoping to see how progesterone and estrogen—two female hormones—impacted women's health and their susceptibility to disease. Chemical messengers produced by the human body, **hormones** serve a myriad of vital functions, such as regulating the development of secondary sexual characteristics, boosting cognition, and protecting the brain and heart from degenerative disease. So it made sense to study hormones and their role in eradicating disease.

What could possibly go wrong with a study that had such a humanitarian goal, investigating how these natural substances in the body affect women as they age? Well, for one thing, doctors conducting the WHI study did *not* use real hormones. As unbelievable, illogical, and dangerous as it may sound, the study instead used *horse* hormones. In fact, the substances they administered to unsuspecting women, equine hormones, are produced from the urine of female horses. In addition, scientists administered to these women a substance that had been created in a pharmaceutical laboratory and that *never* appears in the human body: synthetic progestin. Something totally foreign to human biology. But *why*, in heaven's name? *Why* did they use horse hormones and synthetic progestins instead of natural human hormones?

The answer disappoints everyone who understands the way our medical system works. Pharmaceutical companies usually can't make significant profits from selling natural human hormones. Why? Well, such hormones can't be patented. Only human-made substances, created in a laboratory, are afforded patent protection by our legal system. As a result, only these artificial drugs can be manufactured and sold for big bucks. So pharmaceutical companies, which had their fingers deep into the design of the WHI study, made sure that *the chemicals administered to test women included horse estrogen, which they produced in the lab and patented, together with artificial hormone-like substances (synthetic progestins, which they had also patented in hopes of maximizing their profits).*

Now, even a person with no knowledge of chemistry or biology might balk at such a study design. Wouldn't you? I sure would. But these scientists justified their actions and went forward, despite warnings from critics who believed that an unjustifiable risk existed because synthetic substances were being used. The study scientists assumed that horse estrogen worked the same as human estrogen and that synthetic progestins worked the same as human progesterone, but they did not do the due diligence to test these assumptions. After less than six years the WHI scientists had to stop the study prematurely, shamefaced, for they had found to their great dismay that the *women taking these synthetic substances had a higher risk of developing various cancers and strokes than the control group of women who had not taken the drugs and who just had their own natural hormones circulating through their blood.*

If you were to ask every doctor you know about the risk of women taking hormones, they would all claim that hormones increase the risk of women developing breast cancer. These doctors have the flawed WHI results fixed in their mind, which is why they share this common misconception.

As a result of the WHI study, if you were to ask every doctor you know about the risk of women taking hormones, they would all claim that hormones increase the risk of women developing breast cancer. These doctors have the flawed WHI results fixed in their mind, which is why they share this common misconception. We all remember the front-page headlines from 2002 announcing that **hormone replacement therapy** (HRT) causes cancer. At the time, HRT was used primarily by women who wished to alleviate the symptoms of menopause. Today, of course, HRT can be used safely by both men and women to restore youthful vitality, cognition, and health.[1] But those ominous 2002 headlines sounded a death knell for the initial enthusiasm about hormones because something had gone terribly wrong with the Women's Health Initiative.[2] More specifically, study administrators gave 16,608 women either HRT or a placebo. Originally, the study was to last for 8.5 years, but researchers terminated it after a mean of 5.2 years because those women receiving HRT demonstrated a 26 percent higher rate of invasive breast cancer than women taking the placebo. Other adverse health effects were also observed. In 2008 it was demonstrated that the negative effects from the WHI study were the result of using synthetic hormones, but we're getting ahead of ourselves and will come back to this important point shortly.

In 2003 the results of the Million Women Study[3] seemed to verify the dangers uncovered by the 2002 WHI study. There were a total of 1,084,110 women in this new study. The protocol was different from the WHI study. Women who had already been taking various forms of HRT were compared with women who had never taken HRT. The rate of invasive breast cancer was again higher for those women taking the form of HRT used in the WHI study than for those in the control. Women who had taken HRT for less than five years experienced a 60 percent higher rate of invasive breast cancer, and women who had taken HRT for more than five years experienced a 142 percent higher rate.

Most people looking at the results of the above two studies wrongfully concluded that HRT caused breast cancer. However, there were a few doctors who criticized these studies because of the form of HRT that was being used.[4] They argued that the results would be different if hormones that were chemically identical to the hormones found naturally in women, commonly known as **bioidentical hormones**, had been used. For most people, it is obvious what hormone replacement means. Replacing hormones means that you would take a woman of, say, sixty-five years of age and give her enough hormones to get her levels to that of a younger woman, perhaps a thirty-five-year-old. However, both of these studies on HRT used drugs commonly prescribed to women at that time; namely, a combination of horse estrogen and a synthetic progestin called medroxyprogesterone acetate (MPA). Horse estrogen contains significant amounts of certain components not found in humans and lacks other components that are found in significant amounts in humans. MPA is a compound never found in nature in any species. A number of doctors argued (incorrectly, as we found out in 2008) that it made no difference that hormones other than what are found normally in humans were used, since synthetic progestin binding to progesterone receptors should have the same results as human progesterone binding to progesterone receptors. Their argument was bolstered by the fact that the Million Women Study used two other forms of synthetic progestins (norethisterone and norgestrel/levonorgestrel) both of which exhibited results quite similar to MPA. But, oh, how wrong they were!

In looking at the above two studies, the question that has to be asked is, Do the results pass the smell test? Are *hormones* really dangerous to women? Do women actually experience their highest incidence of breast cancer and other diseases when their hormone levels are at their highest, generally in their late teens and early twenties? Obviously, the answer to this question is a resounding *No!* So the question becomes, Would using **bioidentical hormone replacement therapy** (BHRT) eliminate the increased risk observed with HRT (which uses synthetic chemicals)? Put more simply, is bioidentical hormone therapy safe? For many years, these were just hypothetical questions. However, in 2008 the E3N Cohort Study[5] put these questions to rest. This study followed 80,377 women for 8.1 years. It verified that HRT using MPA was dangerous and resulted in a 48 percent increase in the rate of invasive breast cancer when compared to the control. However, its most important finding was that *using bioidentical hormone replacement therapy results in no increase in the rate of invasive breast cancer.*[6] This astounding finding seems to have been totally ignored by the mainstream media. The *New York Times*, for instance, is still mistakenly using the flawed WHI results to claim that hormone replacement is dangerous for women:

> It is, without question, risky for an older woman long past menopause to start hormone treatment to prevent chronic disease. Doing so dramatically increases the risk for heart attack, stroke, breast cancer and other complications.[7]

This 2011 *New York Times* statement, based on the WHI study, is flat-out wrong. The WHI study can be used only to support the contention that synthetic hormones pose a risk. It says *nothing* about the safety of bioidentical hormones. In fact, research conducted after the WHI study demonstrates that *the reason women suffered a slight increase in disease during the WHI study was* not *because they used hormones but because they used* synthetic *hormones.*[8] Unfortunately, you would be hard-pressed to find any doctor in this country who is aware of these findings, unless you are fortunate enough to happen across one who has training in anti-aging hormone therapy.

What does the above analysis mean for women? In plain English, it means wonderful news. It means women can now relieve the symptoms of menopause without worrying about increasing the risk of breast cancer. But it gets even better. Why not relieve the symptoms of menopause and at the same time reduce the risk of breast cancer to near zero—the same as it is for teenagers? In later chapters you'll learn exactly how to do that.

CORRECTING MYTHS ABOUT TESTOSTERONE

Now let's turn our attention to prostate cancer. If you were to ask every doctor you know about the effect of testosterone on prostate cancer, they would all say, "Testosterone causes and feeds prostate cancer. Taking away testosterone kills prostate cancer by starving it. Giving testosterone to a man with prostate cancer is like adding oil to a fire. I learned this in medical school, so it must be right." Unfortunately, what your doctor learned in medical school about testosterone is based largely on outdated research conducted in 1941 by Charles Huggins. Beginning his work with investigations of dog prostates and then turning his attention to humans, Huggins observed that removing testosterone killed most of the prostate cancer cells in his patients.[9] His work convinced doctors that prostate cancer cells starved without testosterone. Huggins was later awarded a Nobel Prize for his work.

In 1977, Robert Noble developed a strain of rat now known as the Noble rat, which developed prostate cancer almost 20 percent of the time after prolonged exposure to very high dosages of testosterone.[10] This experiment convinced doctors that testosterone caused prostate cancer.

In 1981, Dr. Jackson E. Fowler Jr. and Dr. Willet F. Whitmore Jr. published a landmark paper[11] that seemed to support Huggins's findings and that is unfortunately still being relied on by medical schools throughout the world to illustrate the dangers of giving testosterone to men with prostate cancer. Fowler and Whitmore reported that for fifty-two men with prostate cancer, 73 percent of them experienced a noticeable worsening of their symptoms within thirty days of being given testosterone.[12] This experiment convinced doctors that testosterone fueled prostate cancer. Putting all the above studies together *seems* to produce a straightforward argument for the relationship between testosterone and prostate cancer.

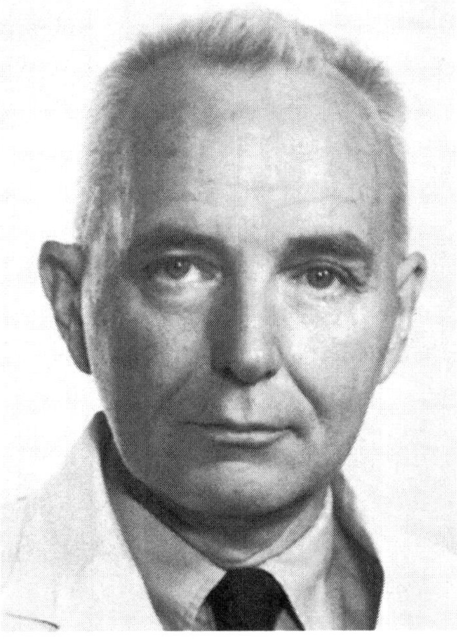

Figure 1.1. Nobel Prize laureate **Charles Huggins** gave testosterone a black eye when he claimed that it enhanced the growth of prostate cancer. Drugs that block the conversion of testosterone to estradiol were never discovered during his lifetime, so he had no way of knowing whether testosterone or estradiol was responsible for the enhanced growth rate.

Testosterone causes and then feeds prostate cancer; increasing the level of testosterone results in prostate cancer growing faster; taking away testosterone starves prostate cancer, which is why so much of it dies when testosterone is taken away.[13]

While this all *seems* to make sense, recent experiments have turned the medical profession's understanding of the relationship between testosterone and prostate cancer on its head. In 2006, Dr. Abraham Morgentaler, associate clinical professor at Harvard Medical School, published a groundbreaking study demonstrating that *prostate cancer is actually present at a much higher rate in men with* low *testosterone.*[14] Morgentaler has published numerous papers over the years confirming and expanding on his original findings. A 2011 paper he coauthored is even more exciting since it actually shows a slight decrease in the **prostate-specific antigen** (PSA), indicating a *reduction* of cancer (about a one-third drop) after an average of 2.5 years for men with untreated prostate cancer who received testosterone replacement therapy.[15] Researchers tend not to consider drops of less than 50 percent significant when treating prostate cancer. PSA is a protein made by prostate cells and prostate cancer cells. For patients who are known to have prostate cancer, a rise in PSA usually indicates an increase in prostate cancer growth. Morgentaler's paper is totally inexplicable by the model that claims testosterone fuels prostate cancer. Other findings also seriously challenge this model, in particular two studies involving the administration of testosterone to men with **castration-resistant prostate cancer** (CRPC) and the finding that none of the men experienced a rapid rise in PSA and that some experienced a drop in PSA.[16] Finally, a new report seems to drive a stake through the heart of this flawed model. Researchers discovered in 2012 that alternating two weeks of ultra-high levels of testosterone with two weeks of near-castrate levels of testosterone reduced the PSA by over 50 percent for two out of four men treated.[17] So today testosterone not only is *not* feeding prostate cancer but *it is being used as an effective tool in its treatment*!

Today testosterone not only is *not* feeding prostate cancer but *it is being used as an effective tool in its treatment*!

Knowing that the traditional model, which has been taught to doctors throughout the world, is fatally flawed raises the question: Is there a model that can explain all these findings, both those of early prostate cancer pioneers and those of current cutting-edge researchers? Actually, there is one such model, namely, the one I published in 2005[18] and refined in 2007,[19] which I refer to as the **Hormone Receptor Model**. This model focuses on the properties of hormone receptors instead of the results of giving hormones and is consistent with all experimental data, not only with those experiments done before the model was published but with all those since. You will learn much more about this model later, but let's look at just one aspect of it to cast new light on the relationship between testosterone and prostate cancer. Let's assume that a hormone receptor known as **estrogen receptor-alpha** is the villain with regard to prostate cancer[20] and not testosterone, then see how this helps us gain some new insight. Estrogen receptor-alpha (ER-alpha) is known to decrease the rate of cell death for prostate cancer.[21] In other words, ER-alpha makes prostate cancer worse. Keep in mind that testosterone can be converted into estrogen in the body, which can then bind to ER-alpha. When lots of ER-alpha is present, then higher levels of testosterone would be expected to result in greater levels of ER-alpha activity, a very bad thing. High-enough levels of ER-alpha should be able to promote cancer cell growth *even in the presence of castrate levels of testosterone.* ("Castrate level" is the level typically achieved when men are physically castrated. There is still a small amount of testosterone being produced by the adrenal glands. Historically, a serum testosterone level of below 50 ng/dL was considered castrate level.)

Modern studies have shown that although normal prostate epithelial cells (the cells that eventually develop into prostate cancer) have almost no detectable ER-alpha,[22] the percentage of cells with this potentially harmful receptor keeps increasing as the prostate cancer evolves, until 94 percent of CRPC has readily detectable ER-alpha activity.[23] Keeping this in mind, let's reexamine the results of the classic Fowler and Whitmore study in more detail. It turns out that 13 percent of the men actually had some relief of their symptoms within thirty days of receiving testosterone.[24] PSA tests were not available when this experiment was done, so the researchers relied on symptoms, namely, intensity of bone pain, appetite, energy level, and sense of well-being. Breaking down the categories of those who received this treatment is even more illuminating. Of the fifty-two men, thirty-four received a reduction of their testosterone to castrate levels, but their symptoms were getting worse in spite of this. If we assume that almost all these men had high amounts of ER-alpha in their prostate cancer, then it should come as no surprise that thirty-two of them did worse within thirty days of receiving testosterone, and none showed improvement. They got worse because testosterone was converted into estrogen, which then triggered ER-alpha activity, a known way to stimulate prostate cancer growth.

There were fourteen men who had castrate levels of testosterone but no worsening of their symptoms. It's safe to assume that none of these men had enough ER-alpha for their cancer to greatly increase its rate of growth with normal levels of estradiol.[25] As we'll see in chapter 2, ER-alpha is proliferative, meaning it helps cancer grow, and it's especially harmful when there's excess estradiol, since estradiol activates the receptor to protect cancer cells from the normal process of cell death (apoptosis). For this group, five men had worsening symptoms within thirty days, as opposed to six whose symptoms improved. Finally, there was a group of four who had never been treated, within which were one man whose symptoms improved and one whose symptoms worsened. If we focus just on the eighteen men who were not in the group who were expected to have had lots of ER-alpha, then 39 percent had their symptoms improve, and 33 percent had their symptoms worsen when given testosterone. This is a finding that is definitely not being taught in our medical schools!

So now we can explain how testosterone feeds prostate cancer. It gets converted into estrogen, which then increases ER-alpha activity. And that, as we have seen, is a very bad thing.

But is there any way to explain why prostate cells die in the *absence* of testosterone other than making the highly unlikely claim that cells are experiencing testosterone starvation?[26] Actually, there is, but it does not involve ER-alpha. It turns out that in the absence of testosterone, prostate cells undergo cell death due to calcium ion overload.[27] Researchers have shown that if you give prostate cells a drug that opens up the calcium channels, those cells die at the same rate as similar cells deprived of testosterone. In addition, in the absence of testosterone, the prostate cells can live if a drug is given that blocks the calcium channels. While this may seem a moot point—who cares whether prostate cancer dies because of starvation or because of calcium ion overload?—it makes a huge difference in treating prostate cancer. Calcium ion overload leads to a type of programmed cell death called apoptosis, and there are known ways for cancer cells to *avoid* apoptosis, such as producing greater amounts of anti-apoptotic proteins. However, if cancer cells required testosterone, then they would need to find some way to create testosterone or to somehow make do with the lower levels of testosterone in order to survive. There is evidence to support both these models, but I don't find the evidence for testosterone being required very convincing. Researchers have shown that they can take prostate cancer cells that need testosterone in order to grow and convert them into cells that can grow in the *absence* of testosterone simply by turning on a gene that makes lots of an anti-apoptotic protein.[28] The point of this discussion is that testosterone didn't cause prostate cancer in these cells. And therapeutically *removing* testosterone kills prostate cancer only because it leads to calcium ion overload, not because testosterone is needed by prostate cancer.

Finally, how does one explain the observation that testosterone *seems* to cause prostate cancer, as doctors still mistakenly believe? It turns out that recent studies have shown that by increasing estrogen levels as well as testosterone levels, 100 percent of Noble rats end up developing prostate cancer.[29] This combination also produces prostate cancer in human prostate tissue cultures.[30] One study used rat prostate tissue cultures with a constant level of testosterone and increasing levels of estrogen. This study demonstrated that *a high level of estrogen was all that was needed to initiate prostate cancer.*[31] As if this weren't enough, a 2008 paper demonstrated that although high levels of testosterone plus estrogen caused prostate cancer 100 percent of the time in mice, *it was impossible to produce prostate cancer in mice that were lacking ER-alpha* no matter how high the levels of hormones used.[32] What this means is simple. It is also paradigm shifting. Because it means that the only way testosterone can cause prostate cancer is if it is first converted to estrogen, which then binds to that villainous ER-alpha! This point bears repeating because it is of vital importance. *Testosterone doesn't cause prostate cancer. Estrogen does.*

The only way testosterone can cause prostate cancer is if it is first converted to estrogen, which then binds to that villainous ER-alpha! This point bears repeating because it is of vital importance. *Testosterone doesn't cause prostate cancer. Estrogen does.*

From what you've learned in this first chapter, I'll wager that you're now quite able to explain to almost any doctor why their beliefs about the relationship between hormones and breast and prostate cancer are wrong. You might think that it's going to be hard to top this revelation, but hold onto your hats. Keep reading, and you will soon be taking the ride of your life and quite possibly a ride that someday may save your life!

CHAPTER 2

HORMONE RECEPTORS: HOW CELLS *TALK* TO ONE ANOTHER, AND HOW *YOU* CAN INFLUENCE THEIR CONVERSATION

- Hormone receptors are complex proteins located within the membrane and the interior of cells.
- These microscopic receptors capture hormones from the bloodstream and then instruct your cells to perform various critical tasks.
- One of the most important tasks hormone receptors perform is instructing defective cells and cancer cells to die.
- The process of instructing cancer cells to die is known as programmed cell death, or apoptosis.
- By manipulating hormone receptors appropriately, we can increase apoptosis and as a result control prostate cancer and breast cancer.

Imagine trying to drive a car with a gas pedal but no brake pedal, or vice versa. In both cases it would be a disaster. In the same way that you control a car with gas and brake pedals, the body controls many internal processes with start and stop mechanisms since there has to be some way to start and stop biological processes. The most obvious example of this is your blood sugar. When there is too much blood sugar, insulin production is increased, driving sugar into cells. Once blood sugar drops to normal, insulin production is shut off.

A similar process occurs *within* cells. In this case, the drivers that are in control are hormone receptors. It turns out that hormone receptors work like gas and brake pedals, turning on and off various critical cellular functions, such as replication and protein synthesis. But before I explain how these vitally important cellular control mechanisms work, I need to set the stage by describing the fascinating cellular environment in which they function.

THE STRUCTURE OF CELLS

Twenty-four hours a day, every day, there is a *lot* is going on inside your cells. There's even a great deal of activity happening on the exterior of cells, the thin membrane surrounding the entire cell. The **cell membrane** is like a wall encapsulating all the other parts of the cell, including the cytoplasm and nucleus (see figure 2.1). In many ways the cell membrane is similar to a bustling city street, with traffic going back and forth and the constant rush of many different vehicles on that street at any given time.

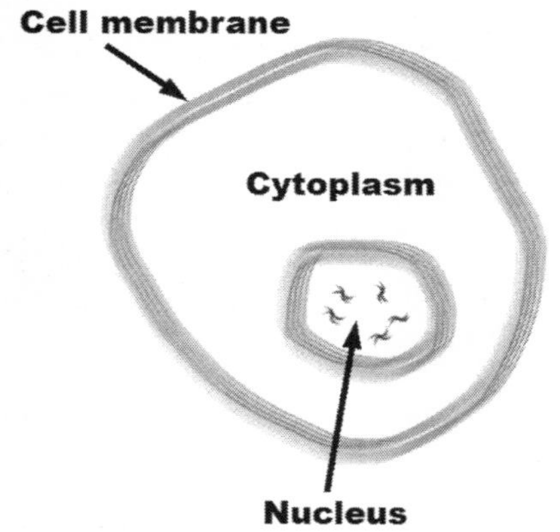

Figure 2.1. The structure of the cell. Three major components of the cell are the membrane, the cytoplasm, and the nucleus. The DNA of most cells is found within the nucleus. Drawing by Michael Christian.

The cell membrane is a complex structure that can be visualized by imagining you're standing under a suspension bridge. Above your head the bridge extends to the left and right. This is a two-level bridge, with traffic ceaselessly moving back and forth at all hours of day and night. The bridge itself is composed of a long chain of phospholipids, which are fat molecules. Lecithin, a major ingredient of chocolate candy, is a phospholipid, so most people are familiar with phospholipids. And phospholipids are very good at what they do—they provide the shell or outer covering of cells.

The phospholipid molecule looks like a circle with two long tails, one of which is a little crooked. The head of the molecule is hydrophilic, meaning it's attracted to water. The tail, however, is repelled by water and so is hydrophobic. As a result, the tail of a phospholipid moves away from water so that all the phospholipid molecules line up with their heads facing out and their tails facing in (see figure 2.2). They form a double layer a mere two molecules thick. This is the thin outer layer of all your cells.

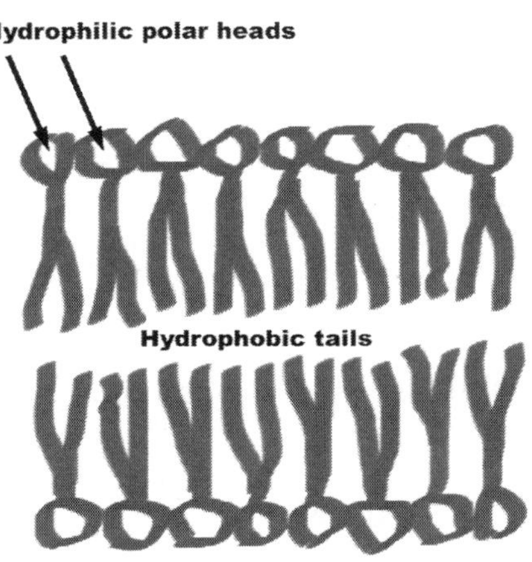

Figure 2.2. Phospholipid bilayer of the cell membrane. Mammalian cells are surrounded by a cell membrane composed of a phospholipid bilayer. Phospholipids are composed of two parts, a hydrophilic section that faces out and a hydrophobic section that faces in. Drawing by Michael Christian.

One of the most interesting properties of the cell membrane is that it isn't a simple covering; instead, it's studded with a myriad of structures, including cholesterol, proteins, and our friends, the hormone receptors.

HORMONE RECEPTORS CONTROL CELLS

Hormone receptors are proteins positioned like sesame seeds stuck into sandwich bread, the bread being the layers of the cell membrane. But these proteins are big enough to extend clear through the slice of bread into the interior of the sandwich. They are complex proteins designed to perform important functions for cells. One of their chief functions is to capture passing hormones, such as testosterone or estrogen, and then send signals down from the cell membrane through the cytoplasm and eventually into the nucleus itself. The signal sent from a hormone receptor in response to capturing a hormone can ultimately instruct DNA to perform various tasks, such as replicating the cell or manufacturing proteins. The technical name for this process is **signal transduction**, and hormones are said to transduce their signals into the cell. The beauty of signal transduction is that the various glands that secrete hormones (such as the pituitary, adrenals, testes, and ovaries) are able to control cells far away from them by sending hormone messengers to instruct cells how to behave.

Because hormone receptors are so important as message conveyors controlling the actions of cells, I'll have a good deal to say in this book about how they work and what they do (see figure 2.3). As we'll see shortly, they can even send signals that cause cancer to grow or to stop growing and die. Clearly, being able to regulate the activity of hormone receptors is going to play a major role in how we prevent and treat certain cancers as well as other diseases.

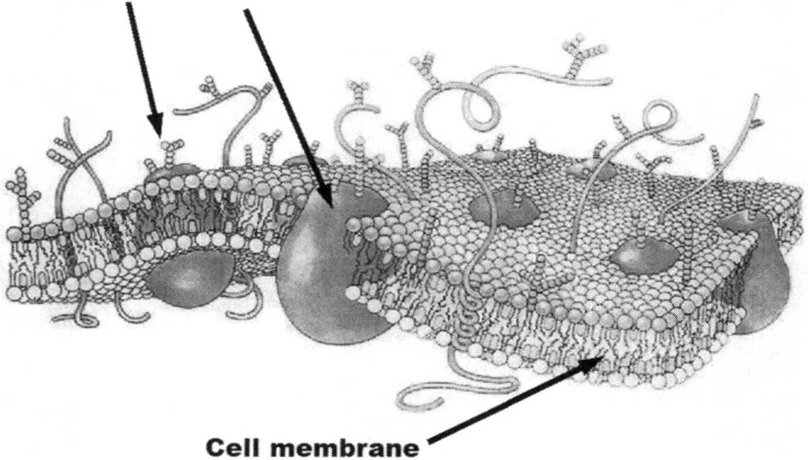

Figure 2.3. Cell membrane. In cross section, a cell membrane resembles two layers of bubbles that are connected by Y-shaped tails. These bubbles are actually densely packed phospholipids. Embedded within the membrane are countless proteins, some of which are hormone receptors. When hormones are captured by the receptors, they release G proteins, which interact with other signaling proteins within the cell and cause specific biochemical reactions. Image courtesy of Dana Burns, National Institute of Standards and Technology (NIST).

Another key aspect of hormone receptors is that their number and placement in the cell membrane is not fixed. In other words, sometimes there are more hormone receptors in a cell membrane, sometimes there are fewer. Various drugs and foods can cause a cell to manufacture more hormone receptors. This fact, too, will play a critical role in how I propose to treat cancer.

Remember the analogy about gas and brake pedals as a way to control a car? Well, it turns out that for each of the sex hormones (estrogen, progesterone, and testosterone), there are at least two receptors that work mostly in opposition to each other, like gas and brake pedals. This was first discovered for the two main estrogen receptors, estrogen receptor-alpha and estrogen receptor-beta.[1] Our discussion will concentrate on the major sex hormone receptors, while keeping in mind that there are minor sex hormone receptors present that may someday be found to have an important role to play.

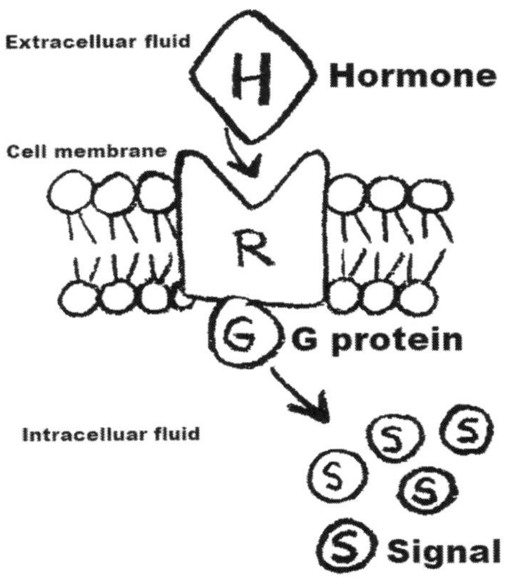

Figure 2.4. Membrane hormone receptor. A hormone binds to a membrane hormone receptor (R), causing the receptor to release a G protein, which in turn sends a signal into the cytoplasm. The signal is amplified so that it takes only a single hormone molecule to cause hundreds of signals in the cell. Hormones also bind to intracellular hormone receptors in the cytoplasm, which then travel into the nucleus to instruct DNA to make proteins, replicate the cell, or make proteins that promote apoptosis (programmed cell death). Sometimes other substances bind to hormone receptors and prevent hormones from binding and doing their job. Drawing by Michael Christian.

Hormone receptors are like locks that can be opened by specific hormones (see figure 2.4). In order to open the lock, you have to have the right key, and you need to turn the key without the key falling out of the lock. The higher a hormone's **binding affinity** to a hormone receptor, the more likely that the key will *stay in the lock* long enough for the lock to open. Lower binding affinities mean the key is more likely to fall out. However, even if you have a hormone with high binding affinity, if you have *lots* of other substances with lower binding affinities, they can interfere with your being able to use the proper key. It is important to understand that hormones aren't the only things that can bind to hormone receptors; other substances can also bind to the receptors, including chemicals in foods and human-made pharmaceuticals. Anything that can bind to a hormone receptor is called a **ligand**. To understand the concept of binding affinity, which describes how likely it is that a particular ligand will stay in a hormone receptor until it causes an effect, just imagine that your four-year-old son or daughter is trying to open the lock to your house's front door with a toy key. Most of the time you can simply wait until your child is finished playing before you get a chance to use your real key, and then you can open the lock and go through the door. But occasionally your child may actually *succeed* in opening the lock with his toy key, especially if you have a cheap lock! Hormone receptors are like cheap locks since lots of different objects can be used to successfully pick them.

The cheap lock analogy also explains why certain foods contain substances that can bind to hormone receptors, especially to estrogen receptors. These ingested substances are called **SERMs**, which stands for **s**elective **e**strogen **r**eceptor **m**odulators. The term *selective* refers to the fact that these substances bind preferentially to receptors in specific tissue, such as breast or brain tissue. Ordinarily, SERMs decrease the activity of estrogen receptors because they interfere with estrogen. In other words, they'll get into the lock first and *prevent* estrogen from binding to the receptor and doing its job. However, if estrogen levels are low enough and SERM levels are high enough, then SERMs can actually increase the activity of estrogen receptors. One of contemporary medicine's major methods of fighting breast cancer is the use of human-made (pharmaceutical) SERMs.

One final point about hormone receptors needs to be introduced before we discuss the specific types of receptors. Hormone receptors aren't found only in cell membranes; they're actually present in three places in the cell: membrane, cytoplasm, and nucleus. Receptors in the membrane are, appropriately enough, called **membrane receptors**, while receptors in the cytoplasm and nucleus are called **intracellular receptors**.[2] As we'll see in chapter 12, exciting new research has demonstrated beyond the shadow of a doubt that manipulating membrane receptors with testosterone is an exceptionally effective method of preventing and destroying prostate cancer.

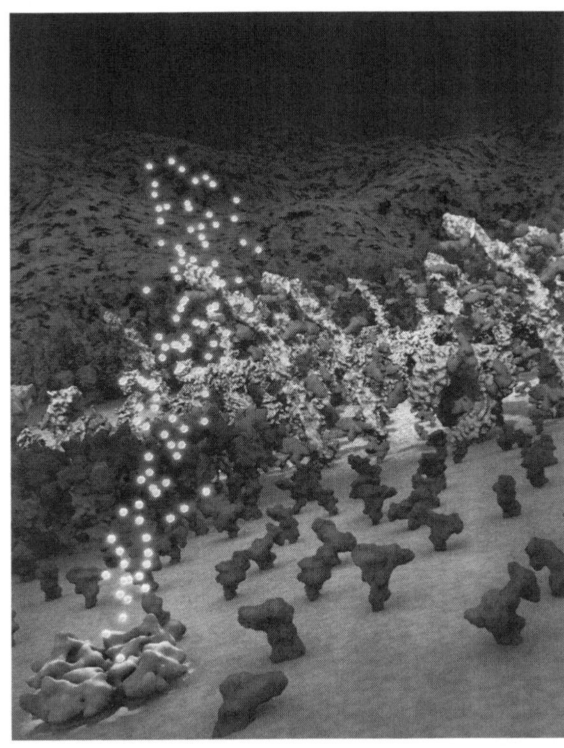

Figure 2.5. Membrane proteins embedded in the cellular membrane. The top parts of the hormone receptors, the parts that catch passing hormones, stick up out of the cell. "Raft Dance" molecular rendering courtesy of SciVis IFC - CNR.

It is well known that cells employ many different types of hormone receptors to carry out their day-to-day activities. One of the most important classes of receptors are **membrane hormone receptors**. Remember, I said that these receptors are analogous to sesame seeds stuck in a slice of bread, but they're large enough to stick up outside the top of the sandwich (see figure 2.5), and they can also penetrate clear through the bread into the interior of the sandwich (the cytoplasm of the cell). In reality this analogy is a slight oversimplification, since the receptors actually loop seven times through the cell membrane.[3] These receptors react quickly by activating G proteins, which are coupled to the receptor on the bottom portion of the receptor located *inside* the cell (see figure 2.4). G proteins affect cell signaling and cause changes rapidly—sometimes within minutes. But the important point is that one G protein and various other response elements usually amplify the hormone signal hundreds of times. Why is this important? Well, because it means that *a single hormone molecule can produce a massive response in a cell within minutes of binding to the hormone receptor.* That's like being broke, getting a dollar, putting it in your left pocket, and a few minutes later taking out five hundred dollar bills from your right pocket. A neat trick if you can do it. And hormone receptors—along with G protein–coupled receptors—do it every day.

A single hormone molecule can produce a massive response in a cell within minutes of binding to the hormone receptor.

Another important class of receptors are **intracellular hormone receptors**, located within the cytoplasm and nucleus. It's all very well, you may be saying, to have hormone receptors inside cells, but how do the hormones get into the cells in the first place to hook up to these intracellular receptors? Although most hormones can't pass through the lipid bilayer of the cell membrane, steroid hormones—like estrogen and testosterone—are exceptions. This is because steroid hormones are highly lipophilic; they have an affinity for fats. As a result, they can slip right through the fatty cell membrane and get inside a cell just as fast as a person passing through a turnstile in a subway. Once inside the cytoplasm, steroids bind to intracellular hormone receptors, causing these receptors to migrate into the nucleus . . . and once inside the nucleus, the receptor attaches to areas of DNA known as hormone response elements. This process of attaching to hormone response elements results in specific genes being turned on or off.

While the mechanism by which hormone receptors operate may seem as complicated as a Rube Goldberg machine, the results are fairly straightforward. To simplify matters, we will talk about hormone receptors increasing or decreasing the production of a protein when in fact the technical terms are **upregulation** for a process that ultimately results in more protein being produced and **downregulation** for a process that ultimately results in less protein being produced. Once you know what the properties of the hormone receptors are and how much of each hormone receptor is present, you can then predict both the effects of hormones that activate these receptors as well as the effects of drugs that block these receptors. Although there are hundreds of proteins being produced by hormone receptors, we are going to focus on those few that affect breast cancer, prostate cancer, and Alzheimer's. The main thing to keep in mind is that hormone receptors do not act in a random manner. If a receptor produces a protein that protects a cell from programmed cell death (apoptosis), then it will produce *many* different proteins (**anti-apoptotic** proteins) that all offer that protection. Similarly, if a receptor produces a protein that causes apoptosis, then it will produce many different proteins (**pro-apoptotic** proteins) that cause apoptosis. In 2007 I detailed the properties of the hormone receptors with regard to apoptosis and pointed out that we can employ our knowledge of the properties of hormone receptors to combat breast and prostate cancer.[4] The basic concept is extremely easy to understand: a combination of drugs is used to *block* receptors that help cancer cells stay alive, along with hormones to increase the activity of receptors that help kill cancer cells. I like to think of it as a one-two punch against cancer, and it turns out to be very effective, as we will demonstrate in the following chapters.

The basic concept is extremely easy to understand: a combination of drugs is used to *block* receptors that help cancer cells stay alive, along with hormones to increase the activity of receptors that help kill cancer cells.

HOW TINY ARE HORMONE RECEPTORS?

Before I talk about the specific types of hormone receptors and what they can do for you, I'd like to share one of the most exciting aspects of my research into hormone receptors. I've always admired Isaac Asimov's novel *Fantastic Voyage*, about scientists who shrink down in size and go into the carotid artery of a dying man to destroy a blood clot. Ever since reading that book as a teenager, the idea of exploring the subatomic world took hold of my imagination. One night as I was drifting off to sleep, I began thinking how amazing it is that hormone receptors have the ability to do so many good—and bad—things for humans and yet these receptors are incredibly tiny, so tiny that you cannot see them with the naked eye or even with a conventional optical microscope. Even electron microscopes have difficulty resolving these mini powerhouses. And why should this be so? It's because hormone receptors are proteins—complex proteins, that's true, but proteins nonetheless—and proteins are strings of amino acids, which are in turn composed of atoms. The estrogen receptor, for example, is composed of 595 amino acids. To give you a sense of its microscopic size, imagine that you are as big as the earth. A cell would be about the size of a football field. The estrogen receptor would be about sixteen feet high. And there might be thousands of hormone receptors embedded in the membrane of the cell and thousands more inside the cell itself.[5] A scanning tunneling microscope, which is more sensitive than an electron microscope, could make a photo of a hormone receptor, but even better images are available via computer simulations based on data entered by many scientists (see figure 2.5).

As I continued to research this intriguing field, I soon discovered to my surprise that some hormone receptors are, as a class, more helpful than others. Put more simply, some receptors prevent cancer in most cases, and these receptors are obviously very good for us. Other less helpful receptors tend to cause cancer to thrive. A third group of receptors has a more ambivalent nature as far as we're concerned and sometimes operates to aid cancer and other times to kill cancer. Probably the best place to start our overview of these three groups of receptors is with the good guys, so we'll turn our attention to them first.

ANTICANCER HORMONE RECEPTORS

Vitamin D receptor

The vitamin D receptor is the only non-sex hormone receptor that will be discussed in this book. However, its anticancer properties are too strong to be ignored. This receptor is extremely simple to understand. The vitamin D receptor is great for you and horrible for cancer. It kills cancer cells in at least four different ways in both breast[6] and prostate[7] cancer, but doesn't harm normal cells.

Ordinarily, the only way for cancer to protect against this good guy is to either have a rare mutated vitamin D receptor that doesn't work right, or to have lots of anti-apoptotic proteins. It is also possible to have multiple specific mutations that result in the vitamin D receptor increasing the rate of growth of the cancer,[8] but this is extremely rare and would not be expected to occur until the very late stages of cancer. Also, in chapter 6 you will learn exactly how vitamin D helps prevent and treat Alzheimer's disease.

Estrogen receptor-beta

Another hormone receptor that is good for you and bad for cancer is estrogen receptor-beta. One of the nice things that estrogen receptor-beta does for you is remove protection from cancer cells, and when the protection is removed, the cancer cells die. The receptor is able to work this miraculous result by decreasing the production of Bcl-2, which means that cancer cells harboring lots of this wonderful receptor don't live very long.

Bcl-2 is the main anti-apoptotic protein produced by cancer cells (see figure 2.6). You might think of it as a shield that cancer cells manufacture to protect themselves in the same way the Invisible Woman deploys a force field in the world of the Fantastic Four to protect herself from outside threats. Don't laugh, but Bcl-2 protects cancer cells by preventing them from committing suicide, which is essentially what programmed cell death, or apoptosis, is. This beneficial receptor (estrogen receptor-beta) makes it very easy for cancer cells to die by stripping away those proteins (such as Bcl-2 and others) that protect cancer from apoptosis.[9]

Bcl-2 protects cancer cells by preventing them from committing suicide, which is essentially what programmed cell death, or apoptosis, is.

Estrogen receptor-beta (ER-beta) also does something else that's quite beneficial for humans: it decreases inflammation.[10] ER-beta is so good that when levels of this receptor drop you ought to be concerned since there is a negative correlation between levels of this receptor and some disease states. For example, as prostate cancer evolves, ER-beta levels decrease.[11] The bottom line is that as this good receptor gets reduced, cancer starts to win the war.

The beneficial effects of ER-beta also apply to breast cancer. The expression (which is the clinician's way of saying production) of ER-beta is less in breast cancer cells than in normal breast cells.[12] This is what you would expect if ER-beta helps to kill breast cancer. But since ER-beta is not *totally* eliminated routinely as cancer cells evolve, it is possible that it has some *minor* effects that help the cancer population grow, although what that could be is unknown at this time. Also, in chapter 11, you will learn that ER-beta helps prevent and treat Alzheimer's disease.

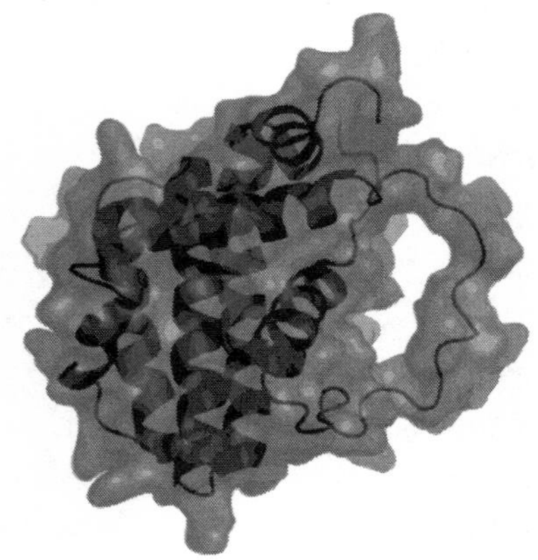

Figure 2.6. Bcl-2 is generally considered one of the bad guys in the cancer world. It's the main protein that helps cancer cells stay alive. Bcl-2 is called an anti-apoptotic protein because it prevents cancer cells from undergoing apoptosis. Image courtesy of Dan Cojocari.

Progesterone receptor B

Progesterone receptor B is good for you and bad for cancer.[13] One of the good things this receptor does—like ER-beta—is decrease Bcl-2.[14] By decreasing Bcl-2, progesterone receptor B encourages cancer cells to kill themselves. And that's really a good thing because the more that cancer cells kill themselves, the less likely they are to kill their hosts—namely, you and me.

DANGEROUS HORMONE RECEPTORS

The more I studied hormone receptors, the more I grew to dislike some of them. You might consider such an emotional reaction unusual in a scientist, but I honestly don't like things—even if they're submicroscopic receptors—that can do so much harm to people. By the time you finish reading this next section, I have a hunch that you'll share my dislike for some of these receptors, too. I have already discussed the main beneficial hormone receptors above, and now I come to the villains of the story. The following hormone receptors all share one thing in common: they contribute to disease more than they contribute to health. Some of them have recently been implicated in serious crimes against humanity. If it were up to me, I would put them on the MOST WANTED LIST of bad receptors that you don't want too much of in your body.

Estrogen receptor-alpha-alpha homodimer

This hormone receptor is especially bad for women because it initiates breast cancer. I know its name sounds complicated, but let's analyze what it actually means. **Dimers** are two receptors attaching to each other to create a new sort of receptor, in which both receptors need the appropriate hormone (in this case, estradiol) attached before they do anything.[15] **Homodimer** means that the two receptors are the same type—in this case, both are estrogen receptor-alpha (see figure 2.7).

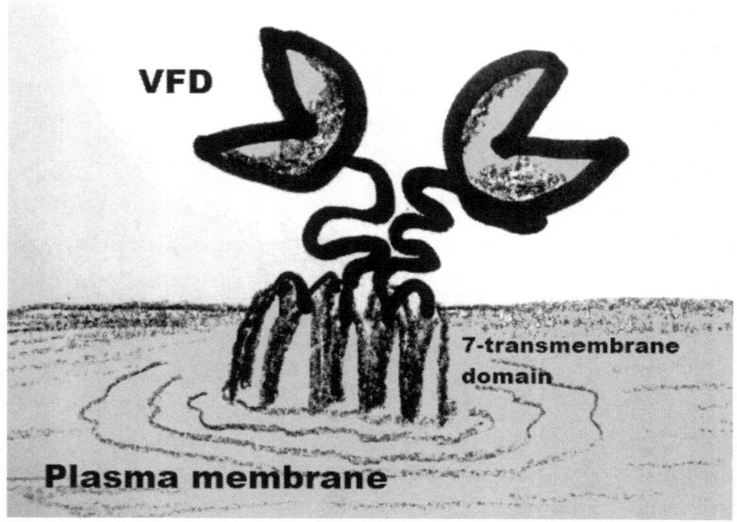

Figure 2.7. The estrogen receptor alpha-alpha homodimer sounds like a monster and also looks like one. It possesses two **Venus Flytrap Domains (VFD)** that rear their gaping jaws over the cell membrane, just waiting to snap up any passing estrogen. The middle part of the receptor (the **7-transmembrane domain**) coils through the membrane seven times like a snake. Down below (not pictured), a G protein–coupled receptor is waiting to send a signal after two hormone molecules are caught in the VFDs above. Drawing by Michael Christian.

Dimers are somewhat fragile since either or both of the hormones attached can fall out before this complex is able to bind to the appropriate hormone receptor element on the DNA in the cell nucleus. Also, the dimers themselves can come apart. The more estrogen receptor-alpha present, the more likely it is that these dimers can be formed. Also, the more estradiol that is present, the more likely it is that the dimers will have both of their ER-alpha receptors bound when they reach the hormone receptor element in the nucleus because estradiol binds with the strength of Krazy Glue®, and once it sticks, it almost never lets go.

Experiments done with both prostate and breast cells[16] have shown that when you add more estradiol, you increase **telomerase** activity. Telomerase is an enzyme that increases the length of telomeres. Telomeres are specific sequences of DNA that exist at the ends of chromosomes and are necessary for cell division to occur properly. Also, when you increase estrogen receptor-alpha, you increase telomerase *activity*. High levels of estradiol are also observed to cause cell division in both breast[17] and prostate[18] cells. There is now convincing evidence that this homodimer, along with high local levels of estradiol, is the initiator of almost all breast cancers. In the case of prostate cancer, it probably is rarely the cause, but only because there is so little estrogen receptor-alpha in normal prostate cells. Bottom line: this hormone receptor needs to be watched like a hawk because it can easily cause a woman lots of problems by initiating breast cancer.

Estrogen receptor-alpha-beta heterodimer

This hormone receptor pair is particularly bad for men. Its name also sounds pretty complicated, but once you understand what it means, it's easy to understand the way it is structured. In this term, the word **heterodimer** means that the two hormone receptors are different. So we are talking about one estrogen receptor-alpha combining with one estrogen receptor-beta. Again, it's a two-headed monster, but this time the two heads are different: one eats its estradiol a little differently than the other, so to speak.

Researchers have demonstrated that increasing estrogen receptor-beta increases telomerase activity in prostate cells but not in breast cells.[19] Increasing estrogen receptor-beta results in more estrogen receptor-alpha-beta heterodimers, as well as more estrogen receptor-beta-beta homodimers (which you will learn more about shortly). Since there was no increase in telomerase activity for breast cells when more estrogen receptor-beta was produced, neither of these dimers (estrogen receptor-alpha-beta, estrogen receptor-beta-beta) can be considered responsible for the initiation of breast cancer. But researchers have shown that prostate cancer *cannot* be caused in mice lacking ER-alpha,[20] so estrogen receptor-beta-beta homodimers can be ruled out for the initiation of prostate cancer. In the normal prostate epithelial cell there is much more ER-beta than ER-alpha,[21] so there will be many more estrogen receptor-alpha-beta heterodimers present than estrogen receptor-alpha-alpha homodimers. Therefore I believe that it has been convincingly demonstrated that the presence of estrogen receptor-alpha-beta heterodimer along with high local levels of estradiol is the leading way that prostate cancer is initiated.

If the preceding paragraph sounded a little complex on first reading, you're not alone; it took me many hundreds of hours to come to the conclusion that this receptor and estradiol are a lethal combination for men . . . but the takeaway message is very clear. What it all means is that estrogen receptor-alpha-beta heterodimer is dangerous enough to cause men untold problems because the combination of this receptor and high local levels of estradiol leads to the initiation of prostate cancer. Fully understanding the risks of this lethal combination, I explain in chapter 11 exactly how to minimize such a harmful scenario by using FDA-approved drugs to reduce the amount of local estradiol. I will also tell you how to use hormones and other natural substances to increase the rate of cell death if any cancer cells begin to develop. The result: the risk of prostate cancer starting in your body will drop to near zero, the same near-zero risk teenage males enjoy.

Estrogen receptor-alpha

Estrogen receptor-alpha is generally bad for you and good for cancer. It increases Bcl-2 for both prostate cancer and breast cancer.[22] In other words, it helps prostate and breast cancer cells protect themselves from normal cell death, enabling cancer cells to live forever. Another bad thing it does is to increase inflammation.[23] In prostate cancer, there is almost always more ER-alpha activity as the cancer becomes more advanced.[24] Approximately two-thirds of breast cancers are diagnosed as estrogen receptor positive.[25]

Estrogen receptor-alpha is generally bad for you and good for cancer. It . . . helps prostate and breast cancer cells protect themselves from normal cell death, enabling cancer cells to live forever.

Historically, doctors thought there was only one estrogen receptor, which we now refer to as ER-alpha. When they classify breast cancers, they still refer to just estrogen receptor positive or negative, ignoring the fact that it is important to know the concentrations of both ER-alpha and ER-beta.

The mechanism cancer cells use for increasing the amount of ER-alpha as cancer progresses is well understood, too. The more ER-alpha that is present, the more Bcl-2 that is produced. More Bcl-2 means there is less cell death, so some of these cells will be able to divide more often before they die than cells with lesser amounts of ER-alpha. The more ER-alpha (up to some maximum amount), the more rapidly that particular segment of the population will increase. Therefore, if no treatment is given to alter this outcome, the amount of cells with higher levels of ER-alpha will continually increase as a cancer population evolves.

There is an interesting twist with this receptor. It is known that some breast cancers lose their ER-alpha. Since this receptor causes cancer, why would a cancer population *lose* this receptor? I'm used to thinking in terms of classical Darwinian evolution, and for an organism or a cell to lose a feature, there either has to be a selective growth advantage in doing so (in which case you will see this loss quite often), or, at the very least, the feature has to serve no purpose (if you don't use it, you lose it). Having one-third of breast cancers lose their ER-alpha puts this more in the category of there being some advantage to losing it, but the fact that it is only one-third means that only under certain circumstances is there any advantage for this loss. We know that ER-alpha increases Bcl-2, so in order to eliminate this receptor, either Bcl-2 is no longer needed or the cell must have another source of Bcl-2. There are known to be mutations that interfere with the ability of pro-apoptotic proteins to start the killing process, others that provide another source of Bcl-2, and some that even interfere with the process that normally breaks the cell apart when subjected to high enough levels of pro-apoptotic proteins. These other mutations can explain why ER-alpha may no longer be necessary, but they cannot explain what advantage there is in eliminating it. There is no clue at this time as to what property of ER-alpha might hinder the growth of breast cancer or why exactly there is any advantage in getting rid of it. One question that should be asked by researchers is exactly how much ER-alpha is left in breast cancer cells that are classified as estrogen receptor negative? Is there enough left to form homodimers that will continue to produce telomerase activity?

An interesting side note is that there are no known cases in which prostate cancer eliminates ER-alpha once it has started up (unlike breast cancer). This seems to indicate that there may be a minor property associated with ER-alpha that is harmful to breast cancer but *not* to prostate cancer. However, in order to be sure of this, researchers must first identify what that property is and then see if the same property exists in prostate cancer.

It is likely that ER-alpha helps promote Alzheimer's because ER-beta helps prevent Alzheimer's (as explained in chapter 11), and ER-alpha tends to act in direct opposition to ER-beta. The absence of ER-alpha mutations that increase the risk of Alzheimer's for all women is indirect evidence in support of this conclusion.

Membrane estrogen receptor

Membrane estrogen receptor is actually a mix of many different estrogen receptors that all reside on the cell membrane. I refer to it as a single type of receptor because when estradiol is combined with protein (beef serum albumin), it only binds to estrogen receptors on the membrane and produces changes in protein production that can be measured. When I refer to the membrane estrogen receptor, I am referring to the overall changes that occur when estrogen binds to it. It turns out that membrane estrogen receptor is bad for you and good for cancer. It makes more Bcl-2, at least in breast cancer.[26] I have to assume that it behaves the same way in prostate cancer, although hopefully someday researchers will verify this.[27]

Progesterone receptor A

This is another easy one—progesterone receptor A is bad for you and good for cancer. Just like ER-alpha, it increases Bcl-2.[28] Progesterone receptor A is also one of the reasons that the BRCA1 and BRCA2 mutations cause breast cancer so frequently, but we will talk more about that later.

RECEPTORS THAT ARE SOMETIMES GOOD, SOMETIMES BAD, AND OFTEN AMBIVALENT

So far we've looked at rather clear-cut cases where hormone receptors are either helpful or harmful. A third group of receptors are more difficult to classify.

Estrogen receptor-beta-beta homodimer

This is the third type of dimer than can be made from the two estrogen receptors. Although at this point, it appears that it does not have any effect at all on prostate or breast cancer, there is a slight chance that this dimer does increase telomerase activity in prostate cells. Researchers can test this by looking to see if increasing estradiol and estrogen receptor-beta results in an increase in telomerase activity for prostate cells from mice lacking estrogen receptor-alpha. Knowing the answer to this question would be very helpful in completing our understanding of the disease-causing and disease-fighting characteristics of the various hormone receptors. It is, after all, rather difficult to play a game when you don't know all the rules. This game analogy is obviously not meant to minimize the seriousness of our subject; instead, it refers to the fact that once we know the properties of the various hormone receptors, we can manipulate them in predictable ways to fight disease.

Membrane progesterone receptor

Membrane progesterone receptor consists of two main types—one that promotes the growth of cancer and one that inhibits it. There are two different types of progesterone that interact with these receptors. 5alpha-pregnanes ("bad progesterone") bind to the receptor that promotes cancer growth, and 4-pregnenes ("good progesterone") bind to the receptor that inhibits cancer growth.[29] Normally there is much more "good progesterone" than "bad progesterone," but once breast cancer starts up and evolves, the situation reverses.

ESTROGEN

Human estrogen is made up of three major components: estradiol, estrone, and estriol. **Estradiol** binds with equal strength to estrogen receptor-alpha and estrogen receptor-beta. **Estrone** binds 5 times more strongly to ER-alpha than it does to ER-beta. **Estriol** binds 3.2 times more strongly to ER-beta than it does to ER-alpha. Both estrone and estriol are considered "weak" estrogens, since they bind to the estrogen receptors with much less strength than estradiol.

TABLE 2.1. RELATIVE BINDING STRENGTHS FOR ESTROGEN

	Estrone	Estradiol	Estriol
Estrogen receptor-alpha	0.1	1.0	0.11
Estrogen receptor-beta	0.02	1.0	0.35

Table 2.1 shows the relative binding strengths of each estrogen component to each receptor.[30] Assuming that ER-alpha increases Bcl-2 by the same amount that ER-beta decreases it, it is then possible to draw a few important conclusions. First, estradiol will reduce Bcl-2 only if there is

more ER-beta than ER-alpha. Estrone will always increase Bcl-2, except when there is at least 5 times more ER-beta than ER-alpha. Finally, estriol will always decrease Bcl-2, except when there is at least 3.2 times more ER-alpha than ER- beta.

In normal breast tissue, the amount of ER-alpha is roughly the same as the amount of ER-beta.[31] So before breast cancer starts, estradiol is having no major effect on Bcl-2, estrone increases Bcl-2, and estriol decreases Bcl-2. This is why estrone is considered a pro-cancer hormone, and estriol is considered an anticancer hormone with regard to breast cancer. The implications for women are clear: *It would be wise to avoid products containing estrone, such as horse estrogen.*

Intracellular androgen receptor

The intracellular androgen receptor has properties that seem to be identical in both breast cancer and prostate cancer and that are a mixed bag of both good and bad.[32] It decreases the amount of Bcl-2, thus increasing the rate of cell death (which is good for you); it decreases the production of pro-apoptotic proteins, thus decreasing the rate of cell death (which is bad for you); and it increases the production of **AS3**—a helpful protein that prevents cancer cells from undergoing cell division (which is good for you). But it also increases a protein called calreticulin, which protects prostate cancer cells from dying due to calcium overload (which is bad for you).[33] So, if you've been keeping score, you can see that the intracellular androgen receptor does two good things and two bad things.

Membrane androgen receptor

The properties of the membrane androgen receptor differ slightly in breast cancer and prostate cancer.[34] In both cases, this receptor increases the production of pro-apoptotic proteins, as a result increasing the rate of cancer cell death (which is good for you). But this receptor also decreases the production of beneficial AS3, and when you decrease AS3, you effectively allow cancer cell division to occur (which is bad for you). However, in prostate cancer it increases the anti-apoptotic protein Bcl-2 (which is bad news for men), whereas in breast cancer it decreases Bcl-2 (which is good news for women).

Androgen receptor balance

While the above sections describe the properties of hormone receptors, they don't give you a sense of *why* things are the way they are. The properties of hormone receptors are not designed to protect you from cancer or to make you more susceptible to cancer. What the body actually does is set up a mechanism by which cells are *not* killed when they are healthy and functioning. However, defective cells tend to be eliminated whether they are defective at the point of their creation or whether they become defective as they age. So Bcl-2 does not just keep *cancer* cells alive; it also protects noncancerous cells as well. It turns out that androgen receptors are crucial for regulating cell life and death. For example, both breast cancer and prostate cancer cells tend to stay alive as long as there is a relative balance between *intracellular* androgen receptors and *membrane* androgen receptors. An imbalance would be an indication that the cell was defective and therefore had to be eliminated. There are three possible imbalances—too little membrane androgen receptor, too little intracellular androgen receptor, or too little of both. To illustrate how these imbalances eliminate defective cells (those that are out of balance), let's take it to the extreme and examine what happens when we have no androgen receptors instead of too little.

No membrane androgen receptor

The first example would be no membrane androgen receptor present. For more than a decade, it has been known that intracellular androgen receptor increases AS3. Recall that AS3 is a good protein that prevents cancer growth. So if there is no membrane androgen receptor, then intracellular androgen receptor is the only receptor in the cell available to receive androgens, and it has an opportunity to catch all the available androgens. This is like a baseball game where the Yankees are playing with no one in the outfield except one player. If that outfielder were, say, Bernie Williams, then Bernie would be the only guy to catch balls hit into the outfield. Similarly, if there is only intracellular androgen receptor present, then any androgen that gets into the cell is going to be caught by the intracellular androgen receptor. Plus, more androgen will get to this interior receptor from outside the cell since there won't be any interference or diminution of androgen flowing into the cell interior because no membrane androgen receptors exist in our hypothetical to bind the incoming androgens (see figure 2.8).

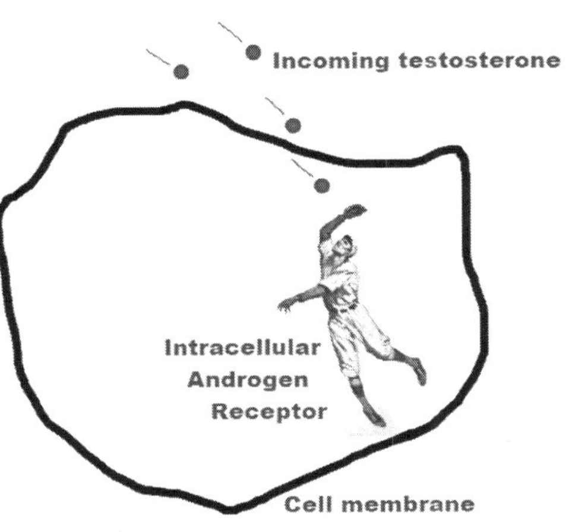

Figure 2.8. When there's no **membrane androgen receptor** to interfere with incoming testosterone, good old **intracellular androgen receptor** can have a field day and catch it all himself. This puts a smile on his face, since he does good things for you with the testosterone he catches, such as manufacturing AS3 protein, which halts prostate cancer in its tracks. Drawing of cell by Michael Christian. Drawing of outfielder by G. P. Hoskins.

It's really to our advantage when the intracellular androgen receptor goes into overdrive, since it does a very good thing, namely, producing beneficial AS3. And when there is an abundance of beneficial AS3, then no more cell division will occur for both breast cancer and prostate cancer. Using a modified human breast cancer cell line with five times more beneficial intracellular androgen receptor than normal, this held true even for the small amount of testosterone normally found in women.[35] Eventually these cancer cells will die out from sources that induce apoptosis other than from the membrane androgen receptor, such as the vitamin D receptor. The important point of this little episode in our story is that if we can manipulate cells so that they eliminate or significantly reduce membrane androgen receptor, then we can enjoy the wonderful benefits that active intracellular androgen receptor conveys: a major reduction in prostate and breast cancer cell division.

No intracellular androgen receptor

Next, let's see what happens when there is no intracellular androgen receptor present. In the case of breast cancer, more pro-apoptotic proteins will be made, but there also will be more Bcl-2 because the intracellular androgen receptor that used to be decreasing Bcl-2 is now gone. So for breast cancer, this situation can be either good or bad. If there is only a little testosterone present, it is bad because you increase Bcl-2 but don't produce enough pro-apoptotic proteins to be effective. As testosterone levels rise, Bcl-2 decreases and pro-apoptotic proteins increase until eventually the cancer cells die off. For younger women, this is not a problem because there is enough testosterone to cause developing breast cancer cells to die. However, as women age and their levels of testosterone drop, they lose their ability to force cancer cells to die in a timely manner. This is one additional reason for women to supplement their hormones as they age, including with appropriate amounts of testosterone, but more about this in chapter 11.

In prostate cancer, the lack of intracellular androgen receptor results in increased Bcl-2, but in addition, more pro-apoptotic proteins are being produced. Studies done in prostate cancer cell lines show that when you add a testosterone protein complex that binds to the membrane androgen receptor only (which is the equivalent of a cell without an intracellular androgen receptor), then the effect of the increase in pro-apoptotic proteins is more pronounced than the effect of the increase in Bcl-2, so that the higher the level of testosterone protein complex present, the more cancer cells die off.[36] In at least one cell line with no intracellular androgen receptor, testosterone alone is sufficient to cause cancer cells to die. Again, high levels of testosterone in young men make it likely that developing prostate cancer cells will die, but when men age and testosterone levels drop, it becomes much more difficult to kill cancer cells.

High levels of testosterone in young men make it likely that developing prostate cancer cells will die, but when men age and testosterone levels drop, it becomes much more difficult to kill cancer cells.

No androgen receptors

Finally, what happens when neither androgen receptor is present? In prostate cancer, reducing both androgen receptors is an effective treatment that tends to cause most of cancer cells to die. Since doctors can't actually eliminate androgen receptors, they lower levels of testosterone in order to achieve the same result. I'll get into the specifics of how this works later in the book. In breast cancer, postmenopausal women already have levels of testosterone lower than the target treatment levels for men, so this does not seem to be a promising avenue of treatment for them.

TABLE 2.2. HORMONE RECEPTOR PROPERTIES

Hormone receptor	Properties
Estrogen receptor-alpha-alpha homodimer	Initiates breast cancer and rarely initiates prostate cancer
Estrogen receptor-alpha-beta heterodimer	Initiates prostate cancer
Estrogen receptor-alpha	Increases Bcl-2 Increases inflammation Helps cause Alzheimer's
Estrogen receptor-beta	Decreases Bcl-2 Decreases inflammation Helps prevent Alzheimer's
Membrane estrogen receptor	Increases Bcl-2
Progesterone receptor A	Increases Bcl-2
Progesterone receptor B	Decreases Bcl-2

Membrane progesterone receptor	Some decreases Bcl-2, some increases Bcl-2
Membrane androgen receptor	Increases pro-apoptotic proteins Decreases AS3 Increases Bcl-2 in prostate cancer Decreases Bcl-2 in breast cancer
Intracellular androgen receptor	Decreases pro-apoptotic proteins Increases AS3 Decreases Bcl-2 Protects calcium overload from killing cell
Vitamin D receptor	Kills cancer cells in many ways Helps prevent Alzheimer's

Table 2.2 summarizes the known properties of the sex hormone and vitamin D receptors for breast cancer, prostate cancer, and Alzheimer's. Almost all the information in this table is nothing more than a summary of existing experimental data published in the literature or logical deductions based on published results. Nevertheless, I am excited to have been able to extract all the key findings and condense them in this way. In looking at this table, it is obvious that the major properties of the hormone receptors with regard to prostate cancer and breast cancer are almost identical. There are only two notable differences: Estrogen receptor-alpha-beta-heterodimer initiates prostate cancer but not breast cancer. Also, membrane androgen receptor increases Bcl-2 in prostate cancer but decreases it in breast cancer. This is why I'm discussing both cancers together in this book—they aren't just *similar* to each other, they're virtually identical.

Table 2.2 represents the essence of my **Hormone Receptor Model**. The most interesting thing is not the facts but how to apply these facts to match up with reality. Think of it like a game of bridge. Once you learn the rules, you can play right away. But it can take you years to truly master the game. In a similar way, this model has existed inside my head for thousands of hours. In some cases it took me months to understand how a single known fact could be explained by the Hormone Receptor Model. However, every time I thought I really understood everything and could explain all the existing experimental results in a straightforward manner,

I would learn something new that forced me to fine-tune my model even more. As you will learn in later chapters, understanding the properties of these hormone receptors means that it is now possible to almost totally prevent prostate cancer, breast cancer, and Alzheimer's. Also, new treatment protocols can be employed that are more effective than what has previously been tried. This is not just theory—a few doctors are actually doing what the Hormone Receptor Model predicts will be extremely effective and, as a result, are observing *excellent* outcomes.

CHAPTER 3

BIOIDENTICAL HORMONES: WHAT WE KNOW AND WHAT WE DON'T KNOW ABOUT THEIR ABILITY TO FIGHT DISEASE

- Bioidentical hormones are safe when used as directed because they work synergistically with hormone receptors.
- Synthetic hormones, on the other hand, can cause life-threatening side effects because they interfere with proper hormone receptor functioning.
- Contrary to popular belief, testosterone doesn't directly cause prostate cancer. It actually interacts with the intracellular androgen receptor, resulting in less protection against apoptosis, and as a result more prostate cancer cells die, which is one of the reasons teenage males almost never get prostate cancer.
- Testosterone improves libido in men and women.
- Testosterone helps prevent type 2 diabetes. It also fights breast cancer by binding to androgen receptors. This binding causes cancer cells to enjoy less protection against apoptosis, so more cancer cells die. This is why young women, who have twice as much free testosterone as middle-aged women, almost never get breast cancer.
- Hormones prevent Alzheimer's and stop it from progressing. Because young people have higher hormone levels than the elderly, they have a near-zero risk for developing Alzheimer's.
- By safely boosting an adult's level of hormones, we can fight prostate cancer and breast cancer, increase libido, fight diabetes, and prevent and halt the progression of Alzheimer's and other diseases.

When the war against cancer is finally won, you might expect that the scientists who discover the cure will receive a Nobel Prize and maybe even a ticker-tape parade. The odd thing is that recent discoveries about testosterone and other hormones—which I discuss in this book—have enabled researchers to take giant strides toward preventing and curing cancer and Alzheimer's, and yet the response from the medical community and the press has been a near-deafening silence.

The story of these exciting discoveries and the reasons for the lack of a ticker-tape parade for the scientists who made them are of interest to me since I've been following this field for many years and I know some of the people who have unearthed the findings that will certainly revolutionize the way we treat cancer and Alzheimer's. I'm sure you'd like to know what the latest discoveries are—and *why* they aren't receiving the press they deserve—but before I get to that, I want to expand on an important point that I touched on in chapter 1: the difference between natural and synthetic hormones.

As I stated earlier, *bioidentical hormones are the exact same molecules as hormones in your body*, and with modern technology we can now synthesize bioidentical hormones in a laboratory. These human-made hormones are very appropriately named because they are identical in every way to the hormones already circulating in your bloodstream. Put more simply, there is absolutely no difference between hormones produced by your body and bioidentical hormones made in a lab. If you were to look at them side by side under a scanning tunneling microscope, you would see the same thing, right down to their identical atomic structure. More to the point, the body reacts to them the same way because . . . well, because they're identical.

THE SAFETY OF BIOIDENTICAL HORMONES

It may sound too good to be true to say that bioidentical hormones are safe, especially in light of all the misinformation published about hormones, but the fact is that bioidentical hormones are not only safe when used properly, they're also vital for good health. Still, let's put the word *safe* in context. It's similar to saying that water is safe. Everyone knows that water is essential for life and that if water comes from a natural source it's safe to drink. The same holds true for hormones: if they're pure; that is, identical to hormones already in the body, then they're safe to use.

When I was in grammar school, we were frightened by rumors about a boy in another school who drank so much water he exploded and died. These folk myths actually reflect a grain of truth. If you drink too much water, you *can* die. The technical term for death by drinking too much water is hyponatremia, or water intoxication. The same considerations hold true for hormone replacement; the levels you achieve in the body when you supplement with hormones should not be higher than those a person typically has in their teens and early twenties.[1] When bioidentical hormones are used in a way that boosts the body's levels to that which they were when we were young adults, we will enjoy some of the same health benefits that we enjoyed when we were younger, such as a near-zero risk for breast and prostate cancer, enhanced cognition, and a near-zero risk of developing Alzheimer's.

Another way to evaluate the safety of bioidentical hormones is to compare their adverse-effects profile to NSAIDs like aspirin and ibuprofen (including Advil® and Motrin®). Although they are widely considered safe, NSAIDs cause ten thousand to twenty thousand deaths a year in the United States,[2] but the FDA admits that it has no reports of any adverse effects from bioidentical hormones.[3]

The negative stories about hormones that are frequently published in the popular press and in scholarly articles are not usually about the adverse effects that result from bioidentical hormones; as I have pointed out, these stories are usually about the harms that result when synthetic hormones are used. Similarly, the negative press associated with baseball players and other athletes who use hormones have primarily been the result of athletes using amounts that are significantly greater than those of people in their teens and twenties. So a person who goes to an anti-aging doctor will have no problems from synthetic hormones and no problems from supraphysiological doses; that is, doses that are larger than would occur naturally in a healthy young person. This is because, as a general rule, anti-aging doctors will not prescribe synthetic hormones and will not allow your levels of bioidentical hormones to become too high.

The safety of bioidentical hormones has been established beyond the shadow of a doubt. A recent meta-analysis of 196 studies concluded that "physiological data and clinical outcomes demonstrate that bioidentical hormones are associated with lower risks, including the risk of breast cancer and cardiovascular disease, and are more efficacious than their synthetic and animal-derived counterparts."

The safety of bioidentical hormones has been established beyond the shadow of a doubt. A recent meta-analysis of 196 studies concluded that "physiological data and clinical outcomes demonstrate that bioidentical hormones are associated with lower risks, including the risk of breast cancer and cardiovascular disease, and are more efficacious than their synthetic and animal-derived counterparts. Until evidence is found to the contrary, bioidentical hormones remain the preferred method of HRT."[4] A 2006 study concluded that bioidentical hormones are safe and that synthetic progesterone is comparatively unsafe and can lead to cancer; in reaching this conclusion, the authors said, "The studies reviewed suggest bioidentical progesterone does not have a negative effect on blood lipids or vasculature as do many synthetic progestins, and may carry less risk with respect to breast cancer incidence. Studies of both bioidentical estrogens and progesterone suggest a reduced risk of blood clots compared to non-bioidentical preparations."[5] In a later section of this chapter, I explain the exciting new research that confirms what anti-aging doctors have believed all along, namely, that it is synthetic hormones that cause problems; and we now know those problems result from the way synthetic hormones interfere with proper hormone receptor function.

The bottom line is that if you are interested in improving your health, you can be confident that, as of 2013, we know that bioidentical hormones are safe when used under the supervision of an anti-aging doctor. If you have normal genetics, they will not increase your risk of getting breast cancer or prostate cancer or any other cancer if you don't already have it.

WHY SYNTHETIC HORMONES ARE DANGEROUS

You've undoubtedly heard the argument that bioidentical hormones are safe and synthetic hormones risky. Suzanne Somers, for example, makes the argument in many of her books.[6] But why are bioidentical hormones safe? And what is it about synthetics that causes the problem? For many years we didn't know the answer to this question. But we do now. And the answer comes down to the different ways that bioidentical and synthetic hormones interact with hormone receptors.

In addition to being able to make bioidentical hormones in the lab, we now also have the ability to manufacture synthetic hormone analogs. Hormone analogs are human-made molecules built on the chassis of human hormones. In order to make synthetic progesterone, for example, technicians add various chemicals and molecules to the human progesterone hormone, creating a new molecule that never existed before. Why would they want to do this? One reason is to make a product that can be patented because human hormones aren't afforded intellectual property protection. Another reason to make synthetic hormones is that sometimes researchers believe they can improve upon nature and make a molecule that works better than a human hormone for a particular purpose. Unfortunately, artificial hormones almost always turn out to be Frankensteins, since they usually have various deleterious side effects. If you recall, it was when women started taking synthetic progestin during the WHI study that they experienced an increased risk of breast cancer.

But let's set the record straight. These synthetic hormones are not really hormones at all. They are never produced by the body. Figure 3.1 illustrates how the natural human molecule progesterone was modified by adding oxygen, carbon, and methyl groups (one carbon atom and three hydrogen atoms) in order to make medroxyprogesterone acetate (MPA), which is sold under the trade name Provera®. MPA is used in birth control pills and also by some doctors (who are not aware of the much higher safety of bioidentical hormones) for hormone replacement therapy for postmenopausal women.

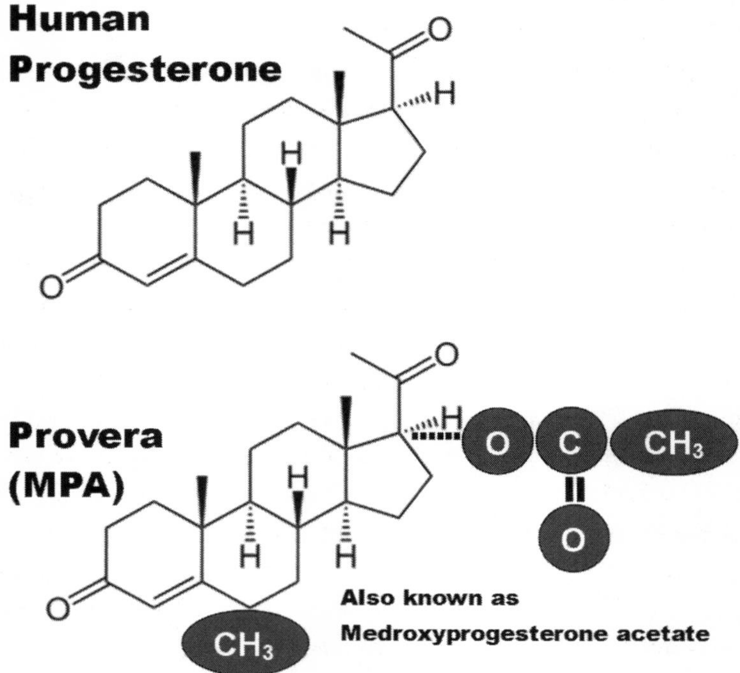

Figure 3.1. In 1956, human **progesterone** was modified by pharmaceutical firms Syntex and Upjohn Company to make progestin (artificial progesterone), also known as medroxyprogesterone acetate (MPA) or Provera. The difference between the real hormone (top) and the synthetic (bottom) is represented by the dark ovals and circles added to the bottom molecule. Diagram of MPA by Michael Christian.

THE RISKS OF PROVERA

The 2002 WHI study found that women who used synthetic progestins, such as Provera, experienced an increased risk for breast cancer compared to women who used no hormone therapy. But how much of a risk did the women using synthetic progestin experience? According to a 2010 analysis, those participants using progestins experienced 20 percent more breast cancer, and they were "twice as likely to die from breast cancer."[7]

Yet as a recent review indicates, "in absolute numbers, the risk remained small: 2.6 breast-cancer deaths per ten thousand women per year in the estrogen-plus-progestin group, compared with 1.6 per ten thousand in the placebo group."[8] Still, the difference was statistically significant.

Separating fact from rhetoric in this area is vital, especially since there is a lot of rhetoric emanating from the desks of pharmaceutical industry public relations firms.[9] But despite how much pharmaceutical firms wanted women to buy synthetic progestin, the product was found to cause an unacceptable increased risk of health problems. If I were reading this book, here's where I'd take out a red pen to underscore the fact that the increased rate of breast cancer experienced by women taking current "hormone" replacement is totally expected due to the properties of the *synthetic* progestin usually prescribed. In fact, everything suddenly made sense in August 2007 when the lead article in the *FASEB Journal* (the journal of the Federation of American Societies for Experimental Biology, one of the leading journals for experimental biologists) revealed that *there is a crucial difference in the way bioidentical progesterone and synthetic progestins affect the androgen receptor.*

There is a crucial difference in the way bioidentical progesterone and synthetic progestins affect the androgen receptor.

I hate to say I told you so on a life-and-death matter like this, but just as I and others had predicted, synthetic progestins help cause breast cancer, while bioidentical progesterone ordinarily does not (if there is more progesterone receptor A than progesterone receptor B, then progesterone can also help cause cancer, but to a lesser extent than the synthetic progestins). In what may be the scientific understatement of the decade, the article's authors said, in rather typical science speak: "We propose that the observed excess of breast malignancies associated with combined HRT may be explained, in part, by synthetic progestins such as MPA acting as endocrine disruptors to negate the protective effects of androgen signaling in the breast." This conclusion should have been front-page news in the *New York Times.* In plain English, it means that synthetic hormones disrupt the protective role of androgens (testosterone). Put even more bluntly, it means that *testosterone powerfully protects against breast cancer and has the potential to save lives.*[10] Just as I have been saying all along. Most importantly, this study also explains exactly *why* synthetic progestin is different from bioidentical progesterone in the effect it produces in the body. We now have a rock-solid understanding of the harm that synthetics do. Because the progesterone molecule was changed so radically to make patentable MPA, the resulting molecule disturbs normal hormone receptor functioning. It essentially gets in the way of testosterone and prevents testosterone from performing its vital role of increasing the rate of cell death for defective cells, such as cancer cells.

Because the progesterone molecule was changed so radically to make patentable MPA, the resulting molecule disturbs normal hormone receptor functioning. It essentially gets in the way of testosterone and prevents testosterone from performing its vital role of increasing the rate of cell death for defective cells, such as cancer cells.

As a result, there is an increased risk of detecting breast cancer experienced by women using synthetic MPA. Recent research has followed this problem even further. As one analyst points out, "However, we now know that these drugs bind not just to the progesterone receptor, but also to the androgen receptor, glucocorticoid receptor, and mineralocorticoid receptor, and most recently, it has been noted that the estrogen receptor is a progestin target as well."[11] What this means is that it is possible that we have not yet seen the end of the adverse side effects that synthetics might cause years from now.[12]

Although synthetics cause problems because they don't work naturally with hormone receptors, just the opposite is true of bioidentical hormones. In fact, if bioidentical hormones are applied in the right combinations and dosages, and at the right time in a person's life, we have before us the real prospect of the end of breast cancer, prostate cancer, and Alzheimer's. It is this conclusion that undergirds my technical publications, and it is this conclusion that has the potential to save hundreds of thousands of lives each year.

It's important to keep in mind that a progestin is a *synthetic* progesterone-like substance; it is not progesterone. I expect it is now clear why the public has a serious misperception about hormones and why a popular source of information like the Wikipedia article on this subject currently misstates the facts when it claims that progestins have "effects similar to progesterone." The effects are decidedly dissimilar. Progesterone typically does not increase breast cancer risk,[13] but progestins do.[14] Let's be even more direct. The fact is that pharmaceutical companies have spent incredible sums of money to manufacture and market synthetic molecules because such products can be patented and sold for substantial profits. Once a pharmaceutical company modifies a natural substance, such as a human hormone, and seeks FDA approval, it merely has to show that this new substance meets the standards of safety and efficacy established by the FDA. While common sense dictates that any such substance should be tested side by side with the unmodified natural substance, this is not the way our current system works. Pharmaceutical companies are selling such drugs to people for one reason only—to make money. If the drug happens to work better than the natural substance, that is fine; if it happens to work less well than the natural substance, that is fine too—so long as money is being made. What is even worse is that the current system allows pharmaceutical companies to file complaints with the FDA about bioidentical hormones because bioidenticals have not undergone the expensive tests that synthetic hormones have undergone. Such complaints can be made without presenting a shred of evidence that the synthetic hormone is in any way superior to (or even as good as) the corresponding bioidentical hormone.

WHY THE PILL IS UNSAFE

The oral contraceptive for women colloquially known as "the pill" is unsafe because it contains synthetic progestin. As such, it confers upon users all the risks that we have discussed in relation to the Women's Health Initiative study, including the increased risk of breast cancer. Because testosterone levels decrease with age, the risk is less in younger women. The bottom line is that the pill does not interact properly with hormone receptors, and as a result it interferes with the body's ability to protect itself against cancer. The same problems are associated with Depo-Provera®, a contraceptive injection for women that is administered once every three months. Contraceptives seem to reduce the risk of endometrial and ovarian cancer while increasing the risk of breast, cervical, and liver cancer.[15] The new birth control pills (such as Yaz® and Yasmin®) are even more dangerous than the old ones.

TESTOSTERONE KILLS PROSTATE CANCER AND COLON CANCER CELLS

A middle-aged man recently visited his doctor to request a prescription for testosterone. But he made the mistake of going to his family doctor.[16] The physician, who was misinformed like most of his contemporaries, told the man, "I won't prescribe testosterone. It makes things grow." Unfortunately, this kind of uneducated response does a serious disservice to male patients, since low testosterone leads to more cancer than high testosterone.[17] As far as testosterone making things grow, testosterone is an anabolic hormone, which means it increases *muscle* mass. But it only increases muscle mass because muscle cells have androgen receptors.[18] Although prostate cells have androgen receptors too, they don't grow under the influence of testosterone.[19] In fact, just the opposite is true; in the absence of excess aromatase (which converts testosterone into cancer-causing estradiol), testosterone is capable of *killing* prostate cancer.[20] As I explain in chapter 4, testosterone kills cancer by binding to the membrane androgen receptor and activating apoptosis.

In the absence of excess aromatase (which converts testosterone into cancer-causing estradiol), testosterone is capable of *killing* prostate cancer.

The same thing happens with colon cancer. Researchers at the University of Tübingen, Germany, and the University of Crete School of Medicine in Heraklion, Greece, are excited to report that they recently demonstrated how testosterone binding to membrane androgen receptor selectively induces apoptosis in colon cancer while not harming normal colon cells.[21] The astonishing message of these European scientists is that the appropriate use of testosterone promises to provide a novel method of fighting prostate and colon cancer. The hormone works within minutes of application to produce pro-apoptotic proteins that eventually kill colon and prostate cancer cells. The researchers concluded that "mAR [membrane androgen receptor] activation [by testosterone] induced profound apoptotic regression of prostate cancer cells *in vitro* and in mouse xenografts *in vivo*."[22] *They further reported that colon tumors in mice were reduced by 65 percent when testosterone was given to the animals.*[23] *More recent evidence shows an 80 percent regression in tumors.*

Controversy rages over the risks and benefits of bioidentical hormones, but one fact stands abundantly clear and is accepted by almost every doctor and researcher worldwide: hormones affect some cancers. It follows logically that the process of appropriately modifying hormones holds the potential to speed or slow cancer progression . . . and also, which is most crucial, to turn cancer on—or off.

TESTOSTERONE BOOSTS LIBIDO

As we have seen, there are numerous benefits of using bioidentical hormones and there are a myriad of diseases than can be prevented and effectively combated by normalizing hormone levels. This improvement in health is the special province of anti-aging medicine.[24]

For women, one of the advantages of using bioidentical testosterone after age forty is that it can boost libido. The APHRODITE study followed 814 women who suffered hypoactive sexual desire (low libido). They were divided into groups receiving testosterone and placebo over the course of a year. Those women who received testosterone reported increased satisfaction with sexual activity.[25] The testosterone cream is usually rubbed into the wrists and is rapidly absorbed into the bloodstream. "My wife, who is fifty, experienced a loss of libido a few years ago, which is not good for us," reported one man. "When she started using testosterone all that changed and she is as responsive now as she was in her teens and twenties. We both find that a very satisfying result."

Men watching television today may be surprised to see ads promising to boost libido with nonprescription drugs. These reports are generally misleading. No sustained boost in testosterone can result from herbs. Herbs such as Eurycoma longifolia (tongkat ali)[26] and Tribulus terrestris[27] may lead to a small increase in testosterone, but the result is not sustained over time and cannot be since a feedback loop prevents it from working. These herbs may provide some boost in dopamine, but even this is a small effect compared to the significant rise in bioavailable testosterone that can easily be achieved through testosterone supplementation.

TESTOSTERONE AND TYPE 2 DIABETES

Through various mechanisms, testosterone combats a major epidemic of our time, the increasing prevalence of obesity and type 2 diabetes.[28] Type 2 diabetes is a disease of carbohydrate metabolism.[29] Testosterone fights this disease by improving insulin sensitivity and glycemic control, thereby reducing cardiovascular risk.[30] In effect, testosterone supplementation works to reverse the risk factors associated with diabetes.[31]

Testosterone supplementation works to reverse the risk factors associated with diabetes.

There is overwhelming evidence that low testosterone is associated with increased type 2 diabetes and that testosterone replacement therapy is a singularly helpful mode of fighting the disease. Researchers today confidently state that "men with lower concentrations of total testosterone and SHBG [sex hormone binding globulin] had a higher likelihood of having metabolic syndrome than those with higher concentrations."[32] While scientists are cautious about claiming that low testosterone causes metabolic syndrome and diabetes, some believe that testosterone replacement therapy, in conjunction with tempering one's carbohydrate intake, can reverse diabetes.[33] But this is only one of the many health advantages of bringing hormones back to youthful levels.[34]

TESTOSTERONE FIGHTS BREAST CANCER

Testosterone also fights breast cancer. It does this by decreasing the protection cancer cells enjoy against apoptosis. Testosterone works by binding to androgen receptors and enabling the normal apoptosis of cancer cells. Although some researchers believe that any increase in sex hormones would increase the risk of breast cancer,[35] more recent studies have demonstrated the fallacy of that oversimplification, pointing out that testosterone powerfully protects from the effect of excess estrogens.[36]

Dr. Rebecca Glaser has shown that using testosterone plus an aromatase inhibitor is effective in treating breast cancer as well as for preventing recurrences.[37] When androgen receptors are blocked, women risk an increase in mammary epithelial proliferation, which can lead to breast cancer.[38] Normally, a woman's androgens will inhibit the initiation of breast cancer by blocking the action of estrogen in breast tissue.[39] The addition of a small amount of testosterone for women receiving estrogen replacement therapy is believed to be sufficient to counter any increased risk of breast cancer associated with the increased estrogen because testosterone reduces harmful estrogen receptor-alpha in breast tissue and simultaneously increases helpful estrogen receptor-beta expression.[40]

So now let's look at the fact that hormone replacement therapy (HRT) increases the risk of breast cancer, but bioidentical hormone replacement therapy (BHRT) does not. As we have seen, MPA (synthetic progestin) increases the risk of breast cancer, whereas progesterone entails no such risk. The dosage of MPA used in the 2002 WHI study blocked the intracellular androgen receptor by 80 to 95 percent.[41] Since the intracellular androgen receptor decreases the production of Bcl-2, blocking the receptor (as progestin does) would increase Bcl-2. More Bcl-2 means less cancer cell death, so tumors would grow more rapidly. According to the Hormone Receptor Model, this would mean that the average tumor size would most likely have been larger for women taking MPA than for those who didn't, and in fact that is precisely what was found.[42]

The effect of blocking the intracellular androgen receptor is almost equivalent to decreasing the amount of testosterone present. If this is the case, then adding testosterone to HRT that includes MPA should negate the increase in Bcl-2 caused by MPA. In fact, this was reported in 2004.[43] Although this study involved only 508 women and had no control, the reported incidence for invasive breast cancer of 293 per 100,000 women-years for women who took testosterone with their HRT was in line with the reported rate for women who had never taken hormones, which was 300 per 100,000 women-years for the 2002 WHI study[44] and 283 per 100,000 women-years for the 2003 Million Women Study.[45] In other words, when used at the right dosage, testosterone supplementation is such a potentially powerful anticancer therapy that it can even protect women from many of the side effects of synthetic progestin.

Suddenly, everything is making sense—the magic and mystery are gone, and logic is taking their place. HRT with MPA is bad because MPA blocks the intracellular androgen receptor. As adult women age, their production of free testosterone continually declines,[46] with the average woman aged forty-five to fifty-four having half as much free testosterone as women aged eighteen to twenty-four. Therefore, the older a woman is, the more we can expect adverse effects from synthetic HRT since older women lose the many health benefits conferred by testosterone. I will explain in chapter 11 how women can enjoy all the advantages of hormone replacement therapy safely by adding testosterone into the mix when using BHRT.

TESTOSTERONE FIGHTS ALZHEIMER'S

Last, but certainly not least, testosterone can prevent Alzheimer's. The way it does this is by allowing excess glucose and oxygen into the brain. It also prevents the tangles and beta amyloid plaque associated with the disease.

By far the most prevalent type of dementia for women over sixty-five is Alzheimer's. There was also an increase in dementia for women over sixty-five years of age shown in the 2002 WHI study,[47] with Alzheimer's being the most common form of dementia observed. Not surprisingly, one study has reported that testosterone improves memory.[48] In addition, researchers have shown a correlation between the increased incidence of Alzheimer's and low testosterone levels in men and women.[49] In later chapters I will discuss why Alzheimer's is a hormone-driven disease that results from low hormone levels, and I will also describe the positive results achieved when hormone levels for Alzheimer's patients are raised even slightly.

HORMONES FIGHT MENOPAUSE AND ANDROPAUSE

What all this means is that men and women no longer have to suffer the adverse effects of menopause and andropause—both the overt adverse symptoms and the hidden adverse effects on overall health—due to a fear of what hormones might do to them. In fact, this book will be making a strong case to show that *there is a very real danger to aging men and women who do* not *replace their hormones.*

There is a very real danger to aging men and women who do not replace their hormones.

PART 2

THE MIRACLE OF HORMONE REPLACEMENT THERAPY

CHAPTER 4

A *NEW* MODEL OF PROSTATE CANCER THAT EXPLAINS EVERY IMPORTANT FACT ABOUT THE DISEASE

- Prostate cells proliferate in response to hormonal stimulation and consequently are more susceptible to cancer than any other part of the body.
- Each prostate cell is surrounded by a cell membrane containing a vast number of hormone receptors. Hormone receptors also abound in the interior of prostate cells.
- Prostate cancer arises as a result of multiple mutations involving several genes, including oncogenes, tumor-suppressor genes, and telomeres.
- Five other factors are also necessary to initiate prostate cancer: testosterone, intracellular androgen receptor, dihydrotestosterone, estradiol, and estrogen receptor-alpha.
- To date, only one theory of prostate cancer can account for all these factors: the Hormone Receptor Model.
- The Hormone Receptor Model predicts that there is a new way to fight prostate cancer safely, effectively and nonsurgically through hormone modulation, with special attention paid to preventing high local levels of estradiol. Researchers and clinicians using elements of this new model are achieving unprecedented success in preventing and treating prostate cancer nonsurgically.

It is one of the great embarrassments of twenty-first-century medicine that none of the current models of prostate cancer can account for all the known significant facts about the disease. Why is it that scientists still can't agree on the cause of—and cure for—the number two killer of men? The answer may surprise you, just as it has surprised many careful thinkers who have looked into the issue.

Without doubt, the biggest source of confusion surrounding prostate cancer stems from the fact that one hormone—testosterone—can both increase and decrease the disease. It is known, for example, that when men with advanced prostate cancer are castrated (either physically or chemically by reducing the production of testosterone), this treatment reduces the severity of the disease for a few years (typically two). But unfortunately, after a few years prostate cancer usually returns in a more aggressive form, and this hormone-resistant cancer grows even in the absence of testosterone. This fact initially caused researchers to conclude that the best they could do was reduce testosterone in men, giving them a few additional years of life before the cancer would come back in a more aggressive form and kill them.

Most doctors still subscribe to this outdated view and believe that because castration reduces prostate cancer for a few years, testosterone must cause prostate cancer. But while testosterone is necessary for the initiation of prostate cancer, this doesn't mean that testosterone *causes* prostate cancer. By analogy, oxygen is *necessary* to start a fire, but no one would argue that oxygen *causes* fires. If it did, then the sky, which is 21 percent oxygen, would always be burning. Similarly, if testosterone *caused* prostate cancer, then all teenage males would have the disease since they have the highest levels of testosterone. But teens almost never get prostate cancer. In fact, this remarkable observation has led researchers to wonder whether testosterone might actually provide protection *against* prostate cancer. After all, if teenage males have the highest levels of testosterone—and there's no argument about that—then maybe testosterone confers some kind of protection *against* prostate cancer. Bolstering this view is the fact that the rate of prostate cancer *increases* as men age and their testosterone level declines. All these observations lead to the logical conclusion that testosterone *doesn't* cause prostate cancer; instead, it fights prostate cancer.

So we have two contradictory views. And scientists have been racking their brains trying to reconcile them. How can one hormone cause prostate cancer to grow (as it sometimes does in men with advanced metastatic prostate cancer) and at the same time confer protection on young men, who almost never get this disease?

As we'll see, there's an exciting new logical explanation for this apparent contradiction—but to fully appreciate it, we first need to take a look at the cells comprising prostate tissue, the hormone receptors embedded in those cells, and the current theories about prostate cancer. In the process, I'll explain how prostate cancer arises, why it's so common in older men, and how logic and recent clinical studies predict that it can be prevented and treated safely and effectively using an inexpensive new hormone-based protocol.

THE STRUCTURE AND FUNCTION OF THE PROSTATE

Everything You Always Wanted to Know About Sex (*But Were Afraid to Ask)* features Woody Allen playing the role of a sperm cell who talks nervously to his buddies as they prepare for ejaculation. In a humorous sequence, he takes his audience into the pleasure centers of the brain and then down into the holding area where sperm are waiting. The sperm, including the one played by Woody Allen, begin moving forward en masse, and finally—despite Allen's nervous comment, "I'm scared. I don't want to go"—they rush down and out to complete the sexual act.

In order to visualize the structure and function of the prostate, it will help to imagine that we're shrinking to similar microscopic size so that we can take a tour of the male reproductive tract, of which the prostate is an integral part (see figure 4.1).

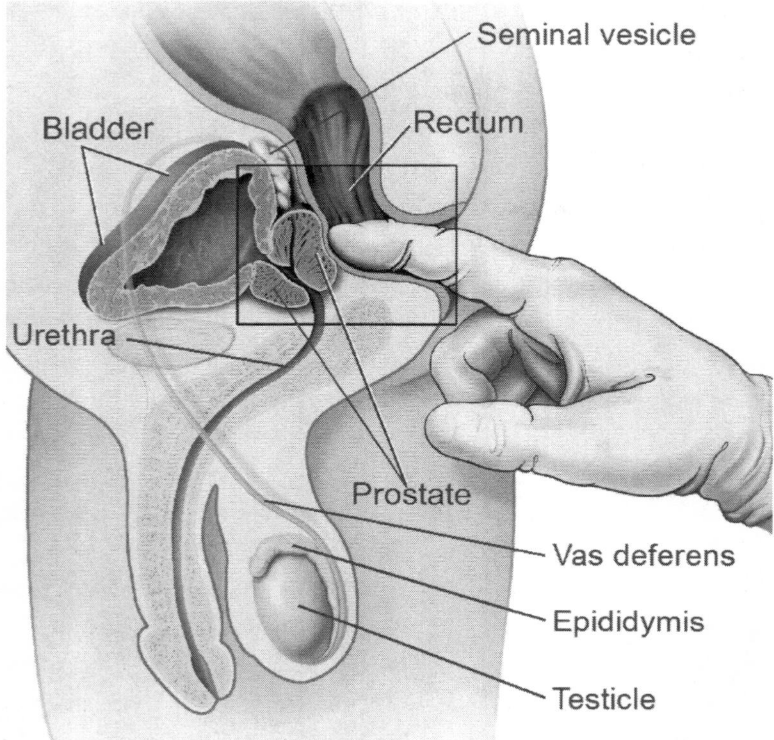

Figure 4.1. The Male Reproductive System. Sperm produced in the testicles is stored in the epididymis for maturation, eventually traveling up the vas deferens tube, through the seminal vesicle, and then through the prostate gland where it enters the urethra for ejaculation. Note that during digital rectal exams, the prostate's posterior lobe can be palpated to check for nodules that may signify prostate cancer. Image courtesy of the National Cancer Institute.

The male reproductive system is like the domino effect, with one thing leading to another. Beginning our tour in the sperm production factory, the testicles, we observe sperm cells being assembled like torpedoes with long serpentine tails. Once outfitted with pointy heads for penetrating the egg, fructose for energy, and powerful tails for propulsion, sperm are sent to a storage center called the epididymis, which is a comma-shaped area sitting on the outside of each testicle. Here sperm wait and mature until needed. During sexual stimulation, the testicles expand and force sperm from the epididymis, propelling them up a long tube called the vas deferens, which leads to the seminal vesicles. After passing through the seminal vesicles, sperm enter the prostate gland, where they receive a series of propulsions forward as the prostate contracts to complete orgasm. These final prostatic contractions send sperm down through the ejaculatory duct, which connects with the prostatic urethra, and from there sperm travel down the final portion of the urethra for ejaculation.[1]

But no tour of the male reproductive system would be complete without mentioning that the prostate gland does more than simply contract and propel sperm forward; it also secretes semen, which is mixed with sperm during ejaculation. Because it secretes fluid through ducts that lead *outside* the body, the prostate is classified as an exocrine gland. The endocrine glands, in contrast, secrete fluids *into* the body, typically into the blood.[2] In addition to the prostate, other examples of exocrine glands include salivary glands, which secrete saliva; lacrimal glands, which secrete tears; and mammary glands, which secrete milk.

It is worth noting that the prostate in men and the breasts in women secrete fluid in response to hormonal stimulation. As we'll see shortly, it is this fact—that the prostate gland secretes fluid in response to hormones—that makes the prostate similar to the female breast and also makes it particularly vulnerable to hormones and cancer.

One final point about prostate anatomy: It's a common misconception that this gland is a discrete oval and that it's defined by a sac, like the bladder. In actuality, the prostate is an undifferentiated mass of tissue about the size of a walnut that hugs the base of the bladder and encircles the neck of the urethra tube, through which urine is excreted. The prostate gland is made up of stromal and epithelial cells. Benign prostatic hyperplasia (BPH) is caused by the inappropriate growth of stromal cells. Prostate cancer involves the inappropriate growth of epithelial cells. Later in this chapter, we'll see that this happens because epithelial cells react to certain hormones and proliferate when they shouldn't.

HOW PROSTATE CANCER ARISES

If researchers knew exactly how prostate cancer started, they would almost certainly be able to prevent and cure it with more success than they're having today. It stands to reason that the more accurate our understanding of the origin of a disease, the more effective our prevention and treatment can be. In this chapter, I'll introduce a new model of how prostate cancer starts, one that is able to account for all the significant facts about the disease. I'm excited about this model because I'm convinced that it's more accurate than any other explanation of how prostate cancer starts. This is the same model I have written extensively about and talked with groups of physicians about since 2005. Many physicians familiar with my work are in agreement with me that this model isn't only more accurate than any previously used but that it also predicts what kind of treatment will be most effective in preventing and fighting prostate cancer.

I'll introduce a new model of how prostate cancer starts, one that is able to account for all the significant facts about the disease.

I believe that the lack of success experienced by mainstream medicine in dealing with prostate cancer is a result of the failure to understand why prostate cancer starts in the first place. The doctors having the greatest success treating prostate cancer, such as Bob Leibowitz, are onto something new and different, and their approach leads me, as a theoretical biologist, to conclude that the cause of prostate cancer is a little different from what most doctors think it is. In the next few pages, I'll explain my understanding of how prostate cancer starts on a cellular and molecular level.

In order to appreciate why prostate cancer is so common, it's important to first understand how cancer arises in other tissues. There are three steps that lead to the initiation of most cancers: (1) excess cell division, (2) defective tumor-suppressor genes, and (3) the lengthening of telomeres that allows cancer cells to replicate indefinitely.

Step 1. Excess cell division. Cell replication isn't perfect, and chemicals and radiation can mix up the structure of DNA so that some of the bases are moved out of sequence.[3] Figure 4.2 illustrates how radiation can cause DNA to undergo such a mutation. Luckily for us, processes to repair cells are constantly fixing out-of-sequence bases. But when this repair process isn't fast enough, problems can accumulate.

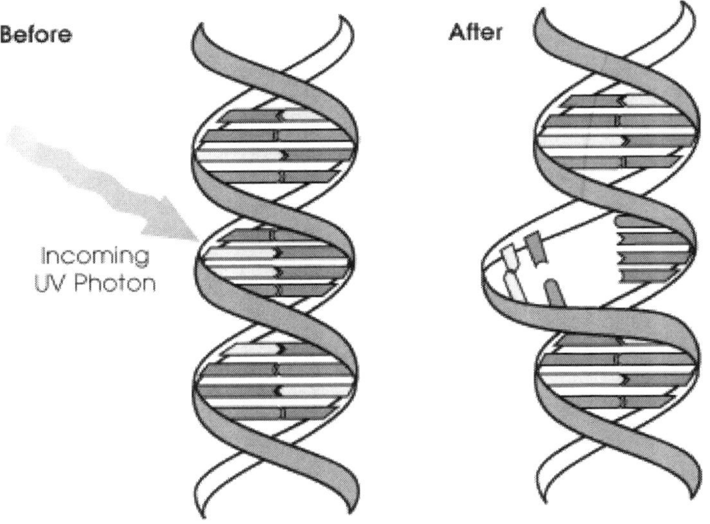

Figure 4.2. DNA undergoing mutation. Mutation in the makeup of DNA can be caused by radiation, chemical carcinogens, or other factors. DNA mutations are usually repaired. If the repairs aren't made, however, mutated DNA can lead to cancer. Image courtesy of NASA/David Herring.

It's a common misconception that all damaged DNA causes cancer, but this isn't so; although damaged DNA may impede the normal function of a cell, it usually doesn't cause cancer. Only certain specific types of DNA damage cause cancer. Usually cancer arises as a result of damage to the specific genes that control a cell's life cycle, that is, genes that control how a cell replicates and divides. The primary type of DNA damage to a cell's life cycle is a mistake in the replication of **proto-oncogenes**.

Proto-oncogenes cause cells to divide. This is a crucial function for life since we need to keep making new cells to replace those that are injured or die. But when proto-oncogenes become damaged, they cause cells to divide too much. In this damaged state, they're referred to as oncogenes or oncoproteins. The excess proliferation caused by oncogenes can be problematic, but even this, in and of itself, isn't usually enough to cause cancer since the body can control such problems through cellular processes that destroy excess cells. In most cases a second step—another mutation—is needed to cause cancer. Often this is a mutation in a tumor-suppressor gene.

Step 2. Defective tumor-suppressor genes. If there's any structure in the cell doing lifesaving work day and night, it's the tumor-suppressor genes. They work round the clock to stop problems from occurring on the molecular level. And without doubt, the hardest-working tumor suppressor is p53. Although it may sound like just a number, p53 is really the workhorse of tumor suppressors. Composed of 393 amino acids divided into several functional regions, p53 performs a series of crucial tasks, including facilitating **apoptosis**, the process whereby cells self-destruct. Apoptosis is a necessary way for the body to make room for other cells. Without apoptosis, cells wouldn't die at a fast enough rate and there would be a buildup of unneeded cells. Because it's so important that apoptosis occur, p53 has several regions that assist in this process. You could think of p53 as a hired assassin, like James Bond, an agent with a license to kill cells that need to be eliminated. p53 also assists in repairing DNA. For example, if there are any bases out of order, p53 binds to the DNA and holds it fast while other cell structures perform the repairs needed to make sure that the DNA's bases are in the proper sequence. Last but not least, p53 works to prevent cancer cells from creating new blood vessels to feed themselves, a process called **angiogenesis**. Put more simply, p53 works to starve cancer cells and prevent them from metastasizing, or spreading. It's no wonder this protein has been called "the guardian angel gene." During times of health, p53 is at low levels in cells, but during stress or when needed, concentrations of p53 increase dramatically in the cell nucleus so that it can perform its vital functions in protecting DNA.[4]

As one researcher recently said, "The p53 pathway is inactivated at one point or another in most and perhaps all human tumors."[5] Tumor-suppressor genes are clearly vital to health because they repair damaged DNA and prevent the uncontrolled division of cells, ensuring that cancer doesn't start (see figure 4.3). They also kill cells that need to die, making way for healthy new cells that strengthen our vitality. Faulty p53 can lead to cancers developing at a younger age than usual.[6]

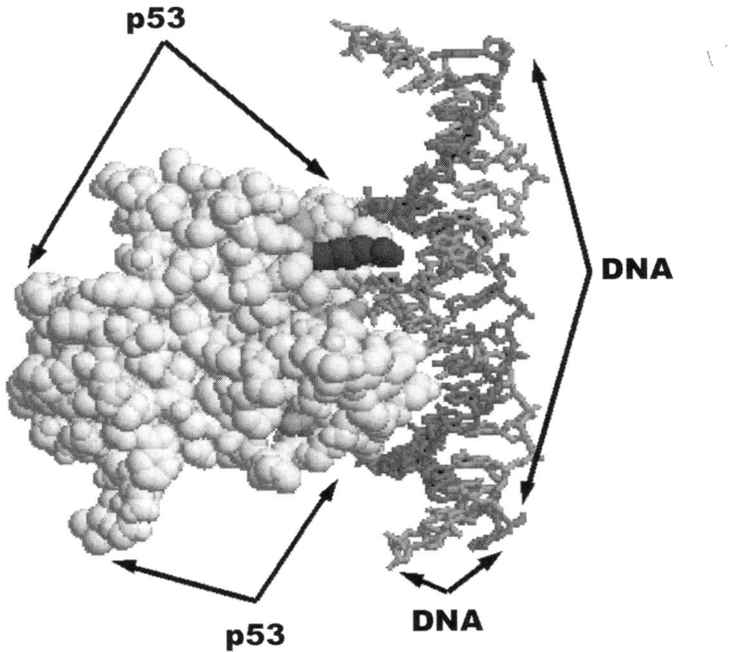

Figure 4.3. The **tumor-suppressor protein** is the large multipart structure on the left. Its DNA-binding domain has seized a DNA strand to facilitate repairing damage sustained by the DNA. Because it works tirelessly in the nucleus of cells to ensure that DNA is replicated correctly, **p53** has been dubbed "the protector of the genome." Image courtesy of RCSB Protein Data Bank, © 2011 David Goodsell.

Step 3. Lengthening of telomeres. A third problem that leads to cancer is one that allows cells to live forever. Some of the cells that are immortal end up becoming cancerous and eventually kill their host.

Once you understand how cells become immortal, I'm sure you'll agree that the process needs to be stopped. There is a region on the end of each strand of DNA called a telomere. It's a pattern of proteins that functions as a cap at the end of the strand. This cap prevents DNA from becoming tangled and mutated. As long as the cap is in place, DNA can replicate over and over again—indefinitely.

In normal healthy cells, every time the cell divides the telomere caps get a little shorter (see figure 4.4). Eventually, after a certain number of replications, the caps get so short they disappear, and as a result the cell can't replicate anymore—if it tries, it dies.

The enzyme telomerase functions to lengthen telomere caps. In other words, the more telomerase enzyme present, the more cells will have long telomere caps, and the longer they will be able to replicate. Telomerase activity—which lengthens telomeres and lets cells live forever—is almost entirely absent in normal prostate cells. But telomerase activity is present in almost all prostate cancer cells.[7] In other words, one of the hallmarks of prostate cancer is long telomeres, which ensure that prostate cancer cells live forever. It should be noted here, however, that as men age, their testosterone levels decline and their estrogen levels increase. High local levels of estradiol cause cell division[8] and lengthening of telomeres[9] in prostate epithelial cells (steps 1 and 3 needed to cause cancer). The age-related decline in testosterone also results in increased levels of anti-apoptotic proteins such as Bcl-2 within the prostate. Anti-apoptotic proteins cancel out the effect of tumor-suppressor genes—thus causing step 2 to occur without the need for defective tumor-suppressor genes. *So all three steps necessary to cause prostate cancer can occur without any mutations.* As you will see in chapter 5, high *local* levels of estradiol result in the mutations that allow steps 1, 2, and 3 to continue in the absence of elevated serum levels of estradiol.

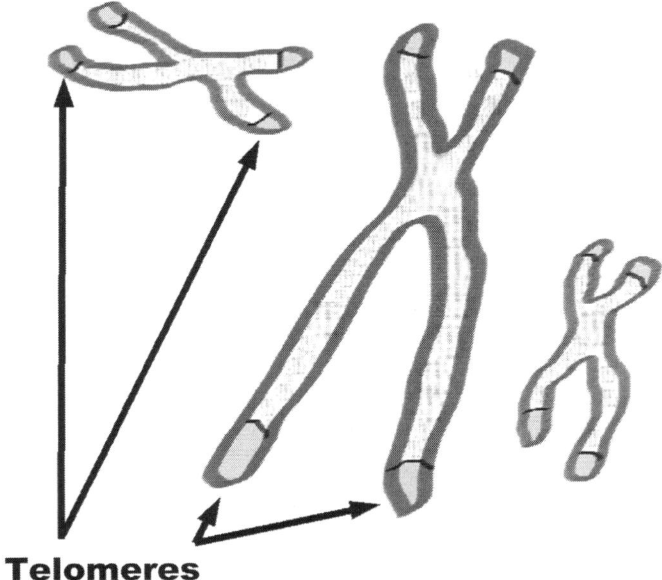

Figure 4.4. Telomeres are structural elements that form caps at the end of chromosomes (chromosomes are comprised mostly of DNA). These caps serve to protect the integrity of DNA so that mistakes (mutations) don't occur during replication. Each time a cell divides and its chromosome replicates, the telomere caps shorten. When telomeres become too short, a cell dies. Conversely, long telomere caps protect chromosomes and prevent cell death. Many cancers have a method of producing long telomeres, which ensures that cancer cells never die. Such cancer cells are immortal. Drawing by Michael Christian.

Let's summarize the steps that lead to prostate cancer: First, there is a high local level of estradiol that causes increased proliferation **(step 1)** and increased telomerase activity **(step 3)**. This is sufficient to immortalize cells unless the rate of cell death is greater than the rate of cell growth. The age-related decline in testosterone results in increased levels of anti-apoptotic proteins, for example, Bcl-2, within the prostate. Anti-apoptotic proteins cancel out the effect of tumor-suppressor genes—thus causing **step 2** to occur. In other words, with prostate cancer we're faced with both an increased proliferation and a reduced rate of programmed cell death (apoptosis), which results in a line of cells multiplying out of control.

Studies indicate that early-stage prostate cancer can experience "a seven- to 10-fold increase in the proliferation rate," and metastatic cancer "also display[s] an approximately 60 percent decrease in the rate of apoptosis."[10] This double whammy of excess proliferation and decreased apoptosis is almost always coupled with increased telomeres, leading to cell immortality or, to put it another way, cancer that refuses to die.[11]

WHY IS PROSTATE CANCER SO PREVALENT?

When I talk with men who have prostate cancer, they ask me, Why is this disease affecting me? What did I do wrong? And why is prostate cancer so common among men my age?

Believe it or not, most men reading this book already have prostate cancer, even if they're in their twenties or thirties.[12] Don't be fooled by the fact that so many men in their fifties are being diagnosed with prostate cancer. It takes about twenty years from the time that the first prostate cancer cell develops until the population is big enough to be detected.

The prostate is a man's Achilles' heel. In fact, the prostate is so vulnerable to cancer that it's the most likely place for a man to get cancer as he ages, not including the skin. But why is this the case? What is it about the prostate that makes it so susceptible to attack by cancer? Why doesn't the brain or the heart or the pancreas get cancer as often as a man's prostate?

The same question could be asked about breast cancer: Why is that the leading cancer among women? As regards prostate and breast cancer, the answer lies in the way the tissues in these organs respond to hormones.

Prostate cancer is more likely to be detected than other cancers in men over fifty because the hormone situation in a man's body is predisposed to protect this cancer as he ages. When you have high levels of testosterone as a teenager, even if prostate cancer does develop in one or two cells, the rate of cell death will be much greater than the rate of cell growth, so it's almost impossible for prostate cancer to survive. But as men age, their hormone levels decline, and at some point if prostate cancer develops, it has about as much chance of succeeding as other tissue cancers. As men get older still, their hormone levels decline to the point where if prostate cancer develops, the rate of cancer cell growth will automatically be greater than the rate of cancer cell death. This is because for men with normal genetics, the hormones that increase the rate of cancer cell death lose to the hormone estradiol, which fosters cell growth and proliferation. In fact, high local levels of estradiol will result in the cell growth of hundreds if not thousands of prostate cells. Also, as you will learn in the next chapter, high levels of estradiol result in more mutations. These mutations result in noncancerous immortalized prostate cells turning into prostate cancer cells. As men age they also have less testosterone, and as a result, in older men, the chance of prostate cancer succeeding is much greater than the success rate for cancers in other non-skin tissues.

When you have high levels of testosterone as a teenager, even if prostate cancer does develop in one or two cells, the rate of cell death will be much greater than the rate of cell growth, so it's almost impossible for prostate cancer to survive.

Many men go through life, at least their later years, worrying about prostate cancer. They know someone who has it or their doctors have told them that they have a precancerous condition. Even men who haven't received such a warning from their doctors may worry that they're at risk because prostate cancer is the second leading cause of cancer death in American men.[13] The American Cancer Society predictions for prostate cancer in the United States for 2011 indicate that 240,890 new cases of prostate cancer will be diagnosed and that 33,720 men will die of the disease. About one man in six will be diagnosed with prostate cancer during his lifetime. More than two million men in the United States who have been diagnosed with prostate cancer at some point are still alive today. But about one man in thirty-six will die of prostate cancer.[14]

Most likely the real reason that breast cancer and prostate cancer are so prevalent is that once you develop a high local level of estradiol to start the immortalization process, unless you have high-enough levels of testosterone (similar to the levels young people have in their teens and twenties), there's no way to stop the process of developing cancer.[15]

HOW IS PROSTATE CANCER DIFFERENT FROM ALL OTHER CANCERS?

It's important to remember that men have both testosterone *and* estrogen in their blood, both being necessary for proper biological functioning. But as men age, the ratio of testosterone to estrogen changes: there is less testosterone and more estrogen.[16] In addition, prostate epithelial cells can develop a condition in which strong **aromatase** (an enzyme that converts testosterone to estrogen) activity is present, whereas normal prostate epithelial cells have no aromatase activity.[17] This increased aromatase activity leads to very high local levels of estrogen. By "high local levels," I mean that the level of estrogen in the prostate is much greater than the blood level. In other words, there's an excess of estrogen in one specific part of the body, and the estrogen isn't flushed away from the site by circulating blood, like other substances might be. Instead, this estrogen remains in the prostate and causes the proliferation and mutation of prostate cells. It is this rapid proliferation and high mutation rate that leads to the increased likelihood of cancer.[18]

The issue is not that other tissues don't have aromatase—in fact many tissues do have plenty of aromatase activity. The real issue is that prostate tissue is susceptible to high levels of estradiol. Both prostate and breast tissue will lengthen their telomeres and divide when subjected to high levels of estradiol—no other tissues in men will do this.[19]

As to why prostate tissue is susceptible to this proliferation by estradiol, we know that the development of the sex organs is determined by hormone levels. From an evolutionary viewpoint, it makes no sense for five-year-olds to have fully functioning sexual organs. I'm not sure that there really is any anatomical necessity for prostate tissue to respond to estradiol; however, there is an anatomical necessity for breast tissue to respond to estradiol since women need functioning breasts to nurse newborn children, so breast tissue grows when estradiol levels become high enough, which they do during puberty. My guess is that prostate tissue is analogous to breast tissue—that is, both organs supply a liquid (breast milk or semen), and from an evolutionary viewpoint, it makes no sense to reinvent the wheel. In other words, once breast tissue is perfected for secreting a liquid, slight modifications result in prostate tissue, which also secretes a liquid.

In short, prostate cancer is different from other cancers because it is sensitive to the effect of hormones, especially estrogen. This insight may sound surprising in light of the fact that the primary male hormone is testosterone. Yet, as we will see, this insight about the crucial role of estrogen in the genesis of prostate cancer will play a pivotal role in our recommendations for how to prevent and treat the disease.

THE DANGER POSED BY IMMORTALIZED CELLS

Most experts will tell you that the first step in cancer formation is the immortalization of the cell. By immortalization they mean the ability of cancer to undergo unlimited cell divisions, not that each individual cancer cell lives forever. The cancer population is then capable of living forever, at least until the person who has the cancer dies. There are other properties of cancer, such as the ability to spread throughout the body by invading nearby and distant tissues and developing new blood vessels. However, if a normal cell were suddenly to take on all the properties of cancer *except* for immortalization, and if it divided ten or so times and thereafter died, then those abnormal cells would never have caused anyone any trouble or be considered cancerous. In short, immortalization is the villain.

Cells become immortal in a variety of ways, primarily through alterations in their DNA. Deoxyribonucleic acid (DNA) is the blueprint for all life. You could think of it as a computer database that contains all the information that makes you what you are physically. Each piece of information is referred to as a gene. One or more genes determine characteristics such as your hair color, eye color, and the shape of your ears. Genes are subject to mutation, or alterations, in their structure. Most mutations reduce a cell's (or organism's) ability to survive, but occasionally a mutation comes along that improves the chance of survival.

As cells divide rapidly, a cancer population becomes more and more diverse, with all sorts of different mutations arising. This diversity is referred to as the heterogeneity in prostate cancer. Put more simply, a prostate cancer mass is composed of cells of different types, and this is one of the primary reasons it's so hard to treat.

For example, imagine a prostate tumor composed of three types of cells. One cell type is able to grow only in the presence of testosterone. A second cell type is able to grow only in the absence of testosterone. And a third cell type is able to grow whether or not testosterone is present. If you try to treat this prostate tumor with testosterone ablation therapy, a common approach whereby a man's testosterone is shut down with drugs, then you will kill most of the first type of cells (the ones that require testosterone). But in doing so, you will leave the second and third type of cells alone, and they will proliferate to take up the space made by the death of the first type of cells. In other words, if you administer a drug that kills one type of cell, you will allow the others to flourish. This is probably the reason that prostate cancer becomes hormone resistant after a number of months of testosterone ablation therapy. The cells that were not killed, those that do not need testosterone to survive, were given a boost when you killed off their competitors, the cells that relied on testosterone. Since most treatments are not able to kill all the cancer cells, typically the treatment will alter the makeup of the cancer population to favor those cells that are best able to survive that treatment (see figure 4.5).

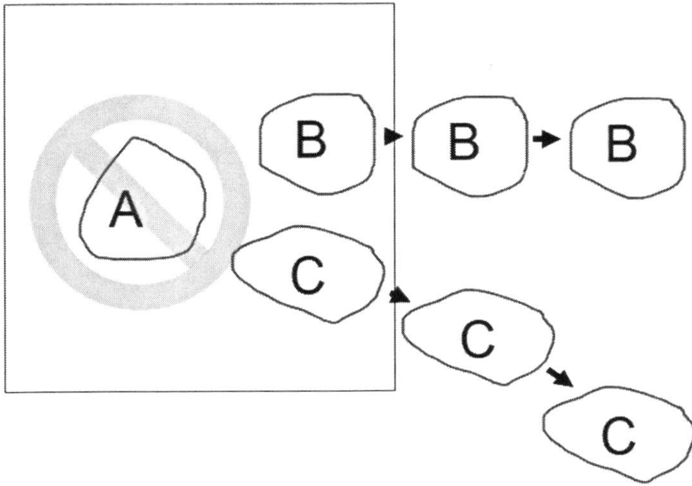

Figure 4.5. Heterogeneous cell populations. Prostate cancer is a heterogeneous disease involving many different types of tumor cells. If a tumor comprised of three types of cancer cells (A, B, and C) is treated with a therapy that kills the predominant Type A cells, then either Type B or C cells will become predominant depending on which population grows faster. In practice, almost any therapy will give a temporary advantage to some subset of cells in a prostate tumor. Drawing by Michael Christian.

It's important to understand the concept of **exponential growth** when discussing cancer. Exponential growth is what makes eradicating cancer so hard, because cancer can always kill you unless you kill *all* the cancer cells first. Take an example in which there are different cancer cells, and one divides every day (Type 1), but the other divides every two days (Type 2). If you start with a single cell of each type, then after sixteen days, you'll have 66,536 cells of Type 1 and 256 cells of Type 2. If a doctor discovered the cancer at this point, you would be told that over 99 percent of the cancer cells were Type 1. And if the doctor then gave you a treatment that killed every one of the Type 1 cancer cells, while not doing anything to the Type 2 cells, you would be thrilled to have 99 percent of your cancer eliminated in a single treatment. However, in just sixteen more days, the Type 2 cancer population would increase to 66,536 cells, and you would have almost as many total cancer cells as you had before treatment started. This is because exponential growth allows the Type 2 cells to multiply to deadly numbers just like the Type 1 cells were doing. It just takes a little longer for the Type 2 cells to kill you.

In real life, we're concerned with the growth rate of cancer populations, not individual cells. The rate of cell division and cell death of each of the individual cancer cells determines the overall growth rate of the population. Also, in real life, treatments are capable of altering the rate of growth of the various segments of the population that make up the cancer. The rate of growth is governed by evolutionary principles; in fact, it's impossible to understand why cancer is so deadly without understanding evolution. The most important evolutionary concept for our purposes is **selective growth advantage**. If a treatment favors one particular segment of a population (or even if it is less harmful to that segment than to other segments), then that treatment is said to give a selective growth advantage to the segment in question. This represents a form of survival of the fittest, whereby those cancer cells able to withstand a particular treatment are the ones that survive. Similar to the above example, if one segment comprised 50 percent of the population prior to treatment, and if the treatment allowed that segment to grow at least twice as fast as any of the other segments (most likely by slowing down the growth rate of the other segments), then after eight doublings of that segment, it would comprise over 99 percent of the overall cancer population. In real life, the doubling time of a population would typically be many days (slow-growing prostate cancer has an average doubling rate of 577 days), not just one or two days. However, the principle remains the same—given enough time, even a single cancer cell is capable of eventually killing you.[20]

If a treatment favors one particular segment of a population (or even if it is less harmful to that segment than to other segments), then that treatment is said to give a selective growth advantage to the segment in question.

MODELS OF PROSTATE CANCER

As we've seen, there are so many scientific articles published each year that nobody can read them all. This means that even scientists doing Nobel Prize–winning work often fail to see the bigger picture. My training as a theoretical biologist, however, prepared me to digest large masses of scientific information and find meaningful patterns, even patterns that might have escaped notice by the authors of the individual studies. Naturally my goal in reading their studies was to discover whether there were any patterns indicating that prostate cancer could be cured. I began by examining the current models of prostate cancer.[21]

In reading the literature, I applied logic to determine which models might possibly be correct and which were definitely wrong. There are numerous models that try to explain how prostate cancer originates. However, there's a funny thing about biology—reality trumps any idea, no matter how neat the inventor of the idea may think it is. What this means in practice is that when you list the known biological facts about the start of prostate cancer, if a fact contradicts a model, then that model must be wrong. Even if the model simply can't explain any of those facts, then the model probably is wrong. Conversely, having a model explain all the facts doesn't necessarily mean that the model is correct. To be correct, a model must not only explain all the facts but also make predictions that can be verified as true. Still, it's not clear that a model is ever really true in an absolute sense because every model is a work in progress, and as new data continues to be collected, the model will evolve to incorporate it. However, it's illogical for medical schools to teach models that are demonstrably false—especially when there's a model available that fits all the known facts—but unfortunately that's exactly what medical schools are doing.

The first known fact about prostate cancer is that it is the most common non-skin cancer in men in the United States. Also, there are a number of mutations (in this case, *mutation* means the gene no longer functions properly) identified in animal and human studies that result in prostate cancer *never* developing. Logically, if a mutation prevents prostate cancer from developing, then either the gene in question is essential for the start of the cancer or the gene is needed to guarantee that the cancer keeps growing. There are many other factors that increase or decrease the *likelihood* of prostate cancer being detected, but those factors won't be discussed here since I'm going to focus on identifying what is *essential* to turn normal prostate cells into cancerous prostate cells.

It's known that the primary male hormone, testosterone, is necessary for prostate cancer to begin. Also, studies show that the intracellular androgen receptor is needed for the initiation of prostate cancer. The androgen receptor is just a fancy name for a testosterone hormone receptor. It's called an androgen receptor because both testosterone and dihydrotestosterone (a modified form of testosterone) are considered androgens, and both bind to testosterone hormone receptors. Androgens are the primary male hormones, just as estrogens are the primary female hormones. We've seen that there are two types of androgen receptors: intracellular androgen receptor, located inside the cell, and membrane androgen receptor, located on the outside surface of the cell. Almost any doctor you meet, including specialists in prostate cancer, will use the term *androgen receptor* to refer only to intracellular androgen receptors, ignoring membrane androgen receptors completely. The important properties of membrane androgen receptors have been uncovered only in the last decade, and as far as I know, facts about membrane androgen receptors are not yet being taught routinely in medical schools around the world. One of the biggest surprises I got when I looked into the literature was that the membrane androgen receptor is one of the most significant discoveries that has ever been made about prostate cancer.[22]

Also, men lacking the enzyme **5-alpha-reductase** type II never develop prostate cancer. Enzymes are proteins that cause biochemical reactions to occur, such as the changing of one biological substance into another. This particular enzyme converts testosterone into dihydrotestosterone (DHT). So let's add DHT to the list of what is essential for prostate cancer development. It's also known that animals lacking the enzyme aromatase never develop prostate cancer. Aromatase converts testosterone into estradiol. Estradiol is one of the three main components of human estrogen, and it binds to estrogen receptors much more strongly than the other two. So we can conclude that estradiol is also essential. (Now you see why even some experts can get confused—we're starting to get complicated here!) Finally, animals lacking estrogen receptor-alpha (ER-alpha) never develop prostate cancer. You'll find out much more about ER-alpha in the next chapter. For now, just keep in mind that it's one of the hormone receptors that estradiol binds to. The logical conclusion is that ER-alpha is also essential for prostate cancer development.

TABLE 4.1. PROSTATE CANCER FACTS

PROSTATE CANCER FACTS
Prostate cancer is the most common non-skin cancer in men in the United States.
Testosterone is essential to initiate it.
Intracellular androgen receptor is essential to initiate it.
Dihydrotestosterone is essential to initiate it.
Estradiol is essential to initiate it.
Estrogen receptor-alpha is essential to initiate it.

Table 4.1 lists all the initiating factors for prostate cancer just discussed. Anyone who is familiar with the biology of the prostate would probably have their eyes popping out of their head at this point because of the last statement in the table. Allow me to clarify this for you. As we've seen, there are two major types of estrogen receptors inside cells: ER-alpha and estrogen receptor-beta (ER-beta). At one time it was thought that normal prostate cells didn't have any ER-alpha, only lots of ER-beta. Later it was discovered that there was actually a little bit of ER-alpha present. However, the amount was so small that it seemed inconceivable that it could possibly affect the growth rate of cancer very much. Then along came a researcher from Australia, Professor Gail Risbridger, who has done amazing award-winning work on prostate

cancer, and she discovered that ER-alpha was necessary for the initiation of prostate cancer.[23]

Upon reading Dr. Risbridger's work, I realized at once that she had discovered a key to understanding this disease. There are two steps in the development of prostate cancer. Think of the analogy of a tree growing. In order for the tree to grow, first you have to plant a seed, then you have to give it water, light, and nutrients from the soil to make it thrive. Now think of the initiation of the cancer as the planting of the seed. Without the seed, nothing else matters—nothing will grow. In the case of prostate cancer, ER-alpha is the equivalent of the seed. If you block ER-alpha, then you stop the planting of the seed, that is, prevent prostate cancer. However, once the tree starts to grow, it is too late to do anything about the seed. Similarly, after prostate cancer starts, eventually some of its cells will have mutations that allow it to grow without needing ER-alpha. I would predict that if you could block ER-alpha at an early enough stage, much earlier than when there are enough cells to be detected, then that should eliminate any prostate cancer that might be developing.

Continuing the tree analogy, think of having enough water, light, and soil nutrients as the equivalent of having a rate of cell growth *greater* than the rate of cell death. In other words, the cancer cell population would get larger and larger. Eliminating any substance that is essential for prostate cancer to start up can stop prostate cancer growth in one of two ways: either it stops the "planting of the seed" or it stops the "water and light" part of the equation. Using logic, we know that ER-alpha must be either the "seed" or the "water and light." But if it represented the water and light part of the equation, that is, if it helped prostate cancer thrive, then it would have to be super-potent because we know that there are just a few ER-alpha receptors in these cells, and this small group of receptors would have to be responsible for guaranteeing that the rate of cell growth was greater than the rate of cell death. If that were the case, then blocking ER-alpha after tumor formation would obliterate most prostate cancer cells, but this is not the case. So if ER-alpha is not the source of the "water and light," then it must be the "seed" part of the equation. The scientific evidence to support this conclusion is that either using more estradiol or increasing the amount of ER-alpha in prostate cells or prostate cancer cells results in increased telomerase activity, and increased estradiol results in more cell division, that is, it immortalizes those cells. Therefore, as a famous fictional detective once said, If you eliminate the impossible, whatever is left, no matter how improbable, must be the answer. In this case, ER-alpha must be the key element for the actual initiation of prostate cancer.[24]

CURRENT MODELS OF PROSTATE CANCER

Do you realize that prostate cancer is so complex that there are numerous competing theories to explain how it starts? I'm going to outline these theories for you in the next few pages. If you like a good murder mystery, you're going to love this discussion. And let's remember, prostate cancer is a real killer. Each one of these theories is trying to tell you that it can point a finger at one culprit and prove beyond a shadow of a doubt that "This is the guilty party! This is the killer." At the end of this review, I think you'll agree with me that each one of these theories is flawed. Moreover, you don't have to be a scientist to follow this discussion. All you have to do is use logic and common sense.

I hate to spoil a mystery, but I want to assure you that after I examine the current models for explaining the initiation of prostate cancer proposed by members of the medical establishment, I won't leave you with an unresolved crime. Although each one of these models is flawed, I will wind up the discussion with an explanation of my model, which I call the Hormone Receptor Model. I'll let you be the judge and jury to decide how well my model stacks up against the others in explaining these known facts. I think you'll be pleasantly surprised at the resolution of this mystery.

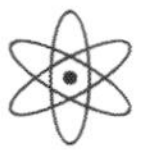

THE TESTOSTERONE MODEL

This model claims testosterone causes prostate cancer

The Testosterone Model is the oldest theory of how prostate cancer occurs. Basically, it states that prostate cancer is caused by testosterone. The only problem with this theory is that autopsy studies show that prostate cancer is virtually nonexistent in teenagers (who generally have high levels of testosterone), but that it occurs with a frequency of over 80 percent in eighty-year-olds (who generally have low levels of testosterone). Since the level of testosterone decreases as we age, the observed facts get in the way of a neat theory. Researchers have tried to explain the observed data by suggesting that it was the prolonged exposure of intracellular androgen receptors of epithelial cells to testosterone over the course of many years that caused prostate cancer. But this hypothesis produced further problems because the average prostate cell lives only five hundred days before dying and being replaced. If prolonged exposure is the culprit, then there has to be some memory. The basic premise of the Testosterone Model is equivalent to saying that your right hand itches because in the past, your great-great-grandfather touched some poison ivy with his right hand. That doesn't make sense, but in medicine, logic sometimes gets pushed aside as researchers cling to what they were taught in medical school.

Another attempt to salvage the Testosterone Model is to postulate that the development of prostate cancer has nothing to do with epithelial cells but rather that it is the years of exposure of *stem cells* to testosterone that initiates cancer. Stem cells are specialized cells in the prostate that keep spitting out additional normal prostate cells as needed. If testosterone somehow mutates stem cells over time, then it just *might* produce prostate cancer cells nonstop. But, believe it or not, Dr. Risbridger is one of the authors of an article that proved that stem cells cannot initiate prostate cancer.[25]

The Testosterone Model does, however, seem to explain why prostate cancer is so common in men, since men have lots of testosterone. If DHT is what is really needed to initiate prostate cancer, then this model also explains why testosterone is needed, since the only way to make DHT is by converting testosterone. However, this model has no explanation at all as to why either estradiol or ER-alpha is essential.

TABLE 4.2. TESTOSTERONE MODEL

PROSTATE CANCER FACTS	EXPLANATION
Prostate cancer is the most common non-skin cancer in men in the U.S.	Men have lots of testosterone, which is why prostate cancer is so common.
Testosterone is essential to initiate it.	Testosterone is needed to make dihydrotestosterone.
Intracellular androgen receptor is essential to initiate it.	This has to happen within 500 days but is contradicted by the fact that teenagers don't develop prostate cancer.
Dihydrotestosterone is essential to initiate it.	Dihydrotestosterone is what really acts on the intracellular androgen receptor.
Estradiol is essential to initiate it.	None.
Estrogen receptor-alpha is essential to initiate it.	None.

As Table 4.2 demonstrates, the Testosterone Model has to be considered a failure because of its inability to account for the necessity of estradiol and of ER-alpha. The Testosterone Model is also a failure because it can't adequately explain why teenagers don't get prostate cancer. Finally, the Testosterone Model must be rejected because it fails to explain why males with the lowest levels of testosterone—aging males—have the highest rate of prostate cancer. The explanation that testosterone needs years and years to produce its effect rings hollow in light of the objection that prostate cells live for only five hundred days.

Please keep in mind that although the Testosterone Model is demonstrably wrong—and it doesn't take a scientist to see this—it also happens to be the model that's most widely embraced by the medical establishment. This is because it's the old model that was taught in medical school. It's like when Copernicus showed that the earth revolved around the sun, while other scientists believed something that was eventually proven false. Even your family doctor probably subscribes to the mistaken view that testosterone causes prostate cancer.[26]

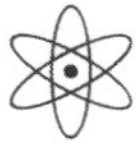

THE INFLAMMATION MODEL

This model claims that inflammation causes prostate cancer[27]

The Inflammation Model emphasizes the fact that there's a correlation between prostate cancer and inflammation. This fairly popular modern model states that changes to cells that undergo inflammation may make conditions more favorable for cancer. However, correlation does not imply causation, and in my opinion it's much more likely that prostate cancer causes inflammation than the other way around. There's no question that men with chronic inflammation are at increased risk of having prostate cancer detected. Also, anti-inflammatory drugs have been shown to decrease the risk of prostate cancer being detected. (The fact that no cancer is detected does not mean that no cancer is present.) In addition, abnormal lesions known as proliferative inflammatory atrophy (PIA) have been associated with chronic inflammation, and some doctors believe these may turn into prostate cancer.

As you may recall, we're *not* looking for factors that simply increase or decrease the *risk* of prostate cancer. If we were, then we would have to include eating broccoli, which has been shown to reduce the risk of prostate cancer being detected. Nobody is seriously saying that since eating more broccoli leads to less prostate cancer, then the initiating step in prostate cancer formation is the absence of broccoli. If that were true, prostate cancer would *never* occur in men who had always eaten lots of broccoli. Similarly, the fact that chronic inflammation increases the risk of prostate cancer being detected is insufficient evidence that inflammation is an essential initiating step. The point is not to find what affects the *risk* of developing prostate cancer but rather to find that which is *essential* for prostate cancer to develop—something whose absence makes it *impossible* for prostate cancer to develop.

Since ER-alpha increases inflammation,[28] it is tempting to say that that might be why this receptor is necessary for the initiation of prostate cancer. However, ER-beta *decreases* inflammation, and there is so much more ER-beta than ER-alpha in the normal prostate cell that any *increase* in estrogen level would lead to a *decrease* in inflammation. Only after prostate cancer develops and evolves to the point where there is more ER-alpha than ER-beta would an increase in estrogen be expected to lead to an increase in inflammation. This model also fails to offer any explanation as to why inflammation would affect only prostate cells, and it doesn't offer any insight into those factors that are essential for prostate cancer to develop. Unfortunately, this flawed model seems to be the one currently in favor with modern researchers.[29]

TABLE 4.3. INFLAMMATION MODEL

PROSTATE CANCER FACTS	EXPLANATION
Prostate cancer is the most common non-skin cancer in men in the U.S.	None.
Testosterone is essential to initiate it.	None.
Intracellular androgen receptor is essential to initiate it.	None.
Dihydrotestosterone is essential to initiate it.	None.
Estradiol is essential to initiate it.	None.
Estrogen receptor-alpha is essential to initiate it.	None.

As Table 4.3 demonstrates, the Inflammation Model has to be considered a failure because it doesn't explain anything, and it's an example of confusing correlation with causality. To explain what this means in simple terms, imagine that every time you wake up in the morning you notice that the sun has already risen. This is a correlation. Now imagine that you propose a model that your waking up is what caused the sun to rise. This would be causality. It would also be wrong, just as claiming that inflammation is the cause of cancer is wrong. The point is that correlation does not prove causation.

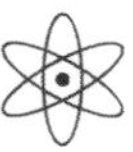

THE GENE FUSION MODEL

This model claims that gene fusions cause prostate cancer

The Gene Fusion Model states that there is a correlation between prostate cancer and gene fusions. While I haven't found any papers in the literature claiming that gene fusions *cause* prostate cancer, I've heard some doctors make this claim. Gene fusions are mutations that result in combinations of more than one gene product being produced when a single gene is expressed. There are particular gene fusions that are found in most prostate cancers. Whenever there's a correlation like this, the question must always be asked, "What causes what?" In other words, does prostate cancer cause gene fusions or do gene fusions cause prostate cancer? Some of the key gene fusions identified involve additional proteins being expressed in addition to those known to be expressed by testosterone. But most gene fusions have no apparent effect on the aggressiveness of prostate cancer; in other words, cancer grows and dies at the same rate as before.[30]

The Gene Fusion Model fails to explain why prostate cancer is so common, unless gene fusions occur only in prostate cells, which is highly unlikely. It does, however, explain why testosterone and the intracellular androgen receptor are both essential: because the gene fusion products are produced by the activation of the intracellular androgen receptor. Dihydrotestosterone binds to the intracellular androgen receptor five times more strongly than testosterone. Going back to the lock and key analogy discussed earlier, if the key slips out of the lock before you succeed in turning it, then you have to start over again. In this case, if the key is testosterone, then it's five times more likely to fall out than if the key is DHT. However, the activation of the androgen receptor is such a common occurrence in prostate cells that even if its rate is reduced fivefold, you still have more than enough opportunity to trigger whatever the initiating step is when the gene fusion products come into being (assuming the initiating step requires a protein not ordinarily expressed by the intracellular androgen receptor). Also, this model has no explanation for why either estradiol or ER-alpha is essential.

TABLE 4.4. GENE FUSION MODEL

PROSTATE CANCER FACTS	EXPLANATION
Prostate cancer is the most common non-skin cancer in men in the U.S.	Gene fusions must only occur in prostate tissue.
Testosterone is essential to initiate it.	Testosterone triggers it by binding to the intracellular androgen receptor.
Intracellular androgen receptor is essential to initiate it.	Testosterone triggers it by binding to the intracellular androgen receptor.
Dihydrotestosterone is essential to initiate it.	None.
Estradiol is essential to initiate it.	None.
Estrogen receptor-alpha is essential to initiate it.	None.

As Table 4.4 illustrates, the Gene Fusion Model is on shaky ground when it tries to explain why prostate cancer is the most common non-skin cancer in men. But the Gene Fusion Model really has to be considered a failure because of its inability to account for the necessity of dihydrotestosterone, estradiol, and estrogen receptor-alpha.

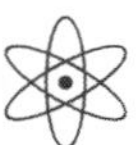

THE COLLAGEN MODEL

This model claims that decreased collagen levels cause prostate cancer

Another model recently proposed in the medical literature is the Collagen Model, which states that prostate cancer somehow arises as prostate cells make less collagen.[31] Collagen is a glycoprotein (an amino acid and sugar combination) that helps cells adhere to neighboring cells and that is the main constituent of connective tissue. There is a correlation between a lack of collagen and the detection of prostate cancer. As men age, their prostate cells produce less collagen, and the likelihood of prostate cancer being diagnosed increases. Also, once a prostate cancer cell metastasizes, that is, breaks free from the prostate and starts growing elsewhere in the body, it produces no collagen at all.

Although the Collagen Model calls attention to the correlation between low collagen and prostate cancer, it fails to explain why *prostate* cancer is so common, since collagen production also decreases with age in tissue other than prostate. Another flaw in this model is that researchers from Johns Hopkins elegantly demonstrated that the first prostate cancer cell typically develops when a man is in his twenties,[32] and it's highly doubtful that collagen production has significantly decreased at the age when the first prostate cancer cell actually arises.

TABLE 4.5. COLLAGEN MODEL

PROSTATE CANCER FACTS	EXPLANATION
Prostate cancer is the most common non-skin cancer in men in the U.S.	None.
Testosterone is essential to initiate it.	None.
Intracellular androgen receptor is essential to initiate it.	None.
Dihydrotestosterone is essential to initiate it.	None.
Estradiol is essential to initiate it.	None.
Estrogen receptor-alpha is essential to initiate it.	None.

As Table 4.5 shows, the Collagen Model also has to be considered a failure, because it doesn't explain any of the known key facts.

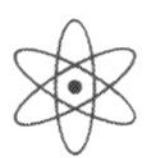

THE INTERNAL SPERMATIC VEIN MODEL

This model claims that faulty internal spermatic veins cause prostate cancer

An extremely new model is the Internal Spermatic Vein Model. This model points out that defects in internal spermatic veins (the veins within the testicles that carry blood back toward the heart) can lead to greatly increased testosterone levels in the prostate—as much as 130 times more than normal. Around 90 percent of this testosterone is converted to DHT, which then binds to the intracellular receptor and causes it to "work" around a hundred times more than it usually does.[33] This is an improved version of the Testosterone Model, in which prostate cancer, instead of developing after years of the intracellular androgen receptors being exposed to normal levels of testosterone, develops soon after being exposed to super-high levels of testosterone. Another supporting fact for this model is that 75 percent of men by age seventy have defects in their internal spermatic veins. However, proponents of this model make no mention of the percentage of men in their twenties (the age when the first prostate cancer cell typically starts up) who have this defect. The model also ignores the importance of estradiol and ER-alpha.

TABLE 4.6. INTERNAL SPERMATIC VEIN MODEL

PROSTATE CANCER FACTS	EXPLANATION
Prostate cancer is the most common non-skin cancer in men in the U.S.	Only if men in their 20s have the same percentage of defects as men in their 70s.
Testosterone is essential to initiate it.	Testosterone is converted to dihydrotestosterone.
Intracellular androgen receptor is essential to initiate it.	Intracellular androgen receptor is the target of dihydrotestosterone.
Dihydrotestosterone is essential to initiate it.	Intracellular androgen receptor is the target of dihydrotestosterone.
Estradiol is essential to initiate it.	None.
Estrogen receptor-alpha is essential to initiate it.	None.

As Table 4.6 shows, the Internal Spermatic Vein Model has to be considered a failure because of its inability to account for the necessity of estradiol and ER-alpha.

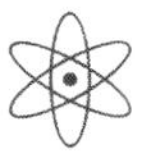

THE HORMONE RECEPTOR MODEL

This model proposes that the aromatization of testosterone into estradiol causes prostate cancer

Finally, let's talk about my model. I call it the Hormone Receptor Model because I'm concerned with the specific properties of each hormone receptor, whereas traditionally, the medical profession is concerned only with the effects of hormones (which often exhibit contradictory results). The Hormone Receptor Model proposes that prostate cancer is triggered by the activation of the enzyme aromatase, which converts testosterone into estradiol. *Ordinary prostate cells don't express aromatase (meaning they don't create this enzyme), but almost all prostate cancers do.*[34] Since the aromatase gene is already present in the prostate cell but is inactivated, all that's needed is for it to become activated in order to cause cells to eventually proliferate out of control.[35] In other words, the activation of just a single gene (which already exists, albeit in a dormant state) in a single prostate cell is all that's required to initiate a chain of events that can ultimately cause prostate cancer.[36]

Researchers have known for about a decade that a high local level of estradiol causes prostate cells to divide[37] and gives them the opportunity to multiply uncontrollably. *Prostate and breast cells are the only cells in men in which this is known to occur.* Cells with high aromatase activity will not only multiply out of control, but the high local level of estradiol will also cause neighboring cells to do the same thing. The higher the level of estradiol being produced, the more neighboring cells that will be affected. So while most cancers have to rely on a single immortalized cell mutating into cancer, prostate tissue contains multiple immortalized cells springing up at the same time, increasing the odds of getting just the right mutation to turn cancerous.[38] This explains why many doctors say that all men will eventually develop prostate cancer if they live long enough.

Once a prostate cell is immortalized, it's just a matter of time before prostate cancer develops. The only defense a man has against this prospect is making sure that he has a rate of cell death *greater* than the rate of cell growth before the errant cell gets a chance to undergo the necessary mutations. It turns out that higher levels of dihydrotestosterone *decrease* the amount of proteins that *protect* prostate cancer cells from dying. In other words, when prostate cancer is initially starting, the more dihydrotestosterone present the greater the chance that the cancer will have a rate of cell death greater than the rate of cell growth.

The only defense a man has . . . is making sure that he has a rate of cell death *greater* than the rate of cell growth before the errant cell gets a chance to undergo the necessary mutations.

So in the late teenage years through the early twenties, the normal balance of hormones means that any prostate cancer cells that start to develop will almost always have a rate of cell death greater than their rate of cell growth. This favorable condition exists because DHT is at its highest level during this time in a young man's life. As men age, however, the level of DHT within prostate cells *decreases*, and potential cancer cells no longer have to worry about having a rate of cell death greater than their rate of cell growth.[39] In chapters 10 and 12, I'll provide specific details about how the Hormone Receptor Model proposes to combat this problem with supplemental testosterone and other therapeutic protocols.[40]

TABLE 4.7. HORMONE RECEPTOR MODEL

PROSTATE CANCER FACTS	EXPLANATION
Prostate cancer is the most common non-skin cancer in men in the U.S.	No mutation is needed for immortalization; multiple immortalized cells appear at once, and as men age, those cells multiply faster than they die.

Testosterone is essential to initiate it.	Testosterone is converted to estradiol.
Intracellular androgen receptor is essential to initiate it.	Intracellular androgen receptor is essential for having a rate of cell growth greater than the rate of cell death.
Dihydrotestosterone is essential to initiate it.	Dihydrotestosterone is essential for initial prostate cancer growth by binding to the intracellular androgen receptor, which results in the cell being protected from the apoptosis caused by androgens binding to the membrane androgen receptor.
Estradiol is essential to initiate it.	High local levels of estradiol immortalize prostate cells.
Estrogen receptor-alpha is essential to initiate it.	Estrogen receptor-alpha is essential for the immortalization of prostate cells.

As Table 4.7 shows, the Hormone Receptor Model is the only model consistent with all the currently known facts about the initiation of prostate cancer. It can also shed some light on the other models. For example, the Testosterone Model is partially correct. Testosterone *is* the cause of the initiation of prostate cancer, but mainly because *it leads to unrestrained cell proliferation when converted to estradiol.*

The Inflammation Model can be explained by prostate cancer itself causing the inflammation. Inflammation increases the chance of prostate cancer being detected, but that's a far cry from saying that inflammation is required for prostate cancer to start up in the first place.

The Gene Fusion Model can be explained by gene fusions conferring some survival benefit on the prostate cancer cells.[41]

The Collagen Model may be correct in suggesting that totally losing the ability to produce collagen is necessary before prostate cancer cells can metastasize. It's also possible that collagen may provide some sort of protective effect against cancer, but the exact biological explanation of how this protection would work has not yet been elucidated.

The Internal Spermatic Vein Model may be correct when it proposes that high enough testosterone levels inside the prostate increase the risk of prostate cancer developing,[42] but this increase in cancer is due only to higher levels of testosterone leading to higher levels of estradiol when high aromatase activity occurs within prostate cells. Remember that aromatase converts testosterone into estradiol, which causes prostate cells to proliferate, leading to the increased potential of cancer starting.[43]

It should be pointed out that one of the primary reasons that doctors are afraid to prescribe testosterone for prostate cancer patients is because of the work of Fowler and Whitmore, published in the early 1980s. Their work is taught in just about every medical school throughout the world to demonize testosterone with regard to prostate cancer. Basically, they claimed that giving testosterone to men who were near death from prostate cancer was almost always bad. Even for those few men (approximately 15 percent) who initially had positive results, continued treatment with testosterone always led to an unfortunate conclusion.[44]

However, what medical schools don't tell future doctors is that in this study, over 45 percent of the men had first been treated with estrogen therapy and had failed that therapy (*failed* here means that estrogen began to speed up the growth of their overall prostate cancer population instead of slowing it down) *before* testosterone was tried. From my point of view, it's much more logical to conclude that the adverse effects demonstrated by Fowler and Whitmore were due not to the action of androgens on the internal androgen receptor but instead to high levels of estradiol that resulted in proliferative estradiol binding to ER-alpha.

Once you understand the logic behind my model of prostate cancer, it might occur to you that if you gave a male animal both testosterone *and* estradiol, you would expect prostate cancer to develop without needing the activation of aromatase. This is because if the level of estradiol you administer is high enough, that level will equal or even surpass the amount of estradiol that would have been produced had aromatase been activated. This hypothetical experiment is what is called a test of a model. If in fact combining these two hormones has little or no effect in causing prostate cancer, then my model would be incorrect. However, it turns out that when this combination is used in mice, prostate cancer almost always develops.[45]

For obvious reasons, this experiment has never been conducted with humans, although recently researchers have demonstrated that treating human prostate cells grown in a tissue culture with testosterone and estradiol always results in prostate cancer starting.[46] Also, research published in 2011 demonstrated that *estradiol alone was sufficient to cause prostate cancer in normal prostate cell cultures derived from rats.*[47] All of this is consistent with high local levels of estradiol being the villain and causing the initiation of prostate cancer for virtually all men who develop this disease.

Thankfully, my model *can* account for every significant fact about prostate cancer, even facts that no other researcher can explain. The Hormone Receptor Model not only identifies the root cause of prostate cancer—amazingly, it also identifies the cause of breast cancer, and it goes on to show that the triggering event for both diseases is essentially the same. For all intents and purposes, high local levels of estradiol in men and women are to blame for initiating both prostate and breast cancer.

The Hormone Receptor Model not only identifies the root cause of prostate cancer—amazingly, it also identifies the cause of breast cancer, and it goes on to show that the triggering event for both diseases is essentially the same. For all intents and purposes, high local levels of estradiol in men and women are to blame for initiating both prostate and breast cancer.

Since knowing the cause is the first step toward developing a cure, this model essentially holds out the promise of a revolutionary new treatment protocol (based on hormone replacement therapy plus the appropriate drugs) for these scourges of humankind, a protocol that can—and must—be put into practice today to save countless lives.[48]

The rest of this book will explore the profound implications of the Hormone Receptor Model for men and women who have prostate cancer or breast cancer, or who want to prevent these diseases in the first place. As you'll see, my treatment plan will also prevent and halt Alzheimer's.

When I first realized that I had essentially solved the mystery of how prostate cancer starts from high local levels of estradiol, I felt elated. At the time I was satisfied to publish my results in professional journals and to speak about my work to doctors. Shortly thereafter I saw how solving the mystery of prostate cancer led logically to important new revelations about treating and preventing breast cancer and Alzheimer's. Naturally I felt obliged to share these discoveries with a wider audience. It's my sincere hope that you'll find the rest of this book as exciting as a good murder mystery because together we're going to track down three killers and do the equivalent of putting them behind bars for life.

CHAPTER 5

HOW BREAST CANCER ARISES FROM ESTROGEN AND HOW HORMONE MODULATION IS CURRENTLY BEING USED TO FIGHT THE DISEASE

- Estradiol is known to cause breast cancer.
- Most researchers mistakenly believe estradiol causes breast cancer through decades of exposure to breast tissue.
- In actuality, breast cancer is caused not by prolonged exposure to estradiol but by exposure to high *local* levels of the hormone. These high local levels of estradiol are in turn caused by high aromatase activity that occurs randomly throughout a woman's life.
- If the Hormone Receptor Model is correct, then inhibiting aromatase will reduce breast cancer, since the inhibition of aromatase will reduce local (in breast tissue) production of estrogen.
- BRCA mutations, which increase cancer risk, are not adequately explained by the standard model.
- The Hormone Receptor Model proposes a more targeted treatment of BRCA mutations by showing how these mutations are dangerous due to progesterone receptor A and B differences.

The cause of breast cancer is no mystery. For decades, researchers have known that estradiol causes breast cancer, but they have never been able to explain exactly how it does so.

In this chapter, I explain for the first time exactly how estradiol causes breast cancer, how current breast cancer treatments try to reduce estradiol, and why the standard approach works fairly well but not perfectly. I also explain a slightly more effective way to limit estradiol based on our model of how breast cancer arises. As a coming attraction for what you will learn in this chapter, I'll tell you up front that the current understanding of breast cancer can be improved upon, and that the Hormone Receptor Model provides a more accurate picture of the origin of breast cancer. My model should therefore allow you and your doctor to have a better chance of treating breast cancer since knowing the precise cause is the first step toward successfully fighting any disease.

HOW BREAST CANCER ARISES

Although estrogen in the form of estradiol is essential for proper development, it can also cause problems, especially with breast tissue. Breast stem cells create breast epithelial cells in response to estradiol, a process responsible for breast development during puberty. But too much estradiol can lead to inappropriate proliferation of breast epithelial cells. If DNA mutations occur (through chance or as a result of exposure to carcinogens or radiation), the proliferation caused by estradiol allows mutant cells to divide and multiply out of control until they become cancerous.[1]

Currently, hormone modulation is used to treat breast cancer by reducing the amount of estrogen in the entire body or by blocking the binding of estrogen to estrogen receptor-alpha (ER-alpha) in breast cells. These methods work because, by reducing the amount of binding to ER-alpha, they reduce Bcl-2 production, telomerase activity, and cell proliferation. But this method, which is currently being used to fight breast cancer, is somewhat ineffective because it ignores the effects that other hormone receptors have on breast cancer.

Studies clearly show that estradiol is responsible for breast cancer. For example, in a study done on a particular strain of rat, five times the normal level of estradiol caused breast cancer in all test subjects, whereas none developed breast cancer when exposed to estriol.[2] Estrone does not cause breast cancer, but it does cause breast tumors. The tumors vanish when the excess estrone is removed.[3] These findings are consistent with ER-alpha being necessary for inappropriate cell division in breast epithelial cells. The fact that estradiol, but not estriol, causes actual breast cancer strongly suggests that estradiol (or one of its metabolites) is mutagenic, in other words, that it is responsible for the mutations needed for changing a benign tumor into a malignant tumor. It is not surprising that saliva levels of estrone were higher in women with breast cancer than in similar women who did not have breast cancer.[4] The point is that estradiol and breast cancer are correlated, and the higher your local estradiol level, the more likely you are to get breast cancer. In fact, the prevailing opinion seems to be that breast cancer in women occurs after decades of breast epithelial cells being exposed to estradiol. The "proof" seems to be that breast cancer is more prevalent in older women than in younger women. The median age of women who develop breast cancer is sixty-one; Table 5.1 shows the distribution of breast cancer according to age.[5] The lifetime chance for a woman to be diagnosed with breast cancer was 12.1 percent in 2006.[6]

TABLE 5.1. DISTRIBUTION OF BREAST CANCER ACCORDING TO AGE

AGE OF WOMAN	BREAST CANCER PERCENTAGE
Younger than 20	0.0
20–34	1.9
35–44	10.6
45–54	22.1
55–64	22.8
65–74	20.4
75–84	16.8
85 or older	5.4

Table 5.2 shows the chance of developing breast cancer within the next ten years for women of various ages.[7] It is clear from Table 5.2 that the risk of being diagnosed with breast cancer increases with age in women, with sixty-year-old women being eight times more likely to develop the disease within the next ten years than thirty-year-old women.

TABLE 5.2. CHANCE OF DEVELOPING BREAST CANCER WITH AGE

CURRENT AGE OF WOMAN	PERCENTAGE CHANCE OF DEVELOPING BREAST CANCER WITHIN THE NEXT 10 YEARS
30	0.43
40	1.45
50	2.38
60	3.45

But is it true that prolonged exposure to estradiol leads to breast cancer? While it is clear that the chance of developing breast cancer increases with age, it does not follow that this is necessarily due to prolonged exposure to estradiol. Since breast cancer occurs in breast epithelial cells and breast epithelial cells are constantly undergoing turnover, it is not clear how prolonged exposure could carry over the effects of estradiol from one generation to the next, especially since breast epithelial cells are produced by stem cells and not by mitosis.

If breast cancer is not caused by prolonged exposure to estradiol, then it must be caused by high local levels of estradiol. Estradiol causes proliferation of breast epithelial cells[8] and increases telomerase activity,[9] both of which are necessary factors for cancer initiation. The question posed by these facts is, *What actually causes estradiol levels in breast tissue to become high enough to initiate cancer?* Measurements of estradiol in blood serum do not show the high levels necessary to cause breast cancer. However, the ratio of serum estradiol to tissue estradiol is around 1:1 in premenopausal women but is 10–50:1 in postmenopausal women. In other words, as women grow older, their serum level of estradiol dramatically decreases, but the level of estradiol around tumors once breast cancer occurs remains constant. This disparity between blood and local levels of estradiol has led researchers to conclude that "*local* concentrations of estradiol in human mammary tissue and in breast tumors depend more likely on the *aromatase activity* of individual mammary cells (autocrine or paracrine action) than on the ovarian hormone supply."[10] In plain English, high local levels of estradiol in breast tissue are caused by local enzyme action rather than by high systemic (blood) levels of estradiol.[11] The bottom line is that aromatase is clearly implicated in the initiation of breast cancer.

The bottom line is that aromatase is clearly implicated in the initiation of breast cancer.

In addition to aromatase within individual breast epithelial cells, there is also aromatase in fat (adipose) tissue within the breast. While I agree with the prevailing opinion that aromatase activity is what raises estradiol levels high enough to cause breast cancer, I disagree with the idea that aromatase within individual breast *epithelial* cells is the sole cause. It turns out that under certain circumstances there can also be significant aromatase activity in fat tissue within the breast. There are regions of DNA called promoters that can affect the production and makeup of aromatase. Normally, there is a low level of aromatase activity in adipose tissue due to a promoter named I.4. However, breast cancer cells produce unknown factors that shut off the I.4 promoter and turn on I.3 and II promoters.[12] The real question is, Did the factors that turn on promoters I.3 and II occur before or after breast cells turned cancerous? If the answer is after, then we still have no idea what initiates breast cancer. However, if the answer is before, then this neatly explains how breast cancer occurs. The very first step is for one or more breast epithelial cells to produce factors that turn on promoters I.3 and II. This does not require a mutation but rather just turning on a gene that is ordinarily turned off in that tissue. Once the factors are produced, surrounding adipose tissue will develop very high levels of aromatase activity resulting in high local levels of estradiol. The estradiol will cause cell division and telomere lengthening in surrounding epithelial cells—not just in the cell that produced those factors. With multiple cells dividing inappropriately coupled with the mutagenic effect of high levels of estradiol, it is just a matter of time before the right mutations occur to initiate breast cancer. And once it is initiated, it will proliferate unless the rate of cell death is greater than the rate of cell growth.[13]

One final issue is relevant for our discussion of the genesis of breast cancer. It is important to consider the rate of growth for breast cancer in order to understand how quickly it can be detected and treated. Typically, the growth rate is faster early on, but then it slows as tumor size increases. Also, as women age, the growth rate tends to slow. Growth is typically measured in terms of the doubling rate, which is the time it takes for a tumor to double the number of cells it contains. Approximately thirty population doublings are needed from the time the first cancer cell arises for breast cancer to grow to a large enough size to be detected, which represents approximately one billion cells.[14] If untreated, then ten more doublings are typically fatal.[15]

By the time breast cancer is large enough to be detected, its doubling rate has been observed to vary between 50 and 400 days, with an average between 200 and 300 days. Researchers used computer simulations and took into account age-appropriate average and standard deviation of the tumor doubling time to determine that 93.3 percent of diagnosed breast cancers in the 2002 WHI study were from occult (hidden) tumors.[16] Their data was consistent with a change in the average doubling time from 200 days for women not taking HRT to 150 days for those who did. In other words, the synthetic progestin used in that study caused breast tumors to speed up their growth. Study scientists predicted that stopping HRT would reduce the overall breast cancer rate by 7 percent in the ensuing five years.[17]

BRCA1 AND BRCA2

There are a number of genetic mutations that increase the risk of developing breast cancer. The most well known of these are mutations in the proteins BRCA1 and BRCA2.[18] Both of these proteins are involved in DNA repair. Instead of the 12.1 percent lifetime chance of developing breast cancer, women with the BRCA1 mutation have a 60 to 80 percent chance of developing breast cancer, with a median age of diagnosis of forty-two, and women with the BRCA2 mutation have a 60 to 85 percent chance of developing breast cancer.[19] Women with these mutations account for about 5 percent of all breast cancer cases.[20]

If a woman is known to have one of these BRCA mutations prior to developing cancer, the current medical options are either maintaining close surveillance or undergoing prophylactic surgery—removal of the breasts (mastectomy), removal of the ovaries (oophorectomy), or both. Those women who undergo both surgeries experience a 3.3- to 6-year-longer life expectancy than those women who choose surveillance.[21] The rationale for removing the ovaries is to greatly reduce the amount of estrogen being produced. But in all likelihood a more effective and less psychologically devastating course of action would be to implement the aggressive prophylactic measures that are recommend in chapter 11.

Researchers also discovered a different approach for preventing breast cancer by working with a particular strain of mice that had the BRCA1 mutation. If untreated, all these mice developed breast tumors within 8.7 months. None of the mice treated with mifepristone, commonly known as RU-486, had tumors after twelve months.[22] RU-486 is known to block progesterone receptor A.[23] This result is not easy to explain using the standard model of BRCA mutations and breast cancer since progesterone should have nothing to do with DNA repair, and it is inconceivable that blocking a progesterone receptor would allow DNA to now be repaired properly.

However, if we consider the Hormone Receptor Model, then everything becomes clear. It turns out that examination of breast tissue from women with BRCA mutations who had prophylactic mastectomies shows that there is almost no progesterone receptor B present.[24] As I noted in chapter 2, progesterone receptor B is good for you because it reduces the production of Bcl-2 (which protects cancer cells from apoptosis), whereas progesterone receptor A is bad for you because it increases the production of Bcl-2, allowing cancer cells to live longer. Therefore, you would expect to find higher than normal levels of harmful Bcl-2 in the breast tissue of women with BRCA1 or BRCA2 mutations. Ordinarily, progesterone decreases the amount of harmful Bcl-2 in breast tissue,[25] which is consistent with there being more progesterone receptor B than progesterone receptor

A present in the breast tissue of healthy women. This explains why women with BRCA mutations are more likely to develop breast cancer—they have high-enough levels of Bcl-2 in their breast tissue so that even if breast cancer starts up at an early age (an age at which the rate of cell death is normally greater than the rate of cell growth), the breast cancer can now take root and grow. If the above assumptions are correct, then progesterone will be *increasing* Bcl-2 in women with BRCA1 or BRCA2, *which is the opposite effect that it has in healthy women.* Increased levels of Bcl-2 will increase the amount of breast tissue, since Bcl-2 decreases the rate of cell death for normal breast cells, not just cancerous ones. In fact, it was shown that for a mouse strain that was lacking normal BRCA1 protein, progesterone greatly increased breast tissue volume, whereas it caused no significant changes in mice that possessed normal BRCA1 protein.[26] What all this means is that women from families with a history of breast cancer or from populations more likely to possess these mutations, such as women of Ashkenazi Jewish heritage, might want to ask their doctor to test for BRCA1 and BRCA2 mutations so that they can take aggressive steps to prevent breast cancer—steps I outline in chapter 11.

In conclusion, the greater incidence of breast cancer in women with BRCA1 or BRCA2 mutations can be attributed to the higher level of Bcl-2 caused by progesterone receptor A. The increase in negative prognostic factors associated with these cancers[27] may well be due to problems with DNA repair. I am convinced that the Hormone Receptor Model explains how to deal with BRCA mutations and points to the most effective method of preventing or mitigating negative outcomes for women who inherited BRCA1 and BRCA2 mutations.

CHAPTER 6

CAN ALZHEIMER'S BE CURED? NEW HOPE FOR THOSE AT HIGH RISK

Sure, I know Alzheimer's results in brain degeneration. I know it results in cognitive decline. And I know it eventually kills the majority of its victims. But here's what bothers me most about Alzheimer's. The fact that patients aren't given hope. The fact that modern medicine seems to just throw up its hands and say, "There's not much we can do." And the fact that the drugs patients are prescribed treat only symptoms, not causes.[1] Worst of all, these drugs don't save lives.

I hate that. And I was determined not to write a word about Alzheimer's . . . unless I could do better.

Well, here's the chapter on the underlying causes of Alzheimer's—and what can be *done* about it using today's technology. I'll let you be the judge whether it makes sense. You don't need a medical degree to understand this chapter. It's as clear as a bell.

Each year, half a million Americans are diagnosed with Alzheimer's, and the number of new cases is increasing at an alarming rate. Most people know that Alzheimer's is a degenerative brain disease, but not everyone understands how often it is fatal—most patients live an average of only four to eight years following diagnosis. Approximately eighty thousand Americans die from Alzheimer's each year, and it is now the sixth leading cause of death. *Officially*, the cause of this disease is unknown, and there is no known cure or effective treatment.

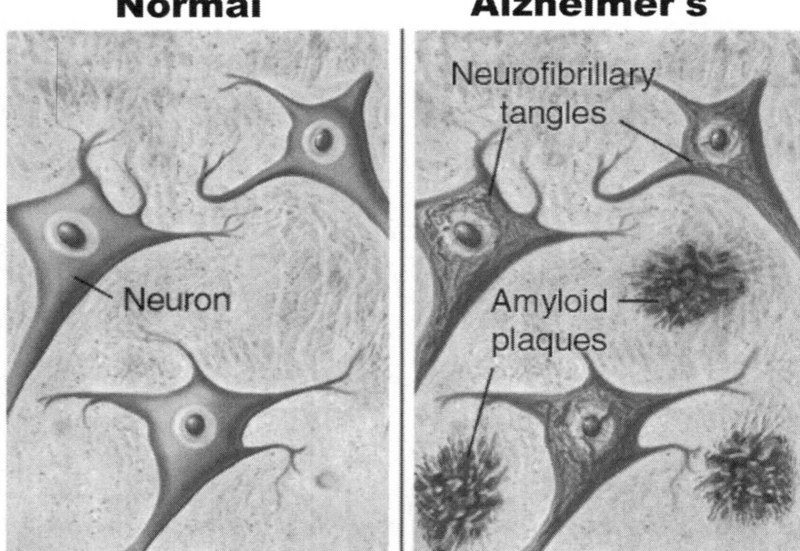

Figure 6.1. Beta amyloid plaques form between neurons. **Neurofibrillary tangles** form inside neurons. The medical illustration is provided courtesy of Alzheimer's Disease Research, a program of BrightFocus Foundation © 2013 http://www.brightfocus.org/alzheimers.

There are two brain anomalies associated with Alzheimer's: **plaques** and **tangles**. Plaques are located between nerve cells (neurons) in the brain and are mostly made up of the protein beta amyloid (figure 6.1). Tangles are located inside neurons in the brain and are mostly made up of **hyperphosphorylated tau protein**. Because of the correlation between excess beta amyloid and Alzheimer's, it has long been suspected that beta amyloid was the *cause* of Alzheimer's. Until recently, however, there was no definitive proof of this. In 2012, more than twenty-five researchers from the United States, Iceland, Germany, Norway, Sweden, and Finland teamed up and discovered a genetic mutation that significantly *decreases* the chance of developing Alzheimer's. This mutation results in an approximately 40 percent *decrease* in the production of beta amyloid. This is a very good mutation to have because it protects against Alzheimer's.

Unfortunately, not everybody has this protective mutation. Researchers observed this mutation in only a fraction of the people (0.13 percent) who have Alzheimer's. In contrast, more people eighty-five and older who are Alzheimer's free (0.62 percent) *do* have this favorable mutation.[2] So, here is the first concrete proof that *reducing levels of beta amyloid can reduce the incidence of Alzheimer's.* Also, this protective mutation was found in 0.79 percent of people who were cognitively intact at age eighty-five. Further evidence that lowering beta amyloid production *protects* against cognitive decline as well as against Alzheimer's.

Naturally, the question we need to answer is, How do we *reduce* beta amyloid? More on this in a moment. First, let's look briefly at other factors associated with Alzheimer's.

A vast amount of research has been devoted to this question, and scientists have identified a number of additional risk factors associated with Alzheimer's. Of these factors, age is the biggest risk. But nothing much can be done about how old you are,[3] so let's press onward. It's also known that having the gene for apolipoprotein E-e4 increases the risk of developing this disease. The apolipoprotein E-e4 mutation *hinders* beta amyloid from leaving the brain.[4] In other words, it makes more of the bad stuff accumulate in your cerebral tissue. Fortunately, vitamin D3 *facilitates* beta amyloid leaving the brain.[5] It's not yet clear to what extent the apolipoprotein E-e4 mutation counters vitamin D3, but it makes sense for everyone—especially anyone with this mutation—to maintain high-normal levels of vitamin D3 in order to help prevent Alzheimer's.

In addition to increased levels of beta amyloid, several other biochemical reactions are known to be associated with Alzheimer's. But as I will demonstrate in the following paragraphs, for every biochemical reaction associated with Alzheimer's, there is almost always at least one hormone that works *against* that reaction as the level of that hormone increases. In other words, optimal hormone levels fight Alzheimer's. For example, both testosterone and estradiol *reduce* the secretion of beta amyloid.[6] Although daily application of progesterone interferes with the ability of estradiol to reduce beta amyloid levels, *when progesterone is applied for ten days every thirty days*, it *enhances* estradiol's reduction of beta amyloid.[7]

The first step in solving the puzzle of Alzheimer's is contained in this intriguing finding about how testosterone, estradiol, and progesterone fight beta amyloid. But before we put the other pieces of the puzzle into place, let's turn our attention to the chief villain of this story, beta amyloid.

Beta amyloid is the Darth Vader of Alzheimer's, the shadowy desperado that lurks behind most of the destruction Alzheimer's causes. Undoubtedly you've heard the term *beta amyloid* in connection with Alzheimer's for years, but what exactly is it? In fact, it's such an important component of Alzheimer's that it deserves to be center stage in this drama. Beta amyloid is a peptide formed from the cleavage of amyloid precursor protein (APP). The number of amino acids that make up beta amyloid peptide is either 40 or 42. Alzheimer's disease results in an *increase* in the ratio of beta amyloid-42 to beta amyloid-40.[8] It follows that an increase in this ratio is a bad sign. Significantly, this ratio is *decreased* by the action of testosterone.[9]

Alpha secretase is an enzyme that cleaves APP in a way that *prevents* the formation of beta amyloid. Today, everyone who works in this field knows that alpha secretase performs a vital function in preventing excess beta amyloid buildup. Ordinarily, there's enough alpha secretase activity to keep beta amyloid at low levels, but alpha secretase activity drops dramatically in the brains of people with Alzheimer's.[10] This is not good. However, both estradiol and testosterone *increase* helpful alpha secretase activity.[11]

Do you see the pattern emerging? Natural hormones are consistently acting *against* key components of Alzheimer's. But we're not through yet. There's more good news.

Beta amyloid is produced from APP, first by the action of the enzyme beta secretase, then by the action of gamma secretase. There are correlations between Alzheimer's and increased beta secretase activity[12] and increased gamma secretase activity.[13] Because gamma secretase is involved in a number of other chemical reactions other than simply producing beta amyloid, it's not an attractive therapeutic target. In fact, the drug Semagacestat®, which targeted gamma secretase, seemed to do more harm than good, and so its clinical trial had to be halted.[14] Clearly, a more appropriate target for therapy would be beta secretase. The logical next question to ask is whether there's anything available to reduce beta secretase. And lo and behold! Testosterone reduces beta secretase activity,[15] as does estradiol.[16] It turns out that our old friends the natural hormones are at it again—working powerfully to *reduce* key components of Alzheimer's.

And it gets even better . . .

Neprilysin is an important enzyme that degrades beta amyloid. Good fellow, neprilysin! Getting rid of excess beta amyloid for us! Reducing the principal component of Alzheimer's! It deserves a round of applause, a big round of applause. Unfortunately, there's significantly *decreased* neprilysin activity in the brain tissue of Alzheimer's patients.[17] Put more simply, people with Alzheimer's don't have the full benefit of this wonderful enzyme. It's as if their brains were hungry for neprilysin, but it's not there . . . it's nowhere to be found. What to do? Can you buy some and ingest it? Can you inject it? Can you inhale it? Of course, people with Alzheimer's would certainly want to know. For heaven's sake, if I had Alzheimer's I would want to know!

Well, it turns out that testosterone increases neprilysin activity,[18] as does estradiol.[19]

Our old friends to the rescue again! Almost too good to be true. Almost hard to believe, too. But documented evidence shows that natural hormones are once more doing double, triple, quadruple duty—like Santa's little helpers. Running hither and thither and patching up problems when things go wrong in the brain. Making sure that this . . . and that . . . and who know what else are all working as they should be.

I ask you, can it get any better than this?

The answer is . . . YES!

But I hesitate to tell you the next piece of the puzzle for fear that you won't believe it.

And yet, how can I not continue, when the evidence is so clear and unequivocal? So, on we go! It is known that tangles, which are made up mostly of hyperphosphorylated tau protein, grow inside brain cells and eventually *kill* them. Bad news. Very bad news. It's perfectly clear that too much hyperphosphorylated tau protein is a very nasty thing. But what can we do? Can we, in fact, do *anything* to stop this unsavory protein from doing its dastardly misdeeds in our brains? I know what you're thinking. "It can't be the hormones again, can it, Dr. Friedman? Are you going to tell me that hormones—natural hormones, like testosterone and estrogen—can work this miracle? Are you *really* going to slap me in the face again with that wake-up call to action?" Come, come, my friends! I'm not making this up. All you have to do is look up the article in the next footnote yourself and then *you'll* be telling people the good news. You'll be shouting it from the rooftops. You'll be clamoring for it to be emblazoned across the front pages of our national tabloids—yes, testosterone decreases the hyperphosphorylation of tau protein.[20] "What about estrogen?" you ask. "Does estrogen do it too?" Well, in this case, although estradiol does not decrease the hyperphosphorylation of tau protein, progesterone does.[21]

Hormones to brain: "We've got you covered. Yes, we've got you covered, provided that you have *enough* of us circulating through your brain, my good man (or woman). Provided that you have enough of us. For, after all, we can't do our work unless we're present in the bloodstream, can we?"

Gentle reader, I know you've come a long way in this chapter and have tarried over many an abstruse term, many a multisyllabic moniker that might choke a professor of neurophysiology—not to mention a casual bystander. I realize you deserve a break. And I'm going to give it to you. But first, let me present you with one more teensy-weensy bit of good news. You have time for that, don't you? One last bit of good news about fighting Alzheimer's?

Here it is, then. Short and sweet and to the point. Impaired brain cell *glucose metabolism* is associated with Alzheimer's disease.[22] Meaning what? Meaning, in plain English, that if your brain doesn't have the capacity to metabolize simple sugar in the form of glucose, you're in trouble. Big trouble. In fact, that inability to metabolize glucose contributes to Alzheimer's. Quite a nightmarish scenario, wouldn't you say? Well, to make a long story short, our good friend testosterone significantly *improves* brain cell glucose metabolism[23] . . . as does estradiol.[24] Similarly, Alzheimer's disease is associated with impaired blood flow to the brain.[25] And, again, testosterone improves blood flow to the brain[26] . . . as does estradiol.[27]

Yes, once again, hormones to the rescue.

I know I've given you a lot to digest here. But you saw that it was all good news about how *hormones fight the critical components of Alzheimer's*. Let's put this good news together in a chart so that we can look at it—and marvel at it and digest it visually. Table 6.1 summarizes the biochemical reactions correlated with Alzheimer's and hormones.

TABLE 6.1. THE EFFECT OF HORMONES ON BIOCHEMICAL REACTIONS ASSOCIATED WITH ALZHEIMER'S

	Alzheimer's disease	Testosterone	Estradiol	Progesterone 10 days every 30 days
Beta amyloid	Increases	Decreases	Decreases	Decreases
42/40 ratio	Increases	Decreases	?	?
Alpha secretase	Decreases	Increases	Increases	?
Beta secretase	Increases	Decreases	Decreases	?
Gamma secretase	Increases	?	?	?
Neprilysin	Decreases	Increases	Increases	?
Hyperphos-phorylated tau protein	Increases	Decreases	No effect	Decreases
Brain cell glucose metabolism	Decreases	Increases	Increases	?
Blood flow to the brain	Decreases	Increases	Increases	?

Even a cursory glance at Table 6.1 makes it clear that men can counter all the known biochemical reactions of Alzheimer's—except for increased gamma secretase activity—with testosterone.[28] Women can do the same with estradiol, progesterone, and testosterone.

Now *you* be the judge.

I told you I'd let you decide whether we could do better than what's currently being offered for people with Alzheimer's. And I promised that you wouldn't need a medical degree to understand it. Decide for yourself whether there's not more hope shown on that chart about hormones fighting *all the causal factors associated with Alzheimer's* than in any of the concoctions currently being whipped up for temporary symptomatic relief by a generation of doctors who admit that *current medications cannot cure Alzheimer's or stop it from progressing*. If I, or someone I loved, had early—or even late-stage—Alzheimer's, no one would have to ask me twice which option I would unhesitatingly choose to try first.

One question that remains to be addressed is why there is a higher percentage of people developing Alzheimer's today than there was in the past. The answer that appears most likely to me is that the increased level of air pollution in the modern world is contributing to the increase in Alzheimer's. In fact, exposure to high levels of air pollution is strongly correlated with increased production of the more harmful beta amyloid-42.[29]

But let me end on a positive note. Naturally, the other question that needs to be addressed is, Why has no one used this information about hormones to formulate a treatment plan to counter all these various nasty components of Alzheimer's? Why is Alzheimer's the scourge it has become for our aging population when hormones appear to hold the promise of fighting this dreaded disease? In short, why is Alzheimer's still killing people when we know all these positive and useful things about hormones?

As we'll see in chapter 14, someone *has* developed a treatment plan based precisely on this information. And, by heavens, I'm convinced that such a treatment plan will work.

CHAPTER 7

THE MIRACLE OF TEENAGE HORMONE LEVELS— HOW TO FEEL LIKE YOU'RE NINETEEN AND HAVE THE SAME IMMUNITY TO PROSTATE CANCER, BREAST CANCER, AND ALZHEIMER'S AS TEENAGERS, WHO ALMOST NEVER GET THESE DISEASES

- In addition to fighting many diseases of aging, sex hormones have a beneficial impact on cardiac and vascular health.
- Replacing hormone levels improves cognition and psychological well-being.
- Bringing hormones into the optimal range also increases energy, drive, and motivation while at the same time reducing irritability, apathy, and depression.
- Replacing hormones boosts sex drive.
- Hormone replacement therapy can reduce fear and stimulate an appropriate level of aggression.
- Testosterone cuts body fat.

Throughout this book, I have been demonstrating that treatment with hormones helps prevent and, in many cases, reverse some of the major disease states associated with aging. I know that people with low hormones who bring their levels into optimal ranges can fight diseases like prostate cancer and breast cancer, but I never expected my research to uncover so many impressive studies demonstrating that hormones are beneficial in addressing other diseases too. Compelling evidence now indicates that bioidentical hormone replacement therapy

(BHRT) fights diabetes in men,[1] Alzheimer's, cognitive impairment,[2] depression,[3] low libido,[4] heart problems,[5] skin and blood vessel disorders,[6] motivation deficits,[7] high blood pressure[8] blood lipid imbalances,[9] and the list goes on.[10]

Unlike other therapies recommended by mainstream medicine for prostate and breast cancer—surgery, radiation, and chemotherapy—hormones will not produce scars, burns, or nausea. Instead, BHRT almost always makes people feel good. Middle-aged and elderly individuals who replace diminished hormones have more energy and zest for life.

The specific negative side effects of BHRT are typically minimal, and I review them in the chapters on practice (chapters 12 to 14). What I have only mentioned but need to elaborate on are the significant positive side effects of topping up your hormones. These side effects include a reduction in irritability, a reduction of fear and anxiety, an enhanced and appropriate aggression—the type that helps a person get organized and stay on track toward the accomplishment of tangible goals. There are other related beneficial effects. This constellation of beneficial feelings is one of the pleasant surprises in store for those who adopt proper hormonal supplementation for disease prevention and treatment.

ARE HORMONES A FOUNTAIN OF YOUTH?

You don't need massive epidemiological data (although it does exist) to know that when we were younger, we were healthier. Generally speaking, that is why explorers have sought the fountain of youth. Scientists have been on a similar quest. This modern scientific search has looked for a way to reverse the aging process so that we can return to a time when our bodies enjoyed robust health and energy and our minds were not hampered by cognitive impairment. In short, we dream of finding the youthful condition again precisely because it was during this time in our lives that we enjoyed the good health that one wishes could last indefinitely.

If scientists—or explorers—ever find the fountain of youth, logic tells us that it *must* also include teenage hormone levels. This is because high hormone levels are *necessary* for the maintenance of optimal health. In other words, *you cannot be healthy unless your hormones are at a high enough level.* There is undeniable evidence that low levels of hormones are a marker of disease. People who are afraid of getting their hormones supplemented as they age—and, unfortunately, too many people fall into this category because of media mistakes and misinformation—are on a sure path to cognitive and physical decline[11] that *cannot* be fixed except by increasing hormone levels to what they were in their youth. And this is why it is so unfortunate when people bemoan their fate after they have a stroke; or suffer geriatric frailty and fall repeatedly and break their bones; or develop type 2 diabetes or a heart condition, memory loss, Alzheimer's, prostate cancer, breast cancer, or a host of other ailments. It's too bad that these people don't realize that no matter how many times they visit their doctor's office, they will not get better if they have an uncorrected underlying hormonal deficit like most aging people experience after age forty.

High hormone levels are *necessary* for the maintenance of optimal health.

But even I, who support the practice of returning hormones to their optimal range of levels, even I must admit that hormones are not really a fountain of youth. Teenage hormone levels are necessary for good health, but they are not sufficient. It is still impossible to match exactly the youthful, delicate balance of hormones of the teen years. We can get close, but there is nothing like the finely tuned symphony of a youthful endocrine system working in perfect harmony. We cannot instantly change other degenerative physical processes either, such as arthritis, inflammation, muscle loss, and the loss of brain cells. So while hormone supplementation will make you feel a good deal of the youthful energy and enthusiasm for life that you had in your teens, it will not turn you into a teenager again. Right now, however, it's the closest we can get to reaching this goal of age regression, and people who do replace their hormones will be astounded at their increased energy, motivation, libido, and feelings of physical well-being.

That being said, there are some advantages that a middle-aged or elderly person using hormones experiences that a teenager cannot know. For instance, an adult will not generally experience the crushing self-doubt that strikes most young people in our culture. Nor will he feel the instant disappointment and critical embarrassment that teens experience on an almost daily basis. Yes, having higher levels of testosterone will make you feel more courageous and fearless, but because you have decades more experience, you will most likely be able to handle the stresses of life much better than a teenager.

If you look at the average young man or woman in their late teens and early twenties, you will find that they are usually smiling, laughing, and having a good time. Life is beautiful. They radiate happiness and good health. True, they may periodically slip into depression or self-doubt, but if they feel self-doubt, it's usually gone by the next morning, when the pulsatile cycle of their hormones kicks in.

It is also the premise of this book that when adults use BHRT and bring their hormone levels up to the optimal range, they too will experience all the joy of life and will smile more, have more energy, do better work, and feel that life has more of a purpose. This is the gift of replacing hormone levels. It simultaneously fights disease and makes you feel wonderful.

One final note on the issue of feeling good. Many health-conscious people faithfully take vitamin and mineral supplements—such as vitamin E, vitamin C, lipoic acid, coenzyme Q10—because they know on an intellectual level that these products will help them. But supplements, while important and valuable, don't make people feel different. When was the last time you took a multivitamin and said, "Wow, this makes me feel great!" It doesn't happen. But hormones are different. Hormones make you feel better—usually starting on the day you begin to take them.

HOW HORMONES BOOST ENERGY

In the spring of 2004, I began the kind of dedicated reading that I had not done since graduate school. But now I was pursuing a goal more important than anything I had done in academia. I was trying to find a way to save lives, including those of people near and dear to me. While researching interactions on the molecular level, I came across a wealth of research on how testosterone can boost energy in aging males. It turns out that men with low levels of testosterone have less energy and are more apathetic than their counterparts with normal hormone levels.[12]

It is clear that testosterone levels generally decline as males age, with the peak being reached in the late teen years.[13] Testosterone is measured as total testosterone, free testosterone, and bioavailable testosterone. Most testosterone in the blood is bound to sex hormone binding globulin (SHBG) and albumin. The small percentage that is unbound is available to have a biological effect; this is referred to as free testosterone. But albumin-bound testosterone easily uncouples in capillaries and so can be considered available also. A test for bioavailable testosterone is the gold standard in BHRT; this test measures free and albumin-bound (also called weakly bound) testosterone and is the real measure of what is available for biological processes.[14] Bioavailable testosterone also drops more quickly than total testosterone for men over age thirty.[15] Replacing your testosterone will boost your bioavailable levels and make you feel more energetic with a sustained energy that is nothing like the jittery feeling you get from caffeine; instead it is a calm sensation that will make you feel thirty years younger.

With a loss of testosterone comes a loss of energy and motivation. Animal studies reveal that the administration of testosterone can overcome fatigue in castrated mice.[16] Similar results are achieved in humans. A recent study of eighty-four HIV-positive men demonstrated that they have a lower-than-normal level of energy, but that giving them testosterone increased their mood and energy level with no significant negative side effects.[17] A similar study of 108 subjects found that the men treated with testosterone experienced a "much improved energy level."[18]

In a pilot study with forty-nine men suffering from Parkinson's, researchers noted that low testosterone is associated with numerous negatives, including decreased enjoyment of life and a deterioration in work performance. They found that men with low free testosterone were more apathetic, and researchers speculated that correcting hormone levels is likely to alleviate apathy and give people more energy and motivation.[19]

This hypothesis about the ability of testosterone to fight fatigue was confirmed when Italian researchers discovered that testosterone supplementation reduced fatigue and boosted energy levels in 120 men with a mean age of sixty-six.[20]

Women suffering from androgen insufficiency can also experience symptoms of fatigue, a diminished sense of well-being, decreased libido, and cognitive decline.[21] Treatment is usually initiated only in women who have normal estrogen levels or who have received estrogen to replace depleted estrogen. The 2002 Princeton consensus statement on female androgen insufficiency reported that side effects of androgen replacement are infrequent when androgen levels are brought within normal physiological range.[22]

TESTOSTERONE BOOSTS LIBIDO IN MEN AND WOMEN

It is known that testosterone boosts libido in women.[23] A one-year trial involving 814 women with a patch providing 300 ug of testosterone found a clinically significant increase in desire and sex drive, as well as reduced distress.[24] Another study of 105 women found that those who had low sex drives also had low testosterone and low dehydroepiandrosterone (DHEA).[25] Researchers in Melbourne, Australia, discovered that replacing testosterone and estrogen in twenty women with low libido brought back their sex drive. These researchers concluded that estrogen alone was not sufficient to bring the sex drive back; testosterone was also needed in the mix.[26]

A study of 1,632 men in the Boston area found that subjects with low testosterone had a lower sex drive.[27] Another study of 1,475 men found similar results, including the fact that a constellation of symptoms often accompany low testosterone, including sleep disturbances, lessened interest in sex, and a depressed mood.[28] Replacing testosterone in men with suboptimal levels brings back their sex drive, along with increased vitality and general feelings of well-being.[29]

HOW HORMONES BOOST MOTIVATION AND MOOD AND FIGHT DEPRESSION

My work on hormone receptors predisposed me to investigate *those* mechanisms of accomplishing testosterone's effects in the body, but I was surprised to find that in some cases, testosterone has a direct effect on other parts of the body and brain, specifically the neurons of the central nervous system and the amygdala,[30] a structure in the brain stem. It turns out that testosterone has a direct effect on these brain structures, boosting mood, motivation, and courage.[31] In fact, testosterone is so effective at increasing motivation that many entrepreneurs, CEOs, and senior managers are using it to keep up with younger traders on Wall Street.[32]

There is now unequivocal evidence that women are better than men at judging another person's emotional state of mind just by looking at them.[33] This means men are generally not as good at judging a woman's mood as women are, which may be a vexing observation to some men. Fortunately, however, we now have the ability to measure a woman's mood in a scientific manner. What this means is that we do not have to guess whether an individual is in a certain frame of mind—for example, if she is happy or sad—we can use a mechanical measuring device to make the determination. The value of this technique is that the operator running the machine can be assured that an objective determination of an important element of interpersonal relationships has been made. Nowhere is this more crucial than in the area of sexuality, where people can dissimulate for personal or professional gain. Fortunately, we now have a machine that can accurately measure a woman's emotional state with a degree of objectivity never before achieved. The technique, known as vaginal photoplethysmography, works by measuring vaginal pulse waves. Researchers insert an unobtrusive device into the subject, and the machine collects reflected light from interior and otherwise unviewable capillaries in such a way that it can determine exactly how dilated they become, with dilation, of course, being a measurable sign of arousal. By calculating vaginal pulse amplitude in healthy young women, researchers from the Netherlands recently discovered that their subjects experienced a boost in mood when their testosterone levels rose by even a small amount.[34] Researchers further concluded that improvement in mood is a result of testosterone interacting with the brain in an area of the limbic system known as the amygdala.[35] Testosterone may also boost mood by affecting vasopressin receptors in the hypothalamus.[36] Collectively, these and other studies[37] indicate that testosterone has the ability to improve mood in women. This should be of interest to many women who traditionally considered only estrogen replacement, not realizing that testosterone is also present in females and that it has an important role to play in their psychological well-being.

Low testosterone is correlated with depression in men.[38] Researchers at the University of California–San Diego found that testosterone levels were 17 percent lower for twenty-five men with categorically defined depression than levels observed in all other men. There was no association between total or bioavailable estradiol and depressed mood.[39] These results suggest that testosterone treatment might improve a depressed mood.

Similar results have been observed with testosterone administration to depressed women. A double-blind placebo-controlled crossover design study with fourteen healthy young women found that a single 0.5 mg sublingual dose of testosterone brought women out of their depression.[40] This intervention worked on a part of the brain known as the depression center of the cortex. Researchers found that the administration of testosterone boosted mood and alleviated depression in a rapid and consistent manner by enhancing the ability of the left prefrontal and right parietal cortex to communicate.

Another group of researchers tested the efficacy of testosterone to alleviate depression in men. They first demonstrated that transdermal testosterone gel increased blood levels of testosterone in men with low testosterone.[41] After 180 days of treating 227 men, whose sexual function and mood changes were evaluated by questionnaire, improvements in sexual function and mood were observed within the first month of treatment.[42] These same researchers had discovered as early as 1996 that testosterone replacement therapy improved positive mood characteristics, including energy, feelings of well-being, and friendliness; and decreased negative mood characteristics, including anger, nervousness, and irritability. They further concluded that once an adequate level of testosterone is achieved, adding more of the hormone does not produce improvements in mood or well-being—which argues against the supraphysiological doses employed by some athletes.[43] Significantly, bioidentical hormones even at doses higher than those normally found in the body appear to be so safe that the side effects are a minimal amount of mania in a small percentage of men.[44] It is as if nature designed men to top up their hormones for optimum mental health at the teenage hormone level and not much higher.

As we have seen, researchers have discovered that testosterone works to alleviate depression by affecting the brain's limbic system, which controls the handling of memory and emotional reactions. More specifically, it is known that testosterone interacts with numerous neurotransmitter systems that impact mood and well-being, including serotonin, dopamine, noradrenaline, vasopressin, and cortisol.[45] The path by which testosterone operates in the brain to affect neurotransmitters is worth noting, especially since the typical way steroid hormones operate is by regulating protein production through genomic mechanisms. But steroid hormones also operate through non-genomic actions, including by opening up and making more permeable the nerve cell membranes, presumably through interaction with the membrane androgen receptor.[46] As a result of testosterone's priming action on brain neurons, there may be a change in electrical potential via the release of neurotransmitters into the synapse.[47]

The brain's arginine vasopressin system is also impacted by testosterone.[48] Since the vasopressin system is involved in memory and mood,[49] it may play a pivotal role in the way testosterone boosts feelings of well-being. Furthermore, testosterone is known to increase the "feel-good" neurotransmitter[50] dopamine, which is likely another reason why aging people who use testosterone feel better.

Last but not least, recent evidence implicates not only free testosterone levels in bringing men out of depression but also a man's *sensitivity* to androgens. Sensitivity to androgens can be affected by the interaction between free testosterone and individual variations in the gene that produces androgen receptors.[51] CAG repeats are duplicate segments in a specific area in the gene that codes for the androgen receptor, and variations in this gene are associated with different risks for prostate cancer and different sensitivity to androgens.[52] Presumably men who are more sensitive to androgens will experience less depression.[53]

HOW HORMONES MODULATE AGGRESSION

Both testosterone and estrogen can increase aggression.[54] While testosterone has been linked with aggression in the popular press, this statement is a gross oversimplification. Testosterone does not directly cause aggression; in some cases it may even reduce inappropriate aggression. One way testosterone reduces inappropriate aggression is by producing calmness. Studies in animals have demonstrated that testosterone reduces anxiety and fear.[55] Human studies also indicate that testosterone reduces fear.[56] In aging human men, testosterone can facilitate calmness and eradicate the irritability commonly known as "grumpy old man syndrome."[57] Reducing irritability can produce a significant alleviation of an annoying symptom of low testosterone, and administering testosterone to men with genetic mutations that were caused by low testosterone produces this beneficial reduction in irritability. In a study of testosterone's ability to alleviate irritability, thirty Klinefelter males—males who are genetically unable to make sufficient testosterone—were treated with testosterone and experienced a welcomed reduction in irritability and an improved mood. In addition they had more energy, drive, and motivation, less fatigue, better concentration, and improved relations with other people.[58] These mood-enhancing aspects of testosterone are likely to be of interest to almost all aging males.

It has been proposed that aggression is less a result of testosterone and more a result of a high testosterone-to-cortisol ratio.[59] Other researchers have discovered that high vasopressin and low serotonin facilitate criminal aggression.[60] In addition, many other factors contribute to aggression, including early childhood experiences. Researchers at the University of Texas at Austin recently pointed out that testosterone is not alone in producing aggression, and that other variables are related to testosterone's effects, including monoamine oxidase A (involved in regulating impulse control), aromatization of testosterone to estradiol, the interaction between testosterone and vasopressin production, and the testosterone serotonin system.[61]

It is also important to keep in mind that hormones do not always limit themselves to binding with or affecting a single receptor type. When it comes to affecting social behavior, for example, testosterone has been shown to modulate aggression by activating vasopressin receptors in the hypothalamus.[62] This hypothesis was first tested in animals by researchers at the University of Massachusetts in Amherst. They discovered that testosterone affects vasopressin in the ventrolateral hypothalamus, a brain region that controls aggression in several species of mammals. A team in the Netherlands then discovered that a similar activation mechanism operates in humans. They further suggested that testosterone enhances the potential for aggression by interacting with vasopressin in the amygdala and hypothalamus.[63]

Differences in ER-alpha in mice brains have been linked to different levels of aggression.[64] In fact, increased aromatase activity in the brain has been linked with higher levels of aggression.[65] But estrogen, like testosterone, sometimes increases, and sometimes decreases, levels of aggression, presumably through its interaction with different types of estrogen receptors. Researchers have noted, for example, that ER-alpha is associated with greater intermale aggression, and ER-beta with decreased aggression.[66]

As anyone who has worked with depressed patients can attest, aggression is not an entirely negative aspect of human life. A certain amount of aggression is necessary for motivation and drive toward goal-oriented behavior. Indeed, aggression is a requisite component of normal human sexual interaction. People without appropriate aggressive impulses are perceived as listless and apathetic. Therefore, the association of sex hormones with appropriate levels of aggression is a welcome correlation, and those who bring their hormones into optimal levels usually report an adequate level of aggression—without the 'roid rage associated with those who use excessive steroids in sports. The bottom line is that you don't have to be afraid that you'll become another Rambo if you use testosterone; instead, you can expect a moderate and appropriate increase in aggression that will help you accomplish more and complete tasks in a timely manner.

TESTOSTERONE CUTS BODY FAT

It has been known since at least 1963 that testosterone therapy in men with low levels of testosterone has a favorable impact on body fat composition.[67] According to a recent study conducted on twenty-five hypogonadal (low testosterone) men aged nineteen to sixty-five, researchers at a German medical university found that as these men aged, they became heavier and had more problems keeping the weight off. But when this population received testosterone replacement therapy, they did not undergo the typical increase in body fat that aging men experience. Instead, researchers found that men treated with testosterone exhibited a BMI (body mass index) and fat mass "similar to those of younger . . . men." Researchers concluded that aging men would benefit from testosterone replacement therapy since it would help keep their weight under control.[68]

A recent meta-analysis of 1,083 men with an average age of 64.5 years (range 49.9–77.6) found that testosterone reduced body fat by 3.5 pounds, corresponding to a 6.2 percent reduction of body fat; but there was no reduction in overall body weight, indicating that a more favorable BMI was achieved in men using testosterone. The subjects also experienced improved bone mineral density and reduced cholesterol.[69]

Korean researchers recently compared caloric restriction and testosterone as ways to reduce body fat. Although they found that both methods worked to effectively reduce body fat, caloric restriction worked slightly better.[70] The real conclusion to be taken away from this study, however, is that a combination of the two methods is probably best, with an elimination of junk carbohydrates being a key part of the weight reduction program for aging men[71] together with replacing testosterone.

In 2007, researchers at Boston University demonstrated that eighty-eight overweight HIV-positive men who received testosterone replacement therapy experienced a significant reduction in abdominal fat mass while the control group, which received a placebo, saw a significant increase in whole body and trunk fat. The men treated with testosterone also had a significantly greater increase in lean body mass than the placebo group, indicating that testosterone cuts fat and builds muscle.[72]

It should come as no surprise that most people who begin testosterone replacement therapy report that they feel significantly better. Their mood and energy level improves, depression lifts, and they have more ability to enjoy life. Who could ask for better side effects from a therapy that also eradicates physical ailments?

CHAPTER 8

HOW TO USE HORMONES SAFELY

- Bioidentical hormones are generally safe and health promoting when used in doses that mimic levels found in young adults.
- Working with an anti-aging doctor, getting periodic blood tests, and choosing the right delivery method are important considerations for successful BHRT.
- An aromatase inhibitor can help keep estradiol levels in check.
- Lab numbers are only part of the picture. How you feel is the other half of the equation. When hormone levels are optimal, you'll feel good.
- You and your doctor can monitor side effects and take steps to control them if necessary.

I don't want you to be shocked when you ask for hormones from your doctor, so let me share a true story to help you understand what might happen and how to deal with it.

An eighty-year-old professor suffering from type 2 diabetes visited his family doctor in hope of getting a prescription for bioidentical hormone replacement therapy (BHRT). He was an intelligent man and had done some research before he went. "I've heard that testosterone declines with age and that replacing hormones to youthful levels might help my diabetes," he said. He presented his doctor with two studies that he had found describing how testosterone fights diabetes. The professor even offered to pay his doctor a hundred dollars if he would read the studies.

To his chagrin, his doctor refused to look at the material. "I don't have time," he claimed.

Indignant and humiliated, the professor left the doctor's office, vowing never to return. Eventually, however, he changed his mind and stayed with his doctor, but he also failed to pursue the matter further and never tried to find a doctor who specialized in anti-aging medicine. Instead, he let his family doctor's attitude guide him, even though his doctor had made a serious error by not even considering looking into the issue of testosterone replacement to fight diabetes.

The point of this story is simple. You can ask your family doctor for testosterone blood tests, but don't expect him to do them. Most doctors consider such tests a waste of time. Even if you convince a doctor to do the tests, he'll often order only total testosterone, since most doctors think that's all they need. In actuality, it's also important to look at free testosterone, bioavailable testosterone, estrogen, and more. The bad news is that when they get the test results, 95 percent of the time doctors will tell you that your levels are fine even if they're not optimal. In other words, family doctors aren't trained to help you replace your hormones. I suggest you use them only to obtain free blood tests that your insurance will cover. You may have to go back numerous times with a list of tests in an attempt to convince your doctor to do them all. Then bring those test results to your anti-aging doctor.[1]

HOW TO FIND AN ANTI-AGING DOCTOR

In general, you'll only have success asking for hormones from an anti-aging doctor. These doctors are trained to dispense hormones. I encourage you to find one and work with him or her to optimize your hormone levels. Luckily, it's becoming rather easy these days to find anti-aging doctors; the American Academy of Anti-Aging Medicine has an online directory. When you find a doctor, you might want to ask these questions before you begin:

1. How much do you charge for the first visit?
2. How much do you charge for subsequent visits?
3. What insurance, if any, do you accept?
4. Do you offer transdermal testosterone (or shots, or pellets, or whichever delivery method you prefer)?

5. Do you ever prescribe human chorionic gonadotropin (HCG) in conjunction with testosterone? (You want the answer to be yes.)
6. Do you prescribe *bioidentical* hormones?
7. Do you prescribe estriol and progesterone? (This is a question for women patients.)

For men, I suggest you read Dr. John Crisler's overview of the process, "My Current Best Thoughts on How to Administer TRT for Men. A Recipe for Success. Second Edition" as well as "An Update to the Crisler HCG Protocol."[2] Both documents are written for practitioners; however, an intelligent layperson should be able to understand them and will certainly profit from studying them carefully. They represent a lifetime of work and contain information that is worth its weight in gold.

Unfortunately, the majority of anti-aging doctors don't accept insurance because insurance companies are rather clueless about the value of hormone replacement. But generic bioidentical hormones are inexpensive, and most people can afford to pay for them out of pocket. For example, transdermal testosterone costs about $40 per month from a compounding pharmacy, and HCG costs only about $25 per month. You can save money by avoiding expensive name brands, such as AndroGel®. A compounding pharmacy can provide generic bioidentical testosterone at a fraction of the cost.

Keep in mind, however, that the cost of going to the doctor may vary widely. For example, in New York and New Jersey, you can find excellent doctors who will charge only about $100 per visit. In Manhattan, however, you may pay $2,000 or more for anti-aging doctors who cater to the rich and famous. Of course, at their offices you will often get free wine and cheese.

BLOOD TESTS

A fifty-five-year-old man—let's call him Teddy—noticed that most of the patients in his doctor's waiting room looked like bodybuilders. They could hardly get through the door. One day he asked about this, and his doctor smiled and said, "I make a lot of money treating them." Pressed for more information, the doctor revealed that he was writing prescriptions for testosterone. Teddy asked whether he might try testosterone too, since he didn't have his old get-up-and-go. Without a second thought, or even a blood test, the doctor gave Teddy a bottle of a new underarm testosterone gel.[3] Teddy went home and applied the gel under his arms, expecting to feel better. Within a month, he had discontinued testosterone treatment, claiming, "It did nothing for me."

In contrast to the eighty-year-old professor's doctor, who was too dismissive of BHRT, Teddy's doctor was too accepting of it. But Teddy's doctor could not know that his patient needed hormones unless he tested Teddy's hormone level *prior* to dispensing testosterone. A clinical report (the patient's verbal report about his state of health) is certainly relevant, but it's always best to use that *in conjunction with* hormone level tests. Men seeking testosterone treatment will want, at a minimum, the following tests:

1. Total testosterone
2. Bioavailable testosterone (also known as "free and loosely bound testosterone")
3. Free testosterone (if bioavailable testosterone is not able to be tested)
4. Estradiol (the sensitive assay for males)
5. Complete blood count (CBC) with differential
6. Lipid profile
7. Prostate-specific antigen (PSA)

Better still, also get SHBG, dihydrotestosterone (DHT), luteinizing hormone (LH), follicle-stimulating hormone (FSH), prolactin, cortisol, a thyroid panel, and a comprehensive metabolic panel.[4] With these tests in hand, you can visit your new anti-aging doctor prepared to request testosterone replacement. In fact, if you do your homework, at your first visit to your anti-aging doctor, he or she may offer you a prescription or a shot right then and there. Be prepared to experience a significant boost in mood and vitality.

A few months after your first use of hormones, your anti-aging doctor will ask for follow-up labs. The purpose of the first batch of tests is to see a baseline. The follow-up labs will determine what effect the hormones are having. Thereafter you will have blood tests a few times a year to monitor results. This is the chief difference between the proper and improper use of hormones. Athletes typically get hormones from friends and associates. They usually don't go to a doctor. They rarely get their blood tested. And they tend to use too much of a particular hormone. In this way they jeopardize their health. And yet, even with the mistakes they make and the huge doses they use, there have been relatively few bad side effects experienced by professional athletes. This is because the use of hormones is generally quite safe, even at above-normal levels.

Some doctors don't like the term *steroids* because of the negative connotations associated with the word. Nevertheless, testosterone and estrogen *are* steroids, and your anti-aging doctor will be prescribing steroids for you. It's helpful to get the idea out of your head that steroids are harmful. When used under the direction of a knowledgeable doctor, hormones are the opposite of harmful—in many cases they're lifesaving. At the very least, they'll be invigorating.

When you use testosterone, your body's own production of the hormone will diminish or shut down because there's a feedback loop that causes the body to stop producing testosterone when levels are high enough. This isn't anything to worry about since your body has already failed to produce enough of this vital hormone as you age. In the opinion of most anti-aging doctors, it's important to use exogenous testosterone (testosterone from outside the body) to bring yourself back up to an optimal level.

"Will I have to use this all my life?" men often ask. As one doctor said, "You can stop anytime you want. But once you see how good testosterone makes you feel, you won't *want* to stop." Most women feel the same way about the boost in self-esteem and confidence that they experience when using BHRT.

OPTIMIZING YOUR HORMONE LEVELS

When you order a blood test, the results show your *personal levels* as well as a *range* found in the general population. For example, a blood test for testosterone in a man might be reported as

430 Range 300–1,200 ng/dL

and for a female, it might be reported as

18 Range 15–100 ng/dL

The first number is *your* testosterone level. This is usually reported as ng/dL, nanograms per deciliter. The range indicates what the lab considers normal.

Ignore that.

Labs consider normal what 90 percent of subjects test at. This means they take all their results and discard the lowest 5 percent and the highest 5 percent and call the rest normal. In fact, total testosterone for men is considered suboptimal by most anti-aging doctors unless it's up near the 650 or higher range. It's very important to remember that lab ranges are *not* optimal ranges because they're based on what the average person's levels are, and the average man typically has suboptimal hormone levels unless he's in his teens or early twenties.

The key point is that what you want is not a normal range but an optimal range. As we discussed, your family doctor will not appreciate this distinction. An anti-aging doctor, however, will not only understand but will agree with you when you tell him that you want an optimal level of hormones. Doctors who specialize in bioidentical hormones know that *optimal* means in the high-normal range. For men, that would translate to free testosterone in a range from about 25 to 30 ng/dL. For women, the optimal range would be about 1.4 to 1.9 ng/dL.

When discussing your optimal hormone range, it's important to understand the role that SHBG plays in preventing hormones from being available. SHBG binds to dihydrotestosterone, testosterone, and estradiol and prevents them from entering cells. As men age they usually produce more SHBG, which is not a good thing. So even if your blood tests reveal high *total* testosterone (such as 800 ng/dL), if your SHBG is elevated you won't be able to *use* all that testosterone because it will be bound to SHBG. Clearly, it's important to look at more than total testosterone when trying to figure out whether you have an optimal amount in your body.

Some anti-aging doctors use different tests for measuring hormones, namely, saliva testing or finger-prick blood-spot sampling. Both of these tests give an accurate indication of the levels of hormones entering the cells. The saliva test has been shown to be reliable except in cases where an individual has bleeding gums[5] and finger-prick blood-spot sampling has also been shown to be reliable.[6] As discussed, you would do well to test for free or bioavailable testosterone.[7]

When looking at lab results, be mindful of the fact that hormone levels vary considerably during the day. For example, if your results show that your total testosterone is 600, it might actually have been higher or lower earlier in the day. Because of this variability, it's unwise to give excessive weight to lab test results. They're not irrelevant, of course, but they're also not the final word on the matter. Other factors also need to be considered when making hormone dosage decisions. Probably the most important other factor is how you feel.

While I've naturally been focusing on testosterone because of its vital role in disease prevention and treatment, it would be a mistake to lose sight of the other hormones that play a major role in well-being, most notably, for our purposes, pregnenolone and DHEA, as well as progesterone and estrogen for women. The more we learn about supplementing with hormones, the more we discover how they're like a symphony, working best when they work in concert with one another. Men using supplemental testosterone, for example, report remarkable improvements in their experience of hormone therapy after they add HCG to their regimen.[8] HCG is a gonadotropin analog of LH, and like LH, it stimulates Leydig cells in men, and theca cells in women's ovaries, to produce testosterone. HCG also contributes to balancing hormones by stimulating the

P-450 side-chain cleavage enzyme, which converts cholesterol into pregnenolone, and which paves the way for the enzyme CYP17A1 to convert pregnenolone into 17a-Hydroxypregnenolone and, ultimately, to another "feel-good" hormone, DHEA.[9] Pregnenolone confers multiple beneficial effects, including enhancing the enjoyment of music; improving balance; boosting mood; and increasing the pleasure to be derived from looking at colors, visual patterns, light, reflections, and art.[10]

I recommend that women use estriol since it's a weaker estrogen than estradiol and estrone. It works like a blocker to prevent estradiol from doing damage. In other words, it binds weakly to estrogen receptor-alpha (ER-alpha) and blocks the more harmful estradiol from sending growth signals to tumor cells. It can be applied in conjunction with progesterone for best results.[11] Asian women have more estriol than women from other races, and they also have a lower incidence of breast cancer, suggesting that their favorable hormone mix may be part of the reason they're protected.[12] Although estriol is the hormone of choice to help women prevent and fight breast cancer,[13] care must be taken to use transdermal rather than oral delivery. Research indicates that *oral* estriol slightly increases breast cancer risk—albeit not as much as oral Medroxyprogesterone acetate (MPA). No such risk has been found to be associated with transdermal estriol.[14] It's interesting to note that during pregnancy women produce up to a thousand times more estriol, which may account for their glowing, smooth skin. Estriol also causes breast tissue to differentiate during pregnancy, conferring significant lifelong protection against breast cancer,[15] which is why women who have children at a young age enjoy a reduced incidence of breast cancer.[16]

In summary, you want to avoid the unnaturally high hormone levels that athletes typically achieve when using hormones without doctor supervision, except in cases where fighting disease requires higher-than-normal doses for short periods of time. For optimal health, aim for the hormone levels of a healthy teenager. Balanced hormones at those levels will generally reduce your risk of getting cancer and Alzheimer's to near zero, the same near-zero risk you enjoyed as a young adult.

HORMONE DELIVERY SYSTEMS

"How can I be sure my doctor will prescribe bioidentical rather than synthetic hormones?" This is a fair question that new patients often ask.

Anti-aging doctors generally prescribe only bioidentical hormones. The reason for this preference is that they are aware of the significant difference between synthetic and real hormones. To be sure that you'll be getting only bioidentical hormones, ask your doctor, "Will the testosterone (or estrogen) you prescribe be bioidentical?" You want a doctor who smiles knowingly at this question and responds in the affirmative.

There are many ways to deliver exogenous bioidentical testosterone to the cells, including

1. Transdermal gel
2. Transdermal cream
3. Transdermal patch
4. Subcutaneous pellets
5. Intramuscular shots
6. Subcutaneous shots

AVOID SYNTHETIC HORMONES AND ORAL TESTOSTERONE AND ESTRADIOL

As we discussed in chapter 1, a large part of the bad press hormones have received was a result of the semantic confusion surrounding the Women's Health Initiative study. Scientific papers published in the aftermath of that study—which did *not* use bioidentical hormones—claimed that they were papers about progesterone. Yet these were *not* articles about progesterone; they were instead articles about the synthetic molecule progestin. And yet they contained the word *progesterone* in their titles.[17] Why is this significant? Because in finding that synthetic progestin caused problems, these articles cast an unfair and inaccurate pall over natural progesterone, which has *never* been demonstrated to cause these negative side effects.

Unfortunately, most people have heard only bad things about hormones, such as the incorrect claim that estrogen causes blood clots, or that HRT causes breast cancer, or that testosterone causes prostate cancer. The irony is that these diseases almost *never* occur in people in their late teens through early twenties, when hormone levels are at their highest! Is there supposed to be some magical transformation that occurs within the human body that causes hormones to become harmful as we age . . . or, as is much more likely, is there a straightforward scientific explanation for all the observed results?

When I was an undergraduate, one of my teachers told the class a story about two different research labs that were testing a new drug on the exact same strain of laboratory animals. Each lab produced results that were totally reproducible but that differed dramatically from the results of the other lab. Finally a researcher from one lab went to the other to try to determine what they were doing wrong. To his astonishment, when he administered the drug that he had brought with him exactly as he had done in his own lab, the results magically changed to become what this other lab had been claiming all along. Further examination ended up determining that in one lab the animals lived with incandescent lights and in the other lab they had fluorescent lights. Both labs then verified that the behavior of the drug was dependent on the lighting that the animals received. This story deeply moved me, and its message has guided me ever since. Even though things may seem paradoxical or impossible, there is always a logical explanation for everything. Naturally I reject the idea that a magical transformation occurs that causes hormones to become harmful as we age; instead, I focus on the properties of hormone receptors, using logic to explain all the harmful results attributed to hormones.

Everyone "knows" that administering estrogen causes blood clots in women, but for some strange reason there's *no* epidemic of blood clots among young women (who have the *highest* levels of estrogen). So what really causes the clots? It's tempting to blame *horse estrogen* for the increased rate of blood clots since horse estrogen has components never found in human estrogen. While this is an excellent initial hypothesis, the problem is that researchers have already proven it wrong. In fact, *bioidentical* estradiol (estradiol is the main component of human estrogen) produced four times more blood clots in women who took oral estradiol than in women in a control group, who took no hormones.[18] The answer to this mystery was revealed when researchers reported that there was no increase in the rate of blood clots for women who received *transdermal* estradiol. While it's not obvious to the general public why it should make any difference whether you take a hormone orally or have it absorbed through your skin, doctors know that hormones taken orally pass through your liver before entering your bloodstream, whereas hormones applied transdermally bypass the liver. It turns out that the liver is breaking down some of the estrogen into compounds that apparently result in blood clots. So our first mystery has a straightforward explanation.[19]

As we have seen, bioidentical hormones can be administered orally; sublingually (under the tongue); transdermally (through the skin) with creams, gels, or patches; or under the skin with injections or pellet implants. Because of the adverse effect of increased blood clots observed with oral estradiol, I can't recommend that any bioidentical hormone be taken orally, especially estradiol and testosterone.[20] This is because the purpose of taking bioidentical hormones is to restore hormone levels within your body to what they once were. After a hormone is processed by the liver, there is the possibility that new metabolites will be formed that are not present when hormones are produced naturally within the body. Even if such metabolites aren't harmful in the short term, I see no reason to recommend the oral route when alternatives that bypass the liver are readily available. I also can't recommend taking hormones sublingually just in case part of the dose makes its way into the stomach and then the liver.[21] Pellet implants are in some ways the most attractive delivery system for bioidentical hormones.[22] They last for months and produce a fairly constant release of hormones twenty-four hours a day. However, once pellets are implanted (through minor surgery), they're impossible to remove, so some care must be taken not to receive too much of a hormone when selecting pellets as your delivery system.

Finally, the safety picture is quite clear. There's no question that there are adverse health effects for women taking HRT consisting of horse estrogen and synthetic progestins. However, every single one of these adverse effects can be explained either because the hormones were taken orally or because the synthetic progestin was significantly lowering the activity of the intracellular androgen receptor. At this point, *no scientific study has shown serious adverse effects in women who take bioidentical hormones* unless they take them orally. Of course, some common sense must be applied in interpreting this fact. It does not mean that you can use bioidentical hormones in any dose or any combination without adverse consequences. The studies we discussed were conducted using hormones at the levels normally found in women. Also, if a woman has breast cancer, then taking estrogen, even if bioidentical, is almost certainly liable to increase the rate of cancer growth.[23]

Despite the fact that estrogen can be expected to increase the rate of cancer growth, it's important to keep in mind that there are three estrogens—estriol, estrone, and estradiol—with differing properties and differing affinities for hormone receptors. There is evidence that estriol, because of the way it interacts with ER-alpha and ER-beta, might hold promise as part of an effective anticancer treatment protocol.[24] A 2009 meta-analysis by Dr. Kent Holtorf cites twenty-three articles finding an anticancer effect for estriol and only one (which used breast cancer tissue cultures) finding a proliferative effect.[25] He further points out that because of its ability to work against the more dangerous estradiol, estriol may have a significant role to play in fighting already existing breast cancer.[26]

If a woman with undiagnosed breast cancer were to take estrogen, she would most likely increase the cancer's rate of growth, but that does not mean that she cannot supplement with estrogen, a vital female hormone. It means that when she does use estrogen, she needs to balance it with other hormones to ensure that cancer cells gradually die off. If a woman hasn't been diagnosed with breast cancer but is over the age of forty, there is a real possibility that she has undetected breast cancer cells. This undiagnosed population of cancer cells is either being controlled by her natural hormone levels and is not increasing in size (which is unlikely), is possibly decreasing in size (also unlikely), or is increasing in size (most likely, as women age). In order to make sure this undetected group of breast cancer cells has a rate of cell death that is greater than its rate of cell growth, she will want to follow the prevention protocol outlined in chapter 11.

HOW TO CONTROL ESTROGEN

As you have learned in this book, estrogen is the chief culprit in causing breast and prostate cancer, so estrogen must be controlled. This is especially important when receiving supplemental testosterone. Your hormone doctor will hopefully understand that some testosterone is routinely converted in the body into estrogen. This conversion is accomplished primarily by aromatase, an enzyme present in many tissues and organs. So once you start using testosterone, you will want to monitor estrogen levels to make sure that they don't climb too high. If they remain stable or drop (which can happen), that's fine, provided they're within optimal ranges. According to a recent study published in the *Journal of the American Medical Association*, a male's optimal range for estradiol is between 21.80 and 30.11 pg/mL.[27]

LOCAL VERSUS SERUM ESTRADIOL

Because estradiol is such an important player in this story, it's helpful to differentiate between local and serum levels. First, keep in mind that what causes cancer isn't serum estradiol (that is, the blood level) but rather local levels of estradiol in breast or prostate tissue.

The local level is produced by aromatase converting testosterone into estradiol. Even with all the sophisticated technology we have, during a routine blood test we don't measure the local level of estradiol. In other words, we don't insert a needle into each cell and ask, "How much local estradiol do you have here?" Instead we use a *serum* estradiol level and exert efforts to optimize *that*, even though the *local* level is the critical factor. Luckily, your serum level can give some notion about what is happening locally.

Local estradiol levels are affected to some extent by serum levels of estradiol, but not by that much. Postmenopausal women have serum levels of estradiol around four times lower than what is in their breast tissue. This means that most of a postmenopausal woman's estradiol in her breast tissue is coming not from circulating blood but from aromatase activity in the breast tissue. Premenopausal women have serum levels of estradiol around two times higher than what is in their breast tissue. In spite of the serum level of premenopausal women being around ten times higher than it is for postmenopausal women, the level in their breast tissue is only around 10 percent higher. Once breast cancer develops in postmenopausal women, the level of estradiol in their breast tissue is around ten times higher than it is in their serum.[28] This all illustrates that the serum level of estradiol has very little to do with the estradiol level in normal or cancerous breast tissue.

So what can you do if you notice that estradiol is rising?

We begin with foods and herbs to reduce it. These include aromatase inhibitors like mushrooms, broccoli, tea, and supplements like diindolylmethane (DIM), indole-3-carbinol (I3C), chrysin, and others.[29] Then if we need more help, we turn to an important class of drugs, **aromatase inhibitors**. Aromatase inhibitors (AIs) prevent the conversion of testosterone to estradiol. I'm astounded that in this day and age, knowing the adverse effects of high levels of estradiol, doctors continue to administer testosterone without also measuring estradiol levels[30] and administering AIs when indicated.[31] The necessity of using AIs when testosterone is being administered is part of the theme throughout many of my publications. It is just common sense—administering testosterone raises both testosterone *and* estradiol levels. If you want to observe the effects of testosterone on androgen receptors, then it's essential that you administer enough AI to prevent increased estradiol. Otherwise, the observed results might just be due to the increase in estradiol and have nothing to do with testosterone or the androgen receptors. I sometimes feel like I'm tilting at windmills when I try to convince the medical profession of this obvious point. This is part of the reason I'm writing this book—the right thing to do is so obvious that once the general public learns about it, doctors will be forced to change their ways and stop increasing estradiol levels in men when administering testosterone.

There are two benefits from AIs. First, the systemic reduction of estradiol can improve overall health in men if their estradiol is too high. But the most important thing from our point of view is that local aromatase activity is the cause of carcinogenesis. In prostate cancer, normal prostate epithelial cells have no aromatase activity, but all prostate cancer cell lines have high aromatase activity.

In breast cancer, normal breast tissue has low levels of aromatase activity in neighboring fat cells, but breast cancer tumors have very high aromatase activity in neighboring fat cells. Before you get put on a pharmaceutical AI, you probably want to take note of the fact that mushrooms are about the most potent AI inhibitor of all natural substances. They can inhibit aromatase by a good 50 percent.[32]

The wonderful thing about AIs is that they block both systemic as well as that all-important local aromatase activity. Blocking systemic aromatase helps with overall health. Blocking local aromatase prevents cancer.

YOUR PERSONAL RESPONSE TO HORMONES

Here's a secret only doctors know. They're trained to *observe* you. Yes, they're taught to listen to what you say, but most people don't realize that doctors are also trained to "look beyond the words" and to discern physical and behavioral manifestations of disease. Once you realize this, you'll be more apt to talk with your doctor. If you're not sleeping well, or if you feel depressed, or if you've lost your motivation, let your doctor know. He'll be more likely to help you get the hormones you need to feel better. Naturally, your physician can be expected to pay close attention to clinical reports of well-being, mood, energy level, and motivation to determine whether hormone replacement is recommended and is working satisfactorily.

Probably the biggest mistake men make when receiving BHRT is putting too much emphasis on lab results, especially total testosterone.

For example, one eighty-two-year-old man proudly reported to his friends that his recent testosterone test was "good." That's what his family doctor told him. Meanwhile the man suffered from depression, poor sleep, irritability, gynecomastia (enlarged breasts), and most of the other classic symptoms of low testosterone. Don't be fooled by a family doctor who claims that you're fine or that your testosterone level is normal. Trust your symptoms. In fact, it might be worthwhile to study the list of symptoms and take the time to ask yourself whether they apply to you. Family doctors make this same mistake and place too much reliance on total testosterone. Women may be less prone to make mistakes that are numbers-oriented because, for various reasons, they're more attuned to their feelings and subjective states of mind. There are two points to be made about this overreliance on total testosterone numbers.

First, total testosterone is not the best marker for an older man's hormone level. This is because SHBG increases with age and reduces the amount of total testosterone available. A better test is bioavailable testosterone. This test measures the amount of testosterone that is free (that is, not bound to SHBG) *plus* the amount that is bound to albumin (this latter amount is known as weakly bound or loosely bound because testosterone bound to albumin can rather easily become detached from the albumin protein and used for biological purposes). The bottom line is that your total testosterone number is often a very misleading indicator. Remember, you don't have all that "total" available since most of it is hooked up with SHBG.

The second thing to consider is that total testosterone isn't the last word in whether you need to supplement with hormones. In other words, sometimes a suboptimal number—such as, say, 550 ng/dL—may show up on a blood test (leading you to think that you need testosterone replacement), and yet you may feel fine. In that case, the lab test isn't the only consideration; a doctor can decide that no additional testosterone needs to be prescribed because you feel good.

Here's another secret only doctors know. They carry around in their head a list of symptoms for most diseases. That's what four years of medical school will do. As a result, one of the best ways to communicate with your doctor is to start mentioning items that appear on one of his lists. If you start rattling off items from one of the lists he carries around in his head, he'll conclude that you're suffering from X, Y, or Z disease. This is why it's important for *you* to become familiar with the list of classic symptoms of testosterone deficiency. Not only so that you can recognize these symptoms when they strike you, as they inevitably do to everyone who ages, but more particularly so that you can mention the right words and phrases when talking with your doctor.

Remember, the clinical picture is developed from what you say to your doctor about how you feel. If you have any of these classic symptoms of low testosterone, be sure to bring them to the attention of your MD (or DO, as the case may be[33]). The symptoms of low testosterone include

Low libido
Decreased motivation
Depression
Low energy
Poor sleep
Irritability (Grumpy Old Man Syndrome)
Anxiety
Anhedonia (inability to experience pleasure)
Slow wound healing
Slow recovery from exercise
Loss of muscle mass
Erectile dysfunction in men
Vaginal dryness and hot flashes in women
Abdominal weight gain in men
Weight gain in women
Fatigue
High cholesterol
High blood sugar
Cognitive impairment
Osteoporosis

The first three symptoms—low libido, decreased motivation, and depression—can easily be monitored by comparing how you feel before and after testosterone replacement therapy.

It's also interesting to note that people who aren't familiar with how various supplements and drugs work will usually *not* notice the difference that testosterone causes as much as people who *are* familiar with the psychological and physical changes that supplements can cause. Before starting on testosterone therapy, you might wish to supplement with DHEA and pregnenolone so that you become familiar with some of these clinical changes. It might also help to read about the many positive effects of testosterone so that you can become more aware when these effects occur for you.

SIDE EFFECTS TO MONITOR

As with any course of drug therapy, it's prudent to monitor side effects when using hormones. The usual side effects from hormones are all relatively minimal and manageable. For men, the risks include thicker blood, which rarely happens and which can be remedied with simple medical procedures, including donating blood. Other risks include high estrogen levels, which, as we discussed, can be avoided with herbs and drugs to limit estrogen. Sleep apnea might be worsened in men,[34] but it could also improve, since androgens strengthen muscle tone, a major cause of obstructive sleep apnea. For women, the risks are similarly mild, including developing acne or a small amount of facial hair, which can be addressed by reducing the dosage of hormones. In one interesting study, it was found that HRT was associated with *less* obstructive sleep apnea in postmenopausal women.[35]

There's a common misconception that it's too dangerous to give men testosterone due to an increased risk of their developing prostate cancer. In fact, there is no solid evidence to support this assertion.[36] At this point, the most serious side effect of administering testosterone to men was reported in a 2010 study in which testosterone was given to men whose age averaged seventy-four years. This study was terminated early because of the high number of adverse cardiac events observed in the group receiving testosterone.[37] It certainly sounds scary that a study had to be stopped early because of adverse effects when testosterone was administered, but a closer examination of this study reveals serious flaws in its design. The authors stated that "testosterone and associated increases in estradiol may promote inflammation, coagulation, and platelet aggregation,"[38] yet there is no indication that any of the subjects had measurements of their estradiol level. This study is at odds with previous research indicating that *low levels* of testosterone are associated with cardiovascular disease in men.[39] It is extremely enlightening to examine the association of estradiol levels in men and cardiovascular disease. Researchers have found that *men with coronary heart disease have significantly higher levels of estradiol than men without coronary heart disease.*[40] These researchers found no indication of increased testosterone levels in men with heart disease. Another study found that estradiol levels were approximately twice as high in men who experienced adverse cardiovascular events as in those who didn't.[41] They also noted that the men with high estradiol levels were receiving testosterone. So now we have a complete picture: testosterone seems to prevent adverse cardiac effects, and high levels of estradiol are associated with adverse cardiac effects no matter what the testosterone level. High testosterone levels are not able to counter the adverse effects of high estradiol. So while it is theoretically possible that the 2010 study[42] found adverse cardiac effects because of the testosterone, it's much more likely that the adverse effects were due to the increased estradiol that can result when testosterone is administered.[43] Unfortunately, the design of this study makes it impossible to know for sure.

CONCLUSIONS

How fortunate to be alive in this age, with a new day dawning on modern medicine! The steps I've outlined above are an integral part of this new day. They'll certainly help you when you find an anti-aging doctor to coach you through the process of balancing your hormones. Before long, you'll be telling friends and family what you've discovered—and helping them replenish *their* hormones, too. Despite mainstream medicine's hesitance about jumping on the BHRT bandwagon, the use of testosterone and other hormones is undoubtedly the wave of the future.

In Philip K. Dick's science fiction novel *The Three Stigmata of Palmer Eldritch*, Dr. Denkmal's E therapy accelerates the process of evolution by causing the brain (and skull) to grow larger. While Dick's novel sounds a satiric warning about the hazards of designer evolution, modern anti-aging medicine has a much safer offer for the current generation of baby boomers. You don't have to wait for futuristic health advances. A bold new technology is available today. You can optimize your hormones at teenage levels and recapture some of your lost youth and vitality. If, in the process, you also happen to effectively punch the daylights out of numerous cancers and cognitive impairments, I would say that in the end, it's all for the better.

PART 3

HELPING HORMONES HELP YOU: PREVENTION STRATEGIES TO MAXIMIZE HORMONE HEALTH

CHAPTER 9

THE BIG PICTURE: HOW HORMONES START *AND* STOP CANCER

- Most doctors mistakenly believe that testosterone causes prostate cancer to grow. In fact, testosterone prevents inappropriate cell proliferation in normal prostate cells.
- Estradiol causes inappropriate proliferation of normal prostate cells.
- It can be a matter of life and death in men and women to prevent testosterone from converting into excess estradiol.
- Removing testosterone kills prostate cancer and normal prostate cells through a process of calcium ion overload.
- Teenage males and females enjoy protection from cancer and cognitive decline because their hormones are balanced and plentiful.
- As men and women age, their hormone levels, especially testosterone, become too low to prevent the development of cancer and cognitive decline.
- Supplementing with hormones in the right amounts and combinations can prevent and even reverse many degenerative conditions.

THE BIG PICTURE FOR MEN

A man who was familiar with my research asked his doctor his opinion of testosterone. He informed me that his doctor said, "Taking it will lead to the growth of everything in your body. I think of it as fertilizer. Yes, it grows muscles, but it could also grow tumors." When I heard this, I was speechless. It was not just the enormous ignorance of this doctor, but the arrogant certainty associated with his ignorance. Here was an intelligent man, one who had obtained a medical degree, who had clearly never read any of the articles in the past few years dealing with testosterone and cancer. And it's doctors like this who ordinary people are trusting with their lives. Most people, including doctors, are convinced that testosterone makes all prostate cancer grow, even tumors that are so small they're undetectable. It's funny how wrong the standard model of prostate cancer can be—and how many people, even intelligent people, subscribe to its flawed reasoning. According to the standard model, testosterone increases prostate cancer. But as anyone who looks into the facts can tell you, the effect of testosterone on the intracellular androgen receptor of normal human prostate epithelial cells[1] is to *suppress* inappropriate cell division[2] due to the production of the protein AS3.[3] On the other hand, the effect of *estradiol* on normal prostate cells is to promote inappropriate cell division by a process that involves estrogen receptor-alpha (ER-alpha), intracellular androgen receptor, and the cancer-promoting enzyme Src.[4] Clearly, estradiol is the dangerous hormone, not testosterone. Also, estradiol increases telomerase activity, lengthening telomeres in normal prostate cells.[5] What all this means is that, *for normal prostate cells, testosterone suppresses inappropriate cell division, and estradiol promotes inappropriate cell division.*

Most articles about prostate cancer and testosterone say something like "It is well known that testosterone is needed for prostate cancer growth." In fact, it is so "well known" that the authors don't bother to cite a reference for this assertion. In the last chapter, I explained why I always search for a logical explanation whenever results seem to be contradictory. In this case, the contradiction that has to be explained is, How can testosterone possibly *prevent* inappropriate cell division in normal prostate cells and at the same time *promote* cell division in cancer cells? The answer is it can't—and doesn't. If you still think that testosterone is essential for prostate cancer growth (which the standard model does), then the problem becomes explaining such growth in the *absence* of testosterone (which certain human prostate cancer cell lines are capable of). One possibility is to assume that some mutation allows the intracellular androgen receptor to act on its own, without requiring any hormone to bind to it. This is a known phenomenon for some cancers, but even if you grant that this is possible sometimes, you are left with the problem of explaining the existence of prostate cancer cell lines that contain no intracellular androgen receptor. If there is no androgen receptor, then cell proliferation and tumor growth cannot be affected by testosterone. It's illogical to say that testosterone causes these cancer cells to grow, since testosterone can't bind to nonexistent intracellular androgen receptors. So my logical explanation for all of this is quite simple: prostate cancer doesn't need testosterone to grow; instead, it needs estradiol initially until it mutates enough to be capable of growing even without estradiol.

THE CELLS OF THE PROSTATE GLAND

The prostate is composed mostly of **stem**, **basal**, **stromal**, and **luminary secretory** cells. Luminary secretory cells and basal cells make up the epithelium. Basal cells are undifferentiated cells that later become luminary secretory cells. Stromal cells are the chief constituent of connective tissue. As a man reaches puberty, his prostate gland changes into its adult structure. Testosterone levels increase, and prostate stem cells produce basal epithelial cells. Testosterone also interacts with stromal cells to produce factors called andromedins, which cause some basal cells to eventually change into luminary secretory cells.[6] Luminal secretory cells are responsible for producing prostatic fluid, which helps make up semen. Once the adult prostate is formed, there are roughly equal amounts of basal cells and luminal secretory cells in the epithelium.[7] If prostate cancer develops, it originates in epithelial cells, *not* in stem cells.[8] Both basal cells and luminal secretory cells in the epithelium are capable of becoming cancerous.[9]

But we still have to explain why the medical profession is so convinced that testosterone is essential for prostate cancer growth. There is no question that taking away testosterone kills most prostate cancer cells—and eventually all normal prostate epithelial cells, too. But this is *not* because testosterone is necessary for cell growth or cell division. It is because *a lack of testosterone leads to programmed cell death (apoptosis) from calcium ion overload.*[10] While this may seem like splitting hairs, there is a big difference between a lack of testosterone making it impossible for cell division to proceed and a lack of testosterone causing apoptosis.[11] The evidence indicates that what really happens when testosterone is removed is that apoptosis occurs.

However, I believed that there has to be more to it than this. I have respect for medical researchers, and they would not believe that testosterone was essential for prostate cancer growth without having some serious evidence to back it up. In digging into the literature more deeply, I discovered that when the anti-androgen drug bicalutamide (Casodex®) is used to *block* the intracellular androgen receptor in LNCaP cells (the line of human prostate cancer cells most often used by researchers), then cell division stops.[12] This looks like a slam dunk for the view of the medical profession, doesn't it? What could be more straightforward? Since testosterone binding to the intracellular androgen receptor is essential for cell division (the argument goes), then using a drug to *block* that receptor naturally stops cell division cold. But this is flawed reasoning, as we shall see.

I must admit that finding this article caused me to have some initial doubts about my own views. However, the basic problems I mentioned before still remain—I can't envision a logical explanation for this turnaround from testosterone *preventing* cell division (as we saw it did at the beginning of this chapter) to testosterone *promoting* cell division (as is claimed by the standard model). Looking more deeply into the literature, I found evidence that *estradiol* increases the rate of growth in LNCaP. Moreover, at the ideal concentration of estradiol (0.01 nM, a level within human physiological limits) adding bicalutamide has almost no effect on the increased growth rate caused by estradiol.[13] Now we have a real puzzle. If *testosterone* is essential for prostate cancer cell growth, then how is it possible for *estradiol* to take its place and cause prostate cancer growth? Of course, this *might* occur if estradiol could bind to the intracellular androgen receptor (which it can do if there is a mutated intracellular androgen receptor such as in LNCaP), but if *that* (estradiol binding to the intracellular androgen receptor) were the cause of prostate cancer growth, then bicalutamide should have *prevented* estradiol from binding there and causing cancer to grow—but bicalutamide *doesn't* prevent estradiol from fostering cancer growth. This means that *estradiol* is causing the increased prostate cancer growth directly, not testosterone and not the stimulation of the intracellular androgen receptor by testosterone or estradiol.

The preceding evidence presents us with an interesting dilemma because either testosterone or estradiol is allowing LNCaP cells to grow. But which one is it? With this additional information about the effect of estradiol, it is now possible to envision some models that might explain what is really happening. The most straightforward explanation is that when cancer cells start to undergo apoptosis,[14] cell division stops. When estradiol is administered, Bcl-2 levels increase because of its binding to membrane estrogen receptor and estrogen receptor-alpha.[15] The resulting high levels of Bcl-2 *prevent* apoptosis. In other words, estradiol prevents programmed cell death. And in addition, estradiol promotes cell division, so the net result is that cancer thrives. When testosterone is administered, apoptosis does not occur because high-enough levels of testosterone eliminate calcium ion influx, and LNCaP does not have the androgen receptor imbalance required for testosterone itself to cause apoptosis.

If I am right, then targeting the binding of testosterone to intracellular androgen receptor (which is the direction that current prostate cancer research is headed) is never going to be curative. In my opinion, the only hope for a systemic cure is to minimize the rate of cell growth and maximize the rate of cell death, which requires a multipronged approach that targets all the hormone receptors. Even if such an approach is not curative, it is very likely to allow men to die *with* prostate cancer instead of *because of* it. If I am wrong and a cure *is* ultimately achieved by attacking the intracellular androgen receptor, then that would be wonderful. Unfortunately, untold thousands of men will die in the meantime as multipronged approaches are ignored. So, assuming I am right, I will present my vision of what happens as men age.

WHAT HAPPENS AS MEN AGE

Every time I watch a baseball game, I smile to myself at how interested the commentators are in the age of the players. As professional athletes age, their performance inevitably declines, and knowledgeable sports commentators notice this and mention it. What is happening in most cases is that testosterone levels are dropping, and as a result athletic performance is not what it was in the player's younger years.[16] While we can clearly see athletic performance and other markers of low testosterone, there are some less visible changes that take place as a result of decreased hormone levels.

Initially, high testosterone levels (which I'll call "teenage" levels) that men have from their late teenage years through their early twenties are protective against prostate cancer. For cancer to thrive, it must have a rate of cell growth that is *faster* than its rate of cell death. Normally, prostate epithelial cells have very little membrane androgen receptor, so in the presence of androgen, the *intracellular* androgen receptor dominates, which results in low levels of Bcl-2 and lots of AS3.[17] Both of these scenarios are good for men. There is also very little ER-alpha, but lots of ER-beta present in young men, which means that estradiol will *decrease* the level of Bcl-2. This is also good for men. Some of the testosterone in the serum is converted to estradiol, which also decreases Bcl-2. Typically, there is more progesterone receptor B than progesterone receptor A, which means that progesterone will also lower the level of Bcl-2. Last, but not least, some progesterone is converted to "good progesterone," metabolites of progesterone that bind to membrane progesterone receptors and help prevent prostate cancer growth.[18]

The youthful ratio of hormone receptors is such that testosterone, progesterone, and estradiol all work harmoniously to lower Bcl-2 levels, which in turn creates an environment where the rate of cell death is *greater* than the rate of cell growth—even if a prostate cancer cell happened to develop. This is why prostate cancer is almost never found in men with teenage hormones levels.[19] The cancer just cannot gain a foothold; the rate of cell death always exceeds the rate of cell growth, keeping cancer at bay.

There are other hormone interactions that come into play during youth. Inside prostate epithelial cells, almost all testosterone is converted to dihydrotestosterone (DHT). DHT binds to intracellular androgen receptors five times more strongly than testosterone.[20] More binding means more activity, which means that DHT will lower Bcl-2 levels even more than testosterone. Also, some DHT is converted to 5alpha-androstane-3beta, 17beta-diol (3beta-Adiol). 3beta-Adiol binds primarily to estrogen receptors, with a preference for ER-beta over ER-alpha. The binding strength of 3beta-Adiol is a little weaker than estriol for both ER-alpha and ER-beta.[21] Because of the ratio of the estrogen receptors, 3beta-Adiol also acts to lower Bcl-2 levels. Since normal prostate epithelial cells have no aromatase activity (and hence no local estradiol worth speaking of),[22] 3beta-Adiol is the main ligand for ER-beta. Not surprisingly, since DHT acts protectively both directly on the intracellular androgen receptor and indirectly on ER-beta, higher levels of DHT at the time of diagnosis of prostate cancer are correlated with a greater, fifteen-year survival rate as compared to men with lower levels of DHT.[23]

As prostate basal cells are created, ordinarily a number of genes, including the aromatase gene, are silenced and *not* active. Occasionally, a mistake is made, and a basal cell will be created with an *active* aromatase gene. The basal cell may still be converted to a luminal secretory cell, but now you have either a basal cell or a luminal secretory cell with active aromatase enzyme within it. This results in a high local level of estradiol, which causes cell division, lengthens telomeres, and increases the mutation rate. All the ingredients are in place for this cell to become immortalized (an essential step in becoming cancerous), but it now comes down to the rate of cell *growth* versus the rate of cell *death*. In addition to hormone levels, diet, exercise, and genetics all play a role here. There is now what I call a tipping point involved. If taking everything into account, the rate of cell *death* is greater than the rate of cell *growth*, then the tipping point has not yet been reached. Even if multiple mutations have already occurred so that not only is the cell cancerous but also capable of metastasizing, the cell and its progeny will still all die out (barring an extremely against-the-odds mutation).

If . . . the rate of cell *death* is greater than the rate of cell *growth*, then . . . the cell and its progeny will . . . all die.

Each prostate epithelial cell usually lives an average of five hundred days before dying.[24] As these cells die, new ones are created from stem cells to maintain a constant number of cells within the prostate. Once a potential prostate cancer cell arises, it divides approximately every two months. Eventually its rate of cell death becomes close to that, but the way I visualize it, it takes time to build up the pro-apoptotic proteins that result in apoptosis, and it will initially be five hundred days before cell death occurs. This means that the cell will have an average of eight divisions in that time, so that one cell will turn into 256 cells. However, at a minimum, the cells *around* those cells with aromatase activity will also start to divide. This can be expected to involve at least ten cells, resulting in at least 2,560 cells. None of these cells would have existed if the aromatase gene had not been activated, but if the rate of cell *death* at this point is greater than the rate of cell *growth*, then they can all be expected to die off.[25] However, if the tipping point has been reached,[26] then all these inappropriate cell divisions mean that it is just a matter of time before the right mutations to create prostate cancer occur. It is even possible that prostate cancer can develop in one of the cells that is dividing but does not contain aromatase, so long as the cell remains in proximity to one of the cells that is supplying the estradiol it needs to keep dividing. Eventually the cancer will mutate to no longer require estradiol in order to grow.

The classic horror film *The Blob* (the original 1958 version, starring Steve McQueen) gives me the shivers as I think about how closely the monster parallels the action of a tumor. The story revolves around an amorphous mass that keeps growing larger and engulfs everything in its path. Well, once prostate cancer develops, the ratio of hormone receptors will change in order to benefit the cancer. That's a scary prospect since it enables the tumor to grow, just like the Blob. The amount of membrane androgen receptor increases[27] in order to increase Bcl-2 levels. Also, a decrease in the amount of intracellular androgen receptor will increase Bcl-2. The more membrane androgen receptor, the more aggressive the prostate cancer becomes.[28] Also, there is a correlation between less intracellular androgen receptor and more aggressive prostate cancer.[29] The question becomes, Is there a limit to how much membrane androgen receptor and how little intracellular androgen receptor there can ultimately be? What happens if there is absolutely no intracellular androgen receptor and lots of membrane androgen receptor? Researchers found that when using a human prostate cancer cell line with no intracellular androgen receptor and lots of membrane androgen receptor, *testosterone by itself was able to kill these cells.*[30] This shows that there is a limit to the amount of membrane androgen receptor that can be produced in order to benefit the cancer. If too much is produced, then the amount of pro-apoptotic proteins produced will result in a greater *increase* in the rate of cell death than a *decrease* in the rate of cell death caused by having more Bcl-2, and those cancer cells will be at a selective growth disadvantage when compared with the other cancer cells. I visualize a system in which the higher the level of testosterone present, the worse things will be for the cancer.[31]

The higher the level of testosterone present, the worse things will be for the cancer.

Also, as cancer grows, more ER-alpha is produced and less ER-beta[32] in order to increase Bcl-2 levels and help the cancer survive. Similarly, more progesterone receptor A will be produced and less progesterone receptor B. In addition, more progesterone will be converted to "bad progesterone" and less to "good progesterone," which will help the cancer population grow and eventually metastasize. Also, individual mutations will occur throughout the DNA to speed up the doubling rate of the prostate cancer population. Besides mutations that change a specific protein, there are also deletions (removing a gene entirely) and translocations. In prostate cancer, translocations that move genes from one hormone receptor to another are called gene-fusions. Some gene-fusions, such as *TMPRSS2:ERG*, are known to be dangerous.[33] In my opinion, one of the most important factors in determining the aggressiveness of prostate cancer is the testosterone level, with more aggressive cancers being associated with *lower* levels of testosterone.[34] As we have seen, testosterone decreases as men age, and so does DHT. In fact, it is known that the local level of DHT within prostate epithelial cells decreases with age, and this can cause problems. A typical sixty-year-old will have half the level of DHT within his prostate epithelial cells as a twenty-five-year-old,[35] increasing the older man's risk of developing more aggressive prostate cancer. This is one of the reasons why it is so important for older men to receive testosterone replacement therapy and to get their testosterone levels into the teen range; but, really, any supplementation is better than none, so even if your doctor is not willing to get you into the teen range, at least getting you into the high-normal range is better than not doing anything to correct your declining hormone levels.[36]

Researchers have found that there is a correlation between very *low* levels of testosterone and an increased incidence of prostate cancer.[37] Since prostate cancer starts up because of the conversion of testosterone to estradiol, once the tipping point is reached and the rate of cell growth is greater than the rate of cell death, then higher testosterone levels should result in higher rates of prostate cancer due to higher local estradiol levels.[38] However, because of the slower growth rate associated with high levels of testosterone (due to the lower amount of Bcl-2), many of these cancers never grow large enough to be detected. On the other hand, a lower level of testosterone corresponds to a *faster* growth rate, which makes the cancer easier to detect.[39] In addition, if testosterone levels are low, the tipping point would typically occur at an earlier age, again making cancer more likely to be detected. A study done on the growth rate of prostate cancer estimated that the first prostate cancer cell occurs during a man's twenties.[40] My own opinion is that most prostate cancers start when men are in their late twenties through their early thirties.

As men get older, their free testosterone levels drop an average of 1.2 percent per year.[41] Lower testosterone levels result in reaching the tipping point earlier. Falling testosterone levels result in an increased risk of dying from heart disease,[42] an increased risk of type 2 diabetes,[43] and decreased mental cognitive ability.[44] In addition, lower testosterone levels cause an increase in beta amyloid,[45] which increases the risk of dementia and seems to be essential for the development of Alzheimer's disease.[46] As if this were not bad enough, if the level of total testosterone drops below 250 ng/dL for men over forty years of age, their overall mortality rate increases by 88 percent.[47] Finally, the incidence of breast cancer increases for men with medical conditions that severely reduce their testosterone levels.[48]

It is only fair to point out that when there is a correlation between low testosterone and an adverse health problem, there is always the possibility that the low testosterone is the result and not the cause of that problem. However, when adding testosterone helps to eradicate a health problem, it's hard to see how that problem could have arisen in the first place if the testosterone level had not dropped. Therefore, I discount the possibility that low testosterone levels are the result of the health problems mentioned here. Instead, I am convinced that these health problems are the result of lower levels of testosterone. The numerous health problems observed when men are intentionally deprived of testosterone bear out this view.

What this all boils down to is a rather frightening prospect. As men age, their hormone levels change: protective testosterone decreases, and dangerous estradiol increases. In addition, more time has passed for mutations to occur. The best way to deal with this scenario using the tools available to modern medicine is to replace hormones to make sure that a more youthful balance is reached, one that ensures that the rate of cell death is greater than the rate of cell growth. I explain how to do this in chapter 11.

What this all boils down to is a rather frightening prospect. As men age, their hormone levels change: protective testosterone decreases, and dangerous estradiol increases.

THE BIG PICTURE FOR WOMEN

One of my favorite movies is George Lucas's *American Graffiti* (1973). Suzanne Somers has only a bit part in the story, appearing briefly as the blonde in the T-Bird, but even that fleeting glimpse proved her to be the incomparable desideratum that many a young man longed to take home. Today, she still has that quality of vitality and attractiveness that draws people to her and suggests a healthy lifestyle and good hormone levels.

Her later career has centered around raising people's consciousness about the value of supplementing hormones as we age. And from the level of youthful energy she brings to her media appearances, one might conclude that there really must be some truth to the notion that hormones can keep you looking and feeling younger. But not only is Somers responsible for leading the popular press in a campaign to educate people about the value of hormone therapy, her work is also useful because it counters a real trend in mainstream medicine that shies away from talking about the value of anti-aging therapy.

As a general rule, women are more likely than men to go to a doctor when they have a health problem. Researchers are not sure why this is so, but they believe that men want to maintain a macho image and fear any physical vulnerability. Men are also less likely to ask for directions if they get lost. Women were more likely than men to seek hormone replacement in the years following World War II—perhaps because they were more aware of their hormonal changes because they experienced menopause. So it is really unfortunate that women were frightened by the WHI study and as a result stopped using hormone replacement in droves after 2002, when the study publicized the dangers of synthetic progestins. I say "unfortunate," since the use of bioidentical hormones carries no such risks, as we have discussed earlier.

It is common knowledge that the highest hormone levels occur for women in their late teens through their early twenties, after which levels decrease. It is also known that in the breast tissue of women with normal genetics, there is roughly the same amount of ER-alpha as ER-beta.[49] As a result of this roughly balanced number of hormone receptors, estradiol never has much of an effect on Bcl-2. The presence of progesterone also tends to decrease Bcl-2 levels in young women,[50] indicating that there must be more progesterone receptor B present than progesterone receptor A. Additional good news for young women is that both their intracellular and membrane androgen receptors decrease Bcl-2, so "teenage" levels of progesterone and testosterone make it almost impossible for breast cancer to develop. As in the prostate, estradiol stimulates and testosterone inhibits breast cell proliferation.[51] Also, just as in prostate cells, estradiol increases breast cell telomerase activity,[52] but this potentially deleterious effect is adequately counteracted by a favorable balance of hormones during the teen years.

The initiating step in breast cancer is the production of factors that cause high aromatase activity in the local vicinity.

The initiating step in breast cancer is the production of factors that cause high aromatase activity in the local vicinity. This will affect aromatase in breast epithelial cells as well as in breast adipose cells. The high local levels of estradiol produced by aromatase will cause breast epithelial cells to divide, will increase the rate of mutations, and will also increase telomere length—effectively immortalizing these cells, unless (as in young women) the rate of cell death is greater than the rate of cell growth. Unfortunately, the rate of cell growth and cell death has not been worked out as completely in breast cancer as it has in prostate cancer. However, during the early stages of disease, there will typically be a myriad of cell divisions with a significant number of breast epithelial cells involved. As in the development of prostate cancer, if the tipping point has not yet been reached (that is, if the rate of cell growth is not yet greater than the rate of cell death), then each cell division offers the opportunity for a key mutation to occur that would allow breast cancer to start. If the tipping point has occurred (that is, if the rate of cell growth is *greater* than the rate of cell death), then these cells will be immortalized, and it is just a matter of time before the right mutations occur to produce breast cancer.

It is somewhat frightening to realize that once breast cancer starts, it will typically increase ER-alpha and decrease ER-beta[53] as well as increase progesterone receptor A and decrease progesterone receptor B in order to produce more Bcl-2. In some cases of breast cancer, the relatively friendly and helpful intracellular androgen receptor is totally eliminated, both in women[54] and in men.[55] When the intracellular androgen receptor is missing, high levels of testosterone can be expected to kill these cells because of the pro-apoptotic proteins produced by membrane androgen receptors.

As women age there are numerous disease processes other than cancer that also become more likely. For example, Alzheimer's is especially sensitive to hormone levels in women. Because women have much lower testosterone levels than men, they cannot rely on testosterone alone to prevent Alzheimer's. [56] To make matters worse, by the time a woman is forty-five to fifty-four years old, her average level of free testosterone drops to only half of what it was when she was eighteen to twenty-four.[57] It is true that the primary female hormone, estradiol, reduces levels of beta amyloid, but other factors often work to offset this positive outcome as women age. For example, progesterone also reduces levels of beta amyloid but does so only when there is a cycle of ten days of high levels of progesterone every month.[58] Therefore, as women age and their levels of estradiol, progesterone, and testosterone decrease, and especially when they stop having ten days of high levels of progesterone each month, they are at greater risk of developing Alzheimer's and other forms of dementia.

It is inevitable that as women grow older all their hormone levels decrease and keep decreasing even after the tipping point is reached. This is an extremely dangerous situation because the tipping point is that moment when the rate of cell growth *exceeds* the rate of cell death. High aromatase activity after this time can lead to unstoppable tumors. Factors such as diet, lifestyle, and genetics all affect when a particular woman's tipping point for cancer is reached, but eventually it is reached in all women. This is why I agree with anti-aging doctors who argue that aggressive steps need to be taken to address these dangers of aging.[59] Estriol has been shown to be associated with lower rates of breast cancer.[60] Estriol decreases the cancer rate because it is a weaker estrogen than estradiol and it interferes with estradiol binding to ER-alpha. But once the tipping point is reached and the rate of cell growth is greater than the rate of cell death, then higher levels of testosterone translate into higher local levels of estradiol, resulting in a slightly increased chance of developing breast cancer.[61] I would expect that the doubling time of those cancers with higher levels of testosterone would be slower than for those cancers with lower levels of testosterone, but I have not found any study on this yet.

I'm the first to admit that this overview of the big picture looks rather bleak for men and women as they age. It's as if our hormone systems start to work *against* us instead of *for* us. But I've always had the same philosophy as NASA scientists. Failure is *not* an option. I refuse to accept the limitations of geriatric biology. In the next two chapters, I will look at the many exciting ways that we can now use our knowledge of what happens as we age to literally halt and reverse the degenerative processes that conspire to kill us. And I have no embarrassment about rejecting what happens to us as we get older. I think Woody Allen spoke for us all when he said, "I don't want to achieve immortality through my work. I want to achieve immortality through not dying."[62]

CHAPTER 10

PREVENTION THEORY: INTRACELLULAR PROCESSES THAT SWITCH CANCER OFF

In theory, the prevention of breast cancer and prostate cancer is relatively straightforward. We simply bring all hormones back to teenage levels. This will work just fine if there are no breast cancer or prostate cancer cells already present. But what if you have one cancer cell, or one hundred, or a million? Since breast cancer can't be detected until there are approximately one billion cells present.[1] it's very possible to have millions of cancer cells growing inside you without your even being aware of it.

So for all practical purposes, when we talk about prevention we're really talking about developing protocols that not only prevent cancer when none already exists but that also avoid stimulating the growth of cancer cells that may already be present. And since we're talking about prevention rather than treatment, we also want to make sure we don't decrease the quality of life or increase the risk of any other disease.

In looking at the properties of the various hormone receptors, it is clear that testosterone will *prevent* the formation of breast cancer or prostate cancer, except in the case where testosterone is converted into estradiol. This overriding preventive and powerfully anticarcinogenic function of testosterone is a direct result of the fact that the hormone lowers levels of Bcl-2 and raises levels of AS3. Bcl-2 is an anti-apoptotic protein that prevents cancer cells from dying, so the fact that testosterone reduces this harmful protein is very good for humans. AS3 is a helpful protein that prevents cancer cells from undergoing cell division, so the fact that testosterone increases this good protein is more good news for us.

It's also worth keeping a few other important facts about hormone receptors in mind before I sketch my overview of prevention theory. One of the most intriguing facts to be mindful of is that in normal breast and prostate tissue the ratio of hormone receptors causes progesterone to decrease Bcl-2 levels, which is a very good outcome. Unfortunately, in breast tissue with BRCA1 and BRCA2 mutations, progesterone has an opposite effect and works to increase Bcl-2 levels, which is bad because Bcl-2 protects cancers from programmed cell death.

If you're starting to suspect that we might be able to use our knowledge of how hormone receptors protect or kill cancer, you're entirely on target. In fact, this is precisely what we intend to do. But first, a couple more key facts . . .

Probably the most surprising fact to keep in mind when attempting to develop a prevention theory is that in normal prostate tissue, estradiol decreases Bcl-2 levels. This is surprising because estradiol is generally a proliferation-causing hormone, which leads to cancer. But the fact that estradiol reduces Bcl-2 is good since Bcl-2 protects cancer cells, and reducing it allows more cancer cells to die. In normal breast tissue, however, estradiol has little effect. The weakest estrogen, estriol, in contrast, will decrease Bcl-2 levels in both breast and prostate tissue, which is quite a good thing since when you decrease Bcl-2 you strip protection away from cancer cells, and this results in more cancer cells undergoing the process of apoptosis, affectionately known as programmed cell death.

For both prostate cancer and breast cancer, foods known to help prevent cancer can profitably be added to your diet. Manipulating your hormone levels will probably be enough to prevent these cancers, but it certainly can't hurt to add some healthy food to your diet as added protection. In the next chapter, I'll explain exactly how to make these healthful supplement and dietary choices. In addition, when serum levels of vitamin D3 are maintained at high-normal levels, cancer is at a severe disadvantage. For example, vitamin D3 plays a vital role in the fight against breast cancer by arresting the cancer cell's replication cycle, increasing tumor cell suicide (apoptosis), and preventing metastasis. Recent research indicates that this miraculous vitamin (some call it a hormone) also does three other very good things for us. It suppresses COX-2 expression, increases tumor suppressor 15-PGDH, and reduces the expression of aromatase, the enzyme that boosts harmful estradiol synthesis in breast cancer cells and in surrounding adipose tissue.[2] If this isn't enough to make you want to catch some summertime rays, I don't know what is.

PREVENTING PROSTATE CANCER

If prostate cancer is present and any of its cells have evolved to possess large quantities of harmful ER-alpha, then estradiol will do its nasty work and slow down the rate of cell death for those cells. This is a very bad scenario since you don't want cancer cells to have a *slow* rate of death, you want them to have a very high rate of death. In fact you'd like to guillotine them all. Under those circumstances, testosterone is also likely to slow down the rate of cell death if it's being converted to high local levels of estradiol by aromatase. Therefore, both testosterone and estradiol may increase the rate at which a cancer population grows. There are two different approaches to address this problem. Either you use a drug to block ER-alpha or you use a drug to block the conversion of testosterone to estradiol. In the presence of either such drug, it should be safe to raise testosterone to teenage levels. The main risk of such a protocol would be having insufficient binding to ER-alpha to maintain health. Experimenters observed a 20–25 percent lowering of bone density in ERKO (estrogen receptor knockout) mice that lacked ER-alpha. Similarly, a human male discovered with a defective ER-alpha gene was found to have dramatically low bone density.[3] The point is that we don't want to totally shut down ER-alpha activity.

If a drug is used to block ER-alpha, then the dosage needs to be adjusted so that there is enough ER-alpha activity to maintain bone density. This is only a theoretical problem since currently no FDA-approved drug is available that totally blocks only ER-alpha activity in all tissues.

If a drug is used to block the conversion of testosterone to estradiol (an example of such a drug is anastrozole, trade name Arimidex®, also known as an aromatase inhibitor or AI), then care must be taken to make sure that you don't reduce estradiol too much because some estradiol is needed to maintain health. Alternatively, if the amount of estradiol is too low, supplementation with exogenous estradiol or estriol can alleviate the problem of too little estradiol. Of the two, I would favor the use of estriol because of all of the favorable effects associated with its binding to ER-beta.

PREVENTING BREAST CANCER

Just as in prostate cancer, if any breast cancer cells are present that have plentiful ER-alpha, estradiol can slow down the rate of cell death for those cells. For such cells, testosterone may also decrease the rate of cell death if enough of it is converted to estradiol. Progesterone also may be dangerous for women with BRCA1 or BRCA2 mutations, as well as for women who have breast cancer cells with plentiful progesterone receptor A. For women with BRCA1 or BRCA2 mutations, a drug that blocks progesterone receptor A will be useful. Since the only FDA-approved drug that blocks progesterone receptor A, RU-486, is currently being used to induce abortions, it is quite unlikely that any women regularly taking such a drug would ever become pregnant. However, since the current medical advice for women known to have BRCA1 or BRCA2 mutations is to surgically remove both the breasts and ovaries, some women might find it preferable to take such a drug instead. Women unfortunate enough to have one of these mutations are the only ones who cannot prevent breast cancer while improving their quality of life.

Because of the enormous changes that occur in hormones during normal pregnancy, more research needs to be conducted before hormones are used in women who may become pregnant. When pregnancy is not an issue, women will want to raise their free testosterone to the highest levels observed in teenage women and also take an aromatase inhibitor (AI). Raising estradiol[4] and estriol to their teenage levels along with ten days of the highest teenage levels of progesterone each month will almost totally eliminate the chance of developing breast cancer for women who don't already have it. However, the problem is that this protocol might harm some women who already have breast cancer cells growing within them.

Therefore, the modification that I recommend is to maintain a teenage level of testosterone, take an AI, and raise estriol to teenage levels or even higher. The reason I say higher is that ER-alpha plays more roles in women than in men, and if you are not using estradiol, then you may need more estriol to eliminate symptoms of menopause. Cyclic use of progesterone is also good to add, but it's not clear if it is best to add it immediately. If there are any early-stage breast cancer cells present, then the combination of testosterone, AI, and estriol can be expected to eliminate them, whereas progesterone may help keep them alive. In my opinion, the younger the woman, the less chance that any breast cancer is present, so the less risk there is in using progesterone. The older the woman, the more likely that there are some cancer cells present, so it may be prudent to delay progesterone use for a number of months. More research is needed to determine what the optimal delay would be. I would not be too surprised if the combination of testosterone with an AI is so effective that no delay in the administration of progesterone is needed.

CHAPTER 11

PREVENTION PRACTICE: MAXIMIZE YOUR IMMUNITY TO PROSTATE CANCER, BREAST CANCER, AND ALZHEIMER'S

Prevention is important for two reasons, the most obvious of which is that using supplements, doing exercise, and making lifestyle changes can actually help you avoid certain diseases. What few people realize, however, is that taking positive steps to prevent disease contributes to well-being in another important way, namely, by giving you a sense of control. That feeling of control has been shown to independently contribute to tangible improvements in health.[1]

Many of the measures we're proposing for prevention are based on the Hormone Receptor Model. In each case, I will explain what steps I recommend and also the rationale behind the suggestion. Since we're designing protocols for prevention, and not treatment, whenever possible the protocol ought to improve the quality of life. Naturally, when dealing with someone who *already* has Alzheimer's or cancer, quality of life isn't as important as slowing down, stopping, or if possible reversing the progression of disease. The following prevention protocols, however, are calculated to both improve quality of life and prevent disease. Although they are theoretical only—there have been no clinical tests of most of them as of yet—the theory is based on solid research that validates the proposed protocols. Moreover, the protocols I recommend for men are ones that I myself use, and the ones I recommend for women are protocols that I recommend to family members and friends.[2]

PREVENTING ALZHEIMER'S IN MEN

First, let's determine the optimal treatment to prevent Alzheimer's in men without any regard to its effect on prostate cancer. As we know from the information presented in chapter 6, it is clear that men need to maximize their vitamin D3 and testosterone levels as much as possible. Brain cells contain a considerable amount of aromatase enzyme, which converts testosterone into estradiol. Based on that, I had long assumed that men had to choose between minimizing their risk of prostate cancer by taking testosterone with aromatase inhibitors (AIs) or minimizing their risk of Alzheimer's by taking testosterone without AIs. Then one day I came across a study in which researchers wanted to know whether aromatase in the brain affected testosterone's ability to prevent the biochemical reactions associated with Alzheimer's. They used mice with a genetic mutation that lacked aromatase and discovered that *testosterone was much more effective in preventing the biochemical reactions associated with Alzheimer's when there was no aromatase present in the brain.*[3] Therefore, aromatase *inhibitors* must be added into the mix when using testosterone to fight Alzheimer's in men since this produces a situation that has been shown to be more effective in preventing Alzheimer's, specifically, a brain in which there is a healthy level of testosterone but little or no aromatase activity. However, there is no need to drop estradiol levels to below normal—a low-normal level should suffice.

There is some controversy about the optimal amount of vitamin D3 that's required on a daily basis.[4] Because absorption differs from person to person, I highly recommend that you monitor the levels of 25-hydroxy vitamin D in your blood. Levels between 81 and 100 ng/mL have been correlated with lower risk of high blood pressure. However, levels above 100 ng/mL have been shown to increase the risk of irregular heartbeat.[5] Therefore, in order to maximize benefits while minimizing risk, I believe that 60–90 ng/mL is the optimal target range.

The reference range for free testosterone is 9–30 ng/dL, according to the Mayo Clinic.[6] With this in mind, I believe that the optimal target range for free testosterone is 25–30 ng/dL. If testosterone levels fall below this optimal range, they can be brought up into the optimal range with supplementation.[7] Testosterone supplementation can result in increased red blood count, decreased testicular size, and decreased sperm count.[8] Blood tests can be regularly conducted to make sure that the increase in red blood count does not reach a dangerous level. If too many red blood cells are produced, either your testosterone level can be decreased or your doctor can perform bloodletting.[9] Testicular shrinkage and possible decreased sperm count can be counteracted by administering human chorionic gonadotropin (HCG) in addition to testosterone supplementation.[10]

A recent study indicated that for men with chronic heart failure, too little as well as too much estradiol increases the risk of dying as compared with those men with serum estradiol in the range of 21.8–30.11 pg/mL.[11] While this study applied only to men with chronic heart failure, I think it is safe to assume that the target for the low-normal range is approximately 20 pg/mL. Therefore, regular blood tests should be conducted when taking an AI to ensure that estradiol remains near the target range, perhaps 15–25 pg/mL.[12] Because, as will be noted later in this chapter, estriol seems to be more effective than estradiol in preventing some of the biochemical reactions associated with Alzheimer's, in theory even lower than the target range of estradiol coupled with a significantly increased level of estriol might be even more protective. However, further research is needed to determine how much estriol is required to prevent any harmful effects of having too little estradiol.

People who stay mentally active throughout their lives seem to have less buildup of beta amyloid and therefore may have less risk of developing Alzheimer's.[13] So if you don't have a mentally stimulating job, you might try taking up a hobby that exercises your brain—even if it's just doing crossword puzzles.

Finally, it was recently discovered that the amount of caffeine from three cups of coffee each day protects people with mild cognitive impairment from developing Alzheimer's.[14] It is believed that caffeine is effective because it blocks the action of the enzymes beta secretase and gamma secretase in producing beta amyloid. In my opinion, it is probably not necessary to ingest caffeine every day if hormone levels are raised high enough, but it could be critical for those men who cannot afford, or who choose not to take, hormones.

PREVENTING PROSTATE CANCER IN MEN

Men who wish to prevent prostate cancer need to raise their vitamin D3 and testosterone close to maximum levels, just as they do if they wish to prevent Alzheimer's. Also, it's an extremely prudent step to add an AI to their supplements to reduce estradiol.

In addition to manipulating their hormone levels, men would be well advised to adjust their diets. For example, men will want to avoid sugars and other refined carbohydrates since any existing prostate cancer cells may grow more rapidly when exposed to sugar.[15]

There are a number of foods that have been shown to be useful in preventing prostate cancer. It is especially important to eat such foods if nothing is being done to change one's testosterone level. Even if you are taking testosterone, it can't hurt to add these foods to your diet, and they may help in other ways. One study showed that walnuts reduce prostate cancer tumor size in mice.[16] No specific constituent in walnuts was found to cause the beneficial effect, and scientists speculated that the entire walnut and its many ingredients contributed to the results. So it makes sense for men to eat three ounces of walnuts each day—the human equivalent of what was given to the mice. As William Davis, MD, points out, walnuts also have the added benefit of not raising blood sugar levels.[17]

Most people have heard that eating broccoli helps protect against cancer. It does this through multiple mechanisms. However, eating at least three servings a week of not just broccoli but of any of the cruciferous vegetable reduces the risk of developing prostate cancer.[18] Some examples of cruciferous vegetables include bok choy, broccoli, brussels sprout, cabbage, cauliflower, horseradish, kale, maca, and radish.

Mushrooms may also be useful in preventing prostate cancer. White mushrooms are natural aromatase inhibitors and help prevent breast and prostate cancer by keeping local estrogen levels in check. Mushroom extract has also been shown to inhibit the growth of several human prostate cancer cell lines.[19] As a result, it makes sense to add mushrooms to your diet. Recently some rather remarkable findings were made with a chemical found in turkey tail mushrooms. When that chemical, polysaccharopeptide, was fed to mice genetically bred to always spontaneously develop prostate tumors, *none* of the mice fed this chemical *developed prostate tumors.*[20] Although turkey tail mushrooms are inedible, a number of vendors sell its extract, and this is a very smart addition to any diet designed to prevent prostate cancer.

The effect of soy on prostate cancer is actually fairly controversial. Genistein is considered the main anticancer chemical in soy. Researchers found that giving genistein to mice with human prostate cancer cells implanted within them almost totally prevented metastases.[21] However, a study done in men with localized prostate cancer showed that genistein had no effect on their prostate-specific antigen (PSA) progression.[22] I personally do not recommend soy for the prevention of prostate cancer, mainly because physiological concentrations of genistein increase telomerase activity and the growth rate of several human prostate cancer cell lines. In fact, researchers who discovered this association between soy and prostate tumors pointed out that previous experiments that showed positive effects with genistein and prostate cancer were all using pharmacological levels of genistein—levels that could not be achieved by men eating soy products.[23]

Finally, there are some men who may have been diagnosed with a condition called high-grade prostate intraepithelial neoplasia (HG-PIN), which is considered a precancerous condition. The drug toremifene reduced the percentage of men whose biopsies showed prostate cancer one year after being diagnosed with HG-PIN from 31.2 to 24.4 percent.[24] Toremifene acts to block estrogen receptors in the prostate. At lower concentrations it blocks estrogen receptor-alpha (ER-alpha) more than it does estrogen receptor-beta (ER-beta).[25] According to the Hormone Receptor Model, blocking ER-alpha reduces the amount of Bcl-2 produced and therefore increases the rate of cell death. In some cases this might slow down the growth of any prostate cancer cells present so that there are too few to be detected. The problem with toremifene is that it also blocks ER-beta to some extent. As you will recall, ER-beta is good for you because it decreases Bcl-2 and causes tumors to die, so we don't want to block this helpful receptor. Ideally, a drug that blocks only ER-alpha will someday be available for use.

While the results of toremifene may offer some hope to men with HG-PIN, even better results were obtained by using extract of green tea. Green tea extract reduced the percentage of men whose biopsies showed prostate cancer one year after being diagnosed with HG-PIN from 30 percent to 3 percent.[26] It is possible that using a combination of toremifene and green tea extract may be more effective than either one alone. While toremifene acts to block ER-alpha, at least one compound found in green tea has been shown to cause apoptosis in a cell line of human prostate cancer cells but not in a cell line of normal human prostate cells.[27] Therefore, these two compounds work in different ways against the formation of prostate cancer, and the effect of both together may be additive.

It is important to take vitamin E complex, not just alpha tocopherol (the chemical name for vitamin E). Some studies indicate that taking just alpha tocopherol may actually be harmful. Researchers have also discovered that gamma tocotrienol (tocotrienols are members of the vitamin E family that have much stronger antioxidant activity than the tocopherols) fights prostate cancer.[28] For this reason, a full-spectrum vitamin E complex product is highly recommended.

It is also helpful to take a multivitamin with minerals because 200 mcg a day of selenium is associated with a lower risk of prostate cancer. Brazil nuts are a good source of selenium.

Men who consume lycopene, which is present in tomato sauce, may have a reduced risk of prostate cancer.[29] Lycopene is also present in watermelons, pink grapefruit, and papaya.

Inositol hexaphosphate also demonstrates strong anticancer properties, especially when combined with inositol.[30]

PREVENTING ALZHEIMER'S IN WOMEN

It's tempting to say that women simply need maintain teenage hormone levels in order to prevent Alzheimer's, but it isn't clear that this is in fact the case. Testosterone is certainly very powerful in counteracting the biochemical reactions associated with Alzheimer's, but while the top teenage range of free testosterone is 30 ng/dL in men, it's only 1.9 ng/dL in women. This doesn't mean that there is too little testosterone to have any effect; rather, it suggests that women have less leeway when making sure that they have enough of this vital hormone. Women are more susceptible to Alzheimer's than men, probably because they have less testosterone. There is a correlation between low testosterone levels and the increased incidence of Alzheimer's in women.[31] But if testosterone alone is not sufficient to protect against Alzheimer's, then is there any evidence that including estrogen and progesterone can be protective? The rate of all forms of dementia, including Alzheimer's, doubles in women who undergo hysterectomies with removal of their ovaries and don't replace any of their hormones.[32] A hysterectomy removes the uterus and reduces a woman's ability to make crucial hormones, including estrogen, progesterone, and testosterone. Women who have a hysterectomy need to be on hormone replacement or they will suffer a doubled risk of dying from heart disease, brain disease, and bone disease.[33] These facts indicate that there is an important protective value to estrogen, progesterone, and testosterone.

Researchers have discovered some mutations that affect ER-beta. These mutations have no effect on the incidence of Alzheimer's in men, but they almost double the incidence of Alzheimer's in women.[34] This study reaffirms that testosterone is so effective in preventing Alzheimer's in men that other hormones are of almost no consequence. However, in women ER-beta seems to be an integral factor in protecting against Alzheimer's.

The most convincing evidence to me is actually totally circumstantial. An autopsy study showed that while children growing up in unpolluted areas have no plaques or hyperphosphorylated tau protein present in their brains, a significant number of children growing up in areas with high air pollution had beta amyloid plaques (51 percent) and hyperphosphorylated tau protein (40 percent).[35] The question that immediately popped into my mind was, Why are we not seeing a significant percentage of people who grow up exposed to heavy air pollution developing Alzheimer's by the time that they are thirty or so years old? The only answer I could think of was that as they entered puberty, their teenage levels of hormones protected them from developing Alzheimer's.

Now that we have established that teenage levels of hormones are very likely to be protective, we next have to ask, Is it safe to give women such high levels of hormones? In women, there are two problems to consider: (1) does the individual plan on becoming pregnant in the future, and (2) does she already have some breast cancer within her? The first question is the thorniest. It is known that a woman's hormone levels change dramatically during pregnancy. What is not known is the effect that taking exogenous hormones and/or drugs such as aromatase inhibitors would have on a pregnancy. Until such questions are answered, I don't see how I can recommend using hormones or drugs on women of childbearing age who hope someday to become pregnant.

So let's discuss what women past childbearing age need to do. At this point, there's no way to tell if a woman has a single breast cancer cell within her. There could easily be millions of breast cancer cells, and we still have no way of detecting them. Therefore, we have to assume that some breast cancer cells may be present and that some may have lots of ER-alpha and little ER-beta. Any such breast cancer cells would thrive if teenage levels of estradiol were administered. Therefore, we cannot include estradiol in any protocol for protecting against Alzheimer's, and we have to modify the hormone levels to become something other than simply emulating teenage levels for all the hormones.

To start with, teenage levels of testosterone are pretty much a requirement. Although the enhanced effect of testosterone against Alzheimer's when no aromatase is present has only been established for males, there is no reason to believe that the same won't also be true for females. Therefore, an aromatase inhibitor (AI) should also be used. The next question is whether estriol will be an adequate substitute for estradiol in preventing Alzheimer's. Unfortunately, none of the straightforward experiments that showed that estradiol decreased beta amyloid levels seem to have been performed on estriol. There was one experiment that showed estriol was actually more effective than estradiol in preventing the aggregation of beta amyloid, which is one of the biochemical reactions associated with Alzheimer's.[36] Because of this and because of the harmful effects of mutations to ER-beta, we have to assume that ER-beta is helpful in fighting Alzheimer's and therefore we will want to use estriol. However, because we are not using estradiol, we may actually need higher levels of estriol than what is seen in teenagers in order to avoid bone loss that may occur if there is not enough binding to ER-alpha. How much higher will most likely vary for each individual and will in large part be determined by how much estradiol each person has naturally when this prevention treatment is begun, as well as how much estriol is converted to estradiol. One question that must be asked is, "How effective is estriol in improving a postmenopausal woman's quality of life?" When estriol alone was given to postmenopausal women, 85 percent reported being satisfied with its effects on eliminating the symptoms of menopause.[37] I would expect that percentage to be higher when testosterone and progesterone are added to the protocol.

It makes sense to also administer ten days' worth of teenage levels of progesterone each thirty days. Although no study has yet been done to show whether this enhances the effect of estriol in decreasing beta amyloid (as it does with estradiol), there is no reason to believe that it won't. In any case, the progesterone will decrease the amount of hyperphosphorylated tau protein. Finally, just as men do, women need to keep the 25-hydroxy vitamin D levels in their blood serum between 60–90 ng/mL.

PREVENTING BREAST CANCER IN WOMEN

In the same way that we had to consider possible pregnancy in designing a protocol to prevent Alzheimer's, we have to consider it in preventing breast cancer. At this point, there isn't enough information to justify giving hormones or drugs to women who may become pregnant. However, for women past childbearing years, it makes sense to start with teenage levels of testosterone plus an AI. It also makes sense to use high levels of estriol along with ten days per month of teenage levels of progesterone. In short, everything (including vitamin D3) that we determined will prevent Alzheimer's will also help prevent breast cancer.

In a 2011 study reported in the *New England Journal of Medicine*, researchers tried using an AI to prevent breast cancer in postmenopausal women. They reported a 65 percent reduction after administering it for an average of almost three years,[38] concluding that aromatase inhibitors can help prevent breast cancer. While I agree with their conclusions, I cannot agree with their reasoning that the AI prevented the *initiation* of cancer. As we already observed in our discussion of the genesis of cancer—and how it takes years for tumors to grow to noticeable size—it is highly doubtful that any breast cancers started up and then grew large enough to be detected during the short three-year span of this study. In my opinion, what these researchers actually demonstrated was that AIs can slow the *growth rate* of *existing* breast cancers. Their therapeutic protocol is still praiseworthy, however. In fact, I predict that if AIs are used for a long enough time frame—perhaps ten years—then a much higher percentage of breast cancers will be prevented. In other words, AIs are one of the best ways for postmenopausal women to prevent breast cancer.

AIs are one of the best ways for postmenopausal women to prevent breast cancer.

Women with BRCA1 and BRCA2 mutations present a unique challenge for prevention-oriented doctors. These women also need prevention help much more than average women because BRCA1 and BRCA2 mutations weaken tumor-suppressor genes (those that make non-mutated BRCA1 and BRCA2) that would normally repair DNA and prevent cancer. Unfortunately, it's not clear that giving progesterone to women with these mutations would help prevent Alzheimer's since at this time we still don't know which of the two progesterone receptors (A or B) protects against Alzheimer's. It's important to know which one it is because if it's progesterone receptor B, that's a problem because women with BRCA1 and BRCA2 mutations may have no progesterone receptor B in their brain cells. The point is that progesterone may turn out to *increase* the likelihood of developing breast cancer in women with these mutations because they have lots of progesterone receptor A and no progesterone receptor B in their breasts, and progesterone receptor A increases Bcl-2, the anti-apoptotic protein that protects cancer and allows it to grow unchecked.[39]

In place of progesterone, I would recommend taking RU-486, a drug that totally prevents breast cancer in mice with the BRCA1 mutation.[40] Because RU-486 blocks the intracellular androgen receptor to some extent,[41] I would recommend women achieve a higher-than-teenage level of testosterone to make up for this loss. More research is needed to determine the optimal dosage of testosterone to use. There has been a case in which a woman was safely given RU-486 for eight years for a different medical condition. The woman was on the drug for four to six months, then off it for two months to allow menstrual cycles to occur.[42] I'm not sure this is the optimal number of months to be on and off the drug—more research is needed on this point. Because RU-486 is currently used to induce abortions, women who take it daily would not be expected to become pregnant. However, once the efficacy of RU-486 in preventing breast cancer is established, women will have to decide for themselves whether they want to undergo prophylactic surgery to remove their breasts and ovaries, take RU-486, or use watchful waiting (the only option that would allow them to get pregnant).

Because of the striking similarities between prostate cancer and breast cancer, my view of which food supplements prevent breast cancer is pretty much identical to my recommendations for preventing prostate cancer. Genistein seems to have a similar effect on breast cancer as it does on prostate cancer. Physiological levels of genistein (the levels found in foods, like soy) promote breast cancer growth, whereas pharmacological levels (the levels found in drugs, like Fosteum®) inhibit breast cancer growth.[43] Therefore, I can't recommend taking soy in order to prevent breast cancer, just as I can't recommend it to prevent prostate cancer. Consuming cruciferous vegetables, such as broccoli and cabbage, is a much better way to help prevent breast cancer.[44]

It's not surprising that, as with prostate cancer, mushrooms and green tea can also be used to help prevent breast cancer. A study done in China showed that women who consumed both mushrooms and green tea each day had an 89 percent reduction in the occurrence of breast cancer compared with women who consumed neither.[45] The authors of the study acknowledged that, in part, their findings might be due to the fact that women who eat mushrooms and drink green tea each day have a generally healthier lifestyle and diet than those who don't. Still, there is compelling evidence that green tea[46] and mushrooms[47] have a direct effect in reducing the risk of breast cancer.

Alcohol, even in small amounts (such as moderate consumption of one drink a day) is associated with an increased risk of breast cancer in women.[48] The mechanism by which alcohol increases the risk of breast cancer may involve its impact on the number of estrogen receptors present.[49] It may be prudent to limit or curtail alcohol consumption.

Women of childbearing age are strongly encouraged to avoid the birth control pill since its synthetic progestin has been shown to increase the risk of breast cancer.[50] It's also advisable to use the spice turmeric or the extract curcumin, which have demonstrated anti–breast cancer properties.[51]

Following these recommended steps to prevent prostate cancer, breast cancer, and Alzheimer's can empower you. New discoveries are being made all the time,[52] and subscribing to a health magazine can keep you on top of the news. In my opinion, it is crucial to take control of your health and not leave it up to your doctor to make a last-ditch effort to try to cure you once you get ill. By taking prevention into your own hands, you'll feel a sense of satisfaction in knowing that you're the one in charge of your physical well-being.

PART 4

NEW TREATMENT PROTOCOLS: USING HORMONES TO FIGHT DISEASE

CHAPTER 12

A NEW TREATMENT PROTOCOL FOR FIGHTING PROSTATE CANCER WITH HORMONE REGULATION

- The only cure for prostate cancer is cutting the disease out or radiating it. Both approaches result in permanent side effects, ranging from mild to severe.
- A better approach is the **Systemic Treatment Protocol**, which modulates hormone levels to kill cancer and promote health. Testosterone kills prostate cancer cells by causing apoptosis, programmed cell death. Testosterone accomplishes this by binding to membrane hormone receptors, causing signals to be sent into the cancer cells, commanding them to kill themselves.
- The use of testosterone to fight prostate cancer is safe and effective. Some doctors are using this treatment plan today.
- Current treatments plans, such as those advocated by Dr. Robert Leibowitz, are showing excellent results (much better than surgery) and can be improved upon by preventing the conversion of testosterone to harmful estrogen.

Throughout this book, I've provided evidence that testosterone and other hormones can be safely used to prevent and treat prostate cancer. In this respect, testosterone replacement therapy is truly miraculous because unlike surgery and radiation, it leaves no scars and destroys no healthy tissue. As you'll discover in the next few pages, this hormone-based therapy significantly reduces the size of prostate tumors for some patients.

I believe that nature provided hormones so that they could be used to fight cancer.[1] We now have the ability to use hormones to do just that. And as we have seen, under the right conditions testosterone can increase apoptosis.

In this chapter, I will spell out exactly how to use this miraculous hormone to increase the apoptosis of prostate cancer cells. When I say that testosterone can, under the right circumstances, lead to the apoptosis of cancer cells, that's the equivalent of saying that we will be making cancer cells self-destruct. And if that's not an exciting prospect, I don't know what is!

Of course, the only reason anyone would want treatment for prostate cancer is if they have the disease or suspect they have it. So in the following discussion I'm going to help you cope with the diagnosis by providing what I consider to be the best treatment plan available today. Let me state right off the bat that if I were diagnosed with prostate cancer, I would not opt for surgery or radiation. Instead I would use the treatment protocol based on the Hormone Receptor Model of prostate cancer, which is the treatment plan that I will explain in this chapter. I call it the Systemic Treatment Protocol. But before I get to my treatment protocol—and why it works so well—let me briefly explain what the medical world is offering you today. As I describe their offerings, I'll tell you why I would personally reject each one as inadequate, too risky, or too invasive. Once you hear what is currently available to you, then you can compare that to my treatment plan and make your own decision about which one you would choose. Naturally, when there are a number of options, you will want to select the one that seems best to you.

Kierkegaard worried that we can never be sure our decisions are right in an ultimate sense because every time we decide something, we prevent ourselves from seeing what would have happened had we chosen another option. Nevertheless, when you hear about the treatment plans available today, I'm confident that you'll be able to decide which one would be best for you. You don't need special scientific information, for example, to know that you would not like a scar or a reduction in sexual function or the burns associated with surgery and radiation.

IS THERE A CURE FOR PROSTATE CANCER?

If anyone claims to have a cure for cancer that no other doctors are using, you can be fairly certain that they are making a false claim. If someone had a cure, even an alternative cure that mainstream medicine hadn't yet adopted, then there would be no need to write a book. A doctor would simply use this cure to eliminate cancer, and patients who had been cured would spread the news by word of mouth, generating increasingly larger numbers of patients who would flock to that doctor until the cure became common knowledge.

Although I'm not offering a cure, I will outline my treatment protocol, which is based on the Hormone Receptor Model of prostate cancer, and which has the potential to stop prostate cancer and significantly reduce tumor size. I consider this approach to be better than a cure.

"How could anything be *better* than a cure?" you might ask.

That's easy to explain when you see the side effects of some of the "cures" currently being offered. Yes, doctors can cut prostate tumors out of your body, but these cures—and they certainly *are* cures since they eliminate every single prostate cancer cell if the cancer has not spread and the surgery is done properly—these cures leave men with side effects such as incontinence and the inability to function sexually like they used to. Men who undergo surgery also experience an average of a 1–2 cm shortening of their penis.[2] Other cures, effected by radiation, succeed in burning the living daylights out of prostate cancer, and they too deserve the name *cure*, since all the prostate cancer cells are burned to death (unless the cancer has already spread), but these radiation cures have their own risks, including the very real risk of patients developing other types of cancer as a result of the radiation. A friend of mine was cured of his prostate cancer this way, but then another cancer sprang up a few years later, caused by the radiation, and he passed away. And he was a person who knew all about the treatment options available at the time. So when I say that the Systemic Treatment Protocol that I am offering is better than a cure, I'm sure you can understand what I mean. My protocol has the potential to reduce tumor size to undetectable levels and reduce prostate-specific antigen (PSA) scores, the marker of prostate cancer. And yet it will not have these horrible side effects. Even better, the major side effect of my treatment plan is that patients often feel like they're teenagers again, with the same vitality and joie de vivre.

CURRENT TREATMENT PLANS FOR PROSTATE CANCER

Before I introduce you to the Systemic Treatment Protocol, let me evaluate the strengths and weaknesses of current treatments for prostate cancer to see if there is any logical way to improve upon them. During this discussion, I'll occasionally be referring to rumors. By rumors, I mean that a doctor has informed me of results that have not yet been published and that particular doctor doesn't want the publicity that would result if I used his name, or I mean that there's something I've seen on a prostate cancer support board posted on the Web by a person I consider credible. Unlike the common meaning of *rumor*, which usually applies to that which is false or misleading, I'll mention rumors only when I believe that the information presented is reliable.

The first concept to understand is the difference between the cure rate and the survival rate, which are actually two separate things. If a person is cured of a cancer, then he will not die from that cancer, so all who are cured will survive. However, in seeking a cure, some patients will die sooner than if they had not sought a cure. As a hypothetical example, consider a cancer for which the only known cure is a complicated surgery. Out of every 100 patients, 50 will die during surgery, 10 will live through it and be cured, and 40 will live through it with the cancer still destined to kill them. Assume that everyone who does not undergo the surgery or who lives through the surgery without it curing them will be dead after five years. So now the question becomes, Should you have this surgery or not? Statistically, half of the men who undergo the surgery will be alive after four years, as will all the people who don't have the surgery. Only the 10 percent who underwent successful curative surgery will be alive after six years. Whether to have this surgery or not is a personal decision, and different individuals might have perfectly valid reasons for making different choices. This is just a hypothetical example, but the choice of whether to maximize the chance of a cure or to maximize the chance for longer survival is a very real one. If it were up to me, however, I would unhesitatingly choose longer survival.

Most books on cancer go into great detail in characterizing the classification of prostate cancer or breast cancer. Those authors are concerned with how aggressive a particular cancer is, how invasive it becomes, and what specific hormone receptors are present. I'm taking a totally different approach. Because of all the mutations possible with prostate cancer, the disease soon becomes a mishmash of cells with various properties. I'm always going to assume that at least one cancer cell has already escaped the local tumor and that at least one cancer cell has properties that make it more dangerous than the rest of the tumor. My goal in designing systemic treatments is to help as much as possible while doing no harm. This means that I try to maximize the rate of cell death for almost all the cancer cells, while trying not to decrease the rate of cell death or increase the growth rate for any cancer cell.

What can you do for me, **Mr. Testosterone?** . . . And won't you make me get **prostate cancer?**
Testosterone
I can build muscle for you, pal. I can help you get organized, increase your motivation, calm you down, make you fearless, improve your sleep, and that's just the beginning. I'll also prevent you from getting type 2 diabetes. Nice, huh? On a cellular level I kill cells that need to die. Scientists call this **apoptosis**, but you know how they are, they'll make up big names for anything. Apoptosis is really cool, though, because it prevents cancer by making sure cells die at the right time. And no, I won't give you **prostate cancer**. Prostate cancer isn't caused by me but by **estradiol**. Watch that estradiol, kiddo, you don't want to mess with too much of that stuff!

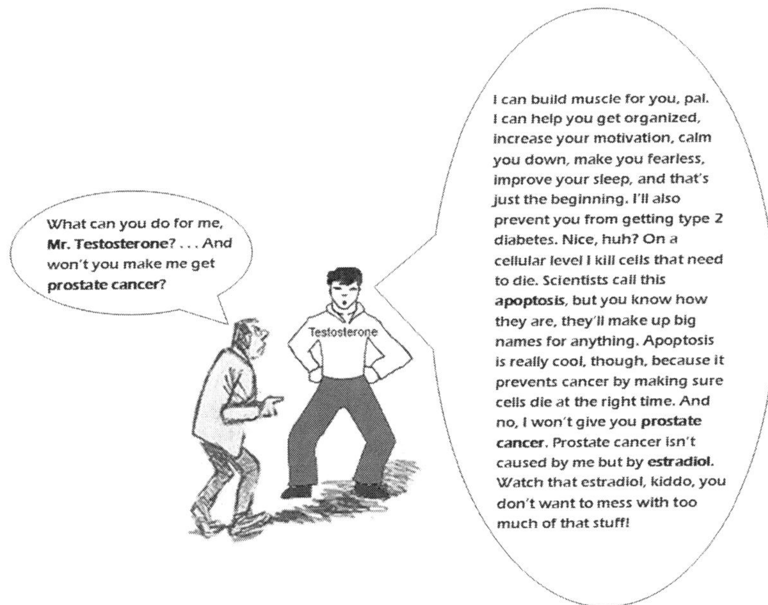

Figure 12.1. Testosterone's rewards. Mr. Testosterone explains some of the many benefits of replacing this marvelous hormone when levels decline.

For all the treatments discussed, it makes sense to take the maximum safe level of vitamin D3.[3] As mentioned in chapter 11, inositol hexaphosphate and gamma tocotrienol can be part of your supplement regimen no matter what treatment is being used. Other nutritional supplements can be useful depending on exactly which treatment is being followed. Finally, whenever 5-alpha-reductase inhibitors are given to reduce dihydrotestosterone (DHT) (by preventing the conversion of testosterone to DHT),[4] your diet needs to be modified to avoid strong selective estrogen receptor modulators (SERMs), such as soy and flaxseed.[5]

Today, newly diagnosed patients are offered two primary options—either local treatment or watchful waiting (also known as active surveillance). Local treatment is typically surgery to remove the prostate, radiation to destroy it, or, less frequently, high-energy radio waves or freezing to destroy it. These local treatments are designed to kill all cancer cells in the prostate. There are books touting the advantages of one local treatment over the other, even the advantages of one type of surgery over the other, but for our purposes, I'll lump all local treatments together into one category and assume that they successfully kill all cancer cells in the prostate.

WATCHFUL WAITING

This treatment plan waits and observes what is happening

Watchful waiting is the option of basically doing nothing except monitoring the PSA and taking further action only if the level becomes too high. It may sound bizarre to do nothing when you have cancer growing inside you, but there's a sound medical reason for this approach. Prostate cancer typically grows so slowly that most men die *with* it, not *because of* it. One of the challenges in modern medicine is to predict at the time of biopsy which cancers require treatment and which can be safely ignored. A meta-analysis of almost sixty thousand men with localized prostate cancer revealed that the percentage who died from prostate cancer within ten years was eleven for those who chose surgery, twenty-six for those who chose radiation, and twenty for those who chose watchful waiting.[6] Comparing surgery to watchful waiting led to the conclusion that in the course of ten years, for every twenty men with prostate cancer treated with surgery, approximately two would have died whether or not they had surgery, two would have lived who otherwise wouldn't have, and the remaining sixteen would have lived even if they did nothing. Partly because of studies like this, many urologists have adopted a ten-year rule, whereby men who have localized prostate cancer but are not expected to live ten more years because of other health problems or advanced age are not initially treated.

SURGERY

This treatment plan cuts the tumor out of the body

The typical course of action for localized prostate cancer when treatment is deemed to be necessary is to start with surgery. This alone is curative approximately two-thirds to three-fourths of the time.[7] All men undergoing prostate removal will experience some side effects. Approximately five in one thousand men will die within one month from complications related to the surgery.[8] Since the prostate makes seminal fluid, men undergoing prostate removal will not produce any semen. The other most common side effects are urinary leakage and impotence. Whether they undergo surgery or radiation, approximately one-third of men will suffer significant side effects.[9] For men who had good sex lives prior to treatment with surgery or radiation, less than half were able to achieve normal erections two years following treatment. Other more serious complications are fairly rare. If the PSA drops to an undetectable level and stays undetectable for the rest of the life of the patient, then the patient is considered cured. On the other hand, if there are three consecutive rises in PSA, then biochemical failure is deemed to have occurred. You may well ask why the term *biochemical failure* is used. I really don't know the answer to that question, although I suspect that it sounds less scary to tell a patient that he has biochemical failure than to tell him that his treatment failed to cure him and he still has prostate cancer.

RADIATION

This treatment plan kills cancer cells with radiation

Typically, salvage radiation will be applied to men who have had biochemical failure. Salvage radiation is external beam irradiation of the prostate bed (the area where the prostate used to be). Side effects of salvage radiation include urinary leakage, rectal bleeding, bowel problems, fistulas, and impotence.[10] The radiation can also cause other cancers to occur since radiation damages DNA. Almost three-fourths of the men who undergo salvage radiation will have some drop in their PSA. After five years, less than one-third of those men will not have an increasing PSA.[11]

ANDROGEN DEPRIVATION

This treatment plan eliminates testosterone

For patients whose PSA is increasing following salvage radiation, treatments that essentially thin the herd of the cancer population are used. Each protocol in this category will kill some cancer cells, but cells that survive will be the strongest and deadliest of the entire population. The next step in treatment is androgen deprivation. This entails using drugs to prevent the production of testosterone in men. Sometimes other drugs are used in combination with this hormone protocol to block the intracellular androgen receptor or to block the conversion of testosterone to DHT. This typically kills most of the prostate cancer cells, although after several years the cancer comes back stronger than ever. At this point, chemotherapy is typically started just to buy the patient a few more months of life. Again, chemotherapy will kill the weakest cells of the cancer population.

DR. ROBERT LEIBOWITZ'S PROTOCOL

This treatment plan uses hormones and drugs to reduce prostate cancer

Let's compare local treatment as reported[12] by a Swedish group in the *New England Journal of Medicine* with systemic treatment as performed by Dr. Robert Leibowitz. Ideally, in order to compare two different treatment methods, a single group of similar patients needs to be treated randomly with one protocol or the other. In this case, this was not done, but the initial description of the two groups' characteristics, such as age, PSA, and the stage of the cancer, were fairly similar. Dr. Leibowitz used an enhanced form of androgen deprivation for thirteen months, followed by administration of finasteride (a 5-alpha-reductase inhibitor) in order to prevent the conversion of testosterone to DHT. According to his website, he also tells his patients to avoid soy, flaxseed, and other strong SERMs. After ten years for men with localized prostate cancer and an average PSA of 10.8, 1.5 percent of his patients died from prostate cancer, and 10.5 percent died from other causes.[13] It is important to include patients who died from other causes because some therapies may lower the chance of dying from prostate cancer while increasing the chance that the treatment itself will kill you. To avoid this misunderstanding, it is useful to consider the overall mortality rate, not just the rate of deaths due to prostate cancer. The breakdown by aggressiveness of the disease is even more interesting. Dr. Leibowitz reported no deaths from prostate cancer for men with low- or medium-risk disease but a 5 percent death rate for men with high-risk disease. The death rate from prostate cancer observed by the Swedish doctors after surgery was 4 percent for men with low risk and 11.6 percent for men with intermediate or high risk.[14] So the death rate from prostate cancer after ten years for men at low or intermediate risk was infinitely better using Dr. Leibowitz's protocol and was at least twice as good for men at high risk. These are statistics that no urologist will ever tell his patients before recommending surgery.

The death rate from prostate cancer after ten years for men at low or intermediate risk was infinitely better using Dr. Leibowitz's protocol and was at least twice as good for men at high risk. These are statistics that no urologist will ever tell his patients before recommending surgery.

So if you happen to be diagnosed with localized prostate cancer with a PSA of a little over 10, the question is, Should you try for a cure or try to maximize your chance of surviving ten years? If your goal is to not die from prostate cancer after ten years, then your chances are around six times greater overall that you will die from it if you use surgery instead of Dr. Leibowitz's protocol. While six times greater sounds like a lot, whether you choose surgery or Dr. Leibowitz's protocol, the chances are over 90 percent that you won't die from prostate cancer within ten years. It is important to keep in mind that none of Dr. Leibowitz's patients were cured. In fact, on his website Dr. Leibowitz makes it clear that his goal is to have his patients die *with* prostate cancer instead of *because of* prostate cancer. So now we have a real-life example of the hypothetical question posed at the beginning of this chapter. There is no right or wrong answer—it is really a matter of what the patient feels comfortable doing. If the goal is to definitely be cured, then the only hope is to undergo surgery (or some other local therapy). There are some men who for psychological reasons cannot bear the thought of having cancer cells growing inside their bodies. However, if the goal is to avoid dying from prostate cancer, then Dr. Leibowitz's protocol is clearly superior.

One obvious question is, What happens when the PSA is much lower before treatment is started? In some cases, men are diagnosed with prostate cancer before their PSA even reaches 4 and are treated at an earlier stage than ever before. Typically, it would take three to five years (or even longer in some cases) before the PSA would rise from below 4 to around 12. For men receiving surgery, the success rate is usually a little higher. Some doctors are claiming only a 5 percent rate of death from prostate cancer for men who start treatment early enough. We can expect there to be a slightly higher percent of men who achieve cures by surgery as well. On the other hand, there still will be no men cured who undergo Dr. Leibowitz's protocol. There would be a lower death rate for ten years, but those deaths may show up three to five years later. A likely possibility would be a 1 percent rate of death for ten years from Dr. Leibowitz's protocol as opposed to a 5 percent rate of death for men undergoing surgery. The basic question remains the same: is it more important to try for a cure or to be alive in ten years?

IMPROVING ON DR. LEIBOWITZ'S PROTOCOL

The Systemic Treatment Protocol improves on Dr. Leibowitz's treatment plan by limiting the harmful effects of estradiol

Although Dr. Leibowitz's work is having wonderful effects, he is first and foremost a clinical physician, and he does not consider the effects of hormone receptors. However, we can use our knowledge of these receptors to improve upon his good work, theoretically making it even more effective.

Dr. Alfred G. Gilman made an important discovery when he found out how cell membrane receptors communicate messages to the interior of cells. He received the Nobel Prize in Physiology or Medicine in 1994 for his work on cell membrane receptors (see figure 12.2). Today we know that certain of these receptors, specifically the membrane androgen receptor (mAR), can be used to kill prostate cancer cells. The way this works is that testosterone binds to the receptor on the cell surface. Then the receptor undergoes a conformational change, meaning it changes shape. When it changes shape, it sends a signal into the prostate cancer cell, telling it to self-destruct (see figure 12.3).

This is very good news, since when prostate cancer cells self-destruct, they commit programmed suicide. In effect, they break apart and die, thereby reducing the overall size of prostate tumors. Recent research indicates that testosterone causes this apoptosis of prostate cancer cells by attaching to the membrane androgen receptors (mAR).[15]

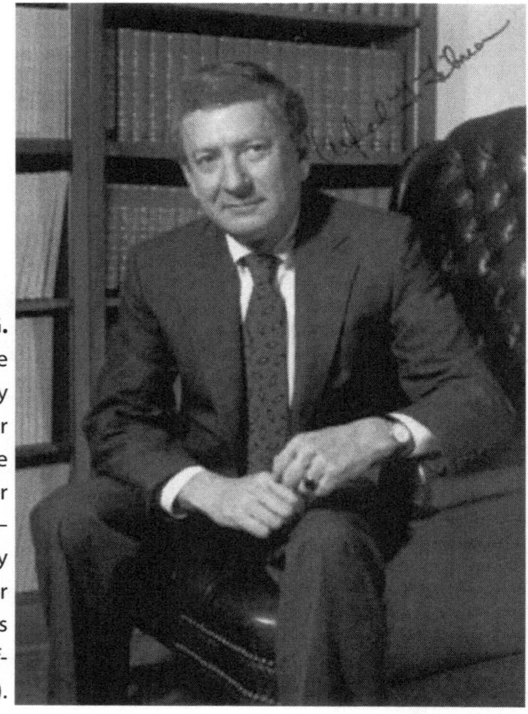

Figure 12.2. Alfred G. Gilman received the Nobel Prize in Physiology of Medicine in 1994 for discovering the membrane hormone receptor. Under the right conditions—when stimulated by testosterone—this receptor causes prostate cancer cells to undergo apoptosis (self-destruction).

Keeping our knowledge of hormone receptors in mind, let's reexamine the logic behind Dr. Leibowitz's protocol. The first question to ask is whether or not his initial androgen deprivation step is necessary. Obviously, performing this step reduces the number of prostate cancer cells, which is a good thing. However, it ends up thinning the herd so that the surviving cancer cells are hardier and more difficult to control. Before androgen deprivation, some dangerous prostate cancer cells had to *compete* with less dangerous cancer cells for nutrition and growing space (think of the difficulty of a cell in the center of a tumor trying to break free), whereas after thirteen months of androgen deprivation, the dangerous cancer cells are free to grow at their maximum rate. On the other hand, androgen deprivation might also kill some of those dangerous cancer cells so that their threat is removed. This is not a cut-and-dried issue, and more research is needed. Dr. Leibowitz cites the case history of a single patient who didn't use androgen deprivation and was treated with teenage levels of testosterone and low levels of DHT (using finasteride) with a resulting PSA doubling time of fifteen years. (The PSA doubling time is the time it takes for the PSA value to double. For a man with an initial PSA of 6, it will take approximately ten PSA doublings to reach a PSA level that is generally known to be fatal.)[16]

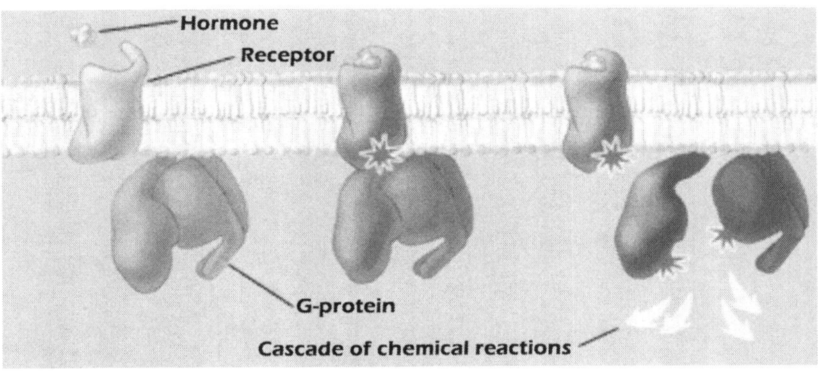

Figure 12.3. G protein hormone receptors. Hormones from the bloodstream bind to cell membrane receptors, causing G proteins to send signals into the cell. Some of these signals instruct a cell to commit programmed cell death. When testosterone binds to the membrane androgen receptors (mAR) it sends self-destruct messages to prostate cancer cells, thereby reducing tumor size. Image courtesy of NIH's National Institute of General Medical Sciences.

Next let's look at the logic of using finasteride following androgen deprivation. This drug reduces the level of DHT, creating an imbalance that increases the ratio of membrane androgen receptor activity to intracellular androgen receptor activity. In theory, this will increase the amount of killers produced by the membrane androgen receptor. By killers, I mean pro-apoptotic proteins.[17] In other words, when there are a great number of membrane androgen receptors then the cell will produce more self-destruct proteins, leading to the likelihood that cancer cells will kill themselves. Pretty neat trick, if you can arrange it. And the good news from the research front is that this is now possible.

Also, finasteride will prevent the conversion of progesterone to "bad progesterone."[18] Side effects from finasteride may include diminished libido or erectile dysfunction.[19]

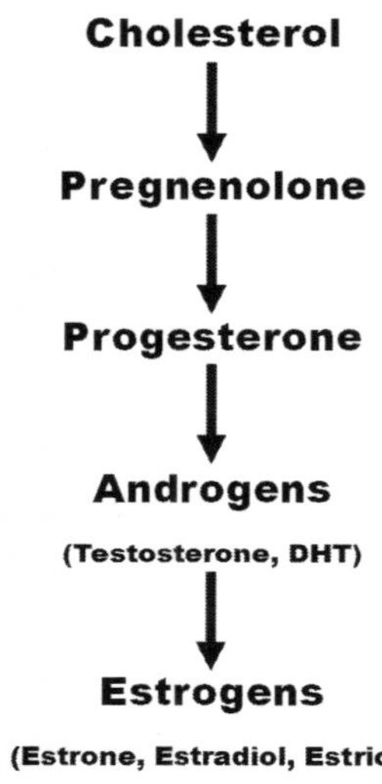

Figure 12.4. Steroid Hormone Chart. This flow chart illustrates how testosterone is derived from cholesterol. It also clearly shows that estradiol can be produced from testosterone, which is why we need to get blood tests when using testosterone replacement therapy to make sure that we do not have too much estradiol, which can cause unwanted cell proliferation. Chart by Michael Christian.

One improvement over giving men only finasteride is to add testosterone. Men given this combination not only don't report the side effects associated with finasteride but actually have an improved quality of life. Dr. Leibowitz achieved this by raising testosterone to teenage levels and even higher. Also, he typically used dutasteride[20] in addition to finasteride in order to counteract the increased amount of DHT that would be expected when testosterone levels are raised. In his published paper he stated that for approximately 40 percent of men, this protocol resulted in stable PSA values for three years.[21] What I found fascinating is why PSA values rose for the other 60 percent and dropped again for almost all of them when the extra testosterone was discontinued. This rise and reversal could be due to any of three different causes. Because of the lack of aromatase inhibitors (AIs), the increased PSA could have been due to the effect of increased estradiol. Another possible cause could have been a high ratio of intracellular androgen receptor to membrane androgen receptor. It is known that prostate cancer cell lines with lots of intracellular androgen receptor grow just fine in the presence of testosterone plus finasteride but don't grow at all in the presence of testosterone alone.[22] Finally, there could have been a mutation on one or both of the androgen receptors that greatly favored the growth of prostate cancer. If the problem was too much estradiol, then adding an AI would stop the rise in PSA. If the problem was too much intracellular androgen receptor, then just using testosterone plus an AI (without using finasteride or dutasteride) would stop the rise in PSA. In the unlikely event that neither of these protocols worked, then you're probably dealing with a mutated androgen receptor, and testosterone and DHT need to be avoided.[23]

For patients whose prostate cancer is already widespread, there's no question that initial androgen deprivation is the proper protocol. Dr. Leibowitz cites the case history of a man whose initial PSA was 3,346 and whose doctors told him he had only a few months to live. Four years after seeing Dr. Leibowitz, his PSA was below 2, and his testosterone level was over 2,000 ng/dL. It's hard to imagine that this man would have been alive at all, let alone with such a low PSA, if he had seen any other doctor in the world.[24]

It's hard to imagine that this man would have been alive at all, let alone with such a low PSA, if he had seen any other doctor in the world.

Dr. Leibowitz gives patients with distant metastases a mixture of anti-angiogenic drugs. **Angiogenesis** is the formation of new blood vessels, a method by which tumors throughout the body are able to get the blood they need to grow larger than about two cubic millimeters. Anti-angiogenic drugs prevent new blood vessels from forming. Dr. Leibowitz is continually trying to fine-tune his anti-angiogenic drug mixture. It has changed over time, and rather than listing it here, I recommend that you go to Dr. Leibowitz's website to find out what the current mixture consists of.[25] So in addition to androgen deprivation, his patients with metastases receive a mixture of anti-angiogenic drugs, which he continues during the testosterone supplementation.

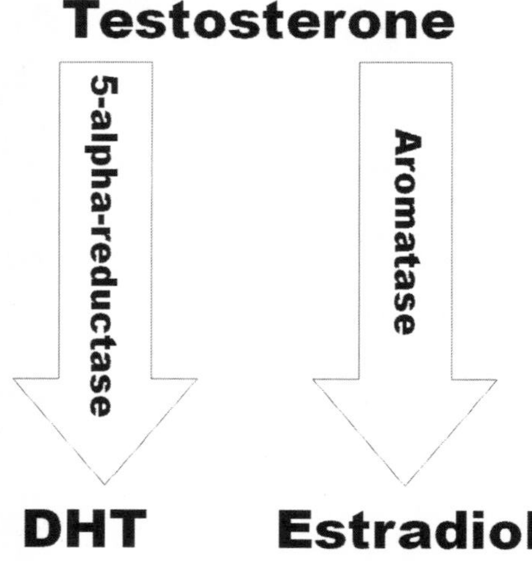

Figure 12.5. Testosterone conversion. The **5-alpha-reductase** enzyme converts testosterone to dihydrotestosterone (DHT), and the **aromatase** enzyme converts testosterone to estradiol. Chart by Michael Christian.

One of the logical questions we need to ask is whether it's a good idea to give an AI to men during androgen deprivation. At first glance, that might seem like an absurd thing to do. Androgen deprivation stops the production of testosterone, and if there's no testosterone then what's the point of administering a drug to prevent the conversion of testosterone to estradiol? Prostate cancer, however, is very similar to breast cancer, especially in the properties of the estrogen receptors. It is known that postmenopausal women typically have lower testosterone levels than those that men achieve during androgen deprivation. Yet even with these low levels of testosterone, AIs have been shown to be very useful in treating and preventing breast cancer recurrence in postmenopausal women. Therefore it would seem to be logical that an AI should always be used in men with prostate cancer—even when they're undergoing androgen deprivation. However, things are never quite as simple as they seem. Since normal prostate cells have lots of ER-beta (a good thing) and almost no ER-alpha, then estradiol would interact with ER-beta and would decrease Bcl-2, which is all to the good, since decreased Bcl-2 means that more cancer cells would die. You could think of Bcl-2 as protection for prostate cancer, so the more we decrease it, the better for us. The problem is that if you continue to allow high local levels of estradiol, those prostate cancer cells with lots of ER-beta will die off (a good thing), but those with lots of ER-alpha will not just live but will thrive because Bcl-2 levels increase when estradiol binds to ER-alpha. If crystal balls worked, then by looking into one you would know just how long an individual with prostate cancer could go before starting to use an AI, but since they don't, we'll have to wait for researchers to determine the optimal time that would help the most people. My best guess is that the time period would be three months—that would allow time for the average prostate cancer cell to die if in fact it is going to die before it divides. This would mean that during the first three months of androgen deprivation no AI would be administered, after which an AI would always be administered, no matter what the subsequent treatment entails.

YOUR FRIENDS (AND ENEMIES) IN THE CELL

Estrogen receptor-beta. Estrogen receptor-beta (ER-beta) is a very good thing. It prevents excess cell proliferation in the prostate. This reduces the chance for cancer. It also encourages prostate cancer cells to undergo apoptosis (programmed cell death). Unfortunately, during most cases of prostate cancer, ER-beta is lessened. The bottom line, however, is that ER-beta provides protection against prostate cancer.

Bcl-2. Bcl-2 is *not* your friend in the cell! It's an anti-apoptotic protein. In other words, it stops cells from dying, including cancer cells. Luckily we now know that the expression of Bcl-2 increases when estradiol binds to ER-alpha and *decreases* when estradiol binds to ER-beta. Just what does this mean for you? It means that if we can find a way to get more estradiol in contact with ER-beta, we're going to kill more prostate cancer.

HOW TO IMPROVE ON LOCAL TREATMENTS

Let's go back to those men who chose local treatment instead of systemic treatment like Dr. Leibowitz provides. Is there anything they can do other than wait to see if their treatment was a success and if they were among the lucky ones who were cured? Since it is known that by the time prostate cancer is detected, it has lots of membrane androgen receptor present, it makes sense to use that imbalance against the cancer by administering teenage levels (or higher) of testosterone, a drug to block the conversion of testosterone to DHT,[26] and some AI to keep estradiol at low-normal levels. This high testosterone, low DHT environment will maximize the production of pro-apoptotic killers caused by the membrane androgen receptors[27] (see figure 12.6).

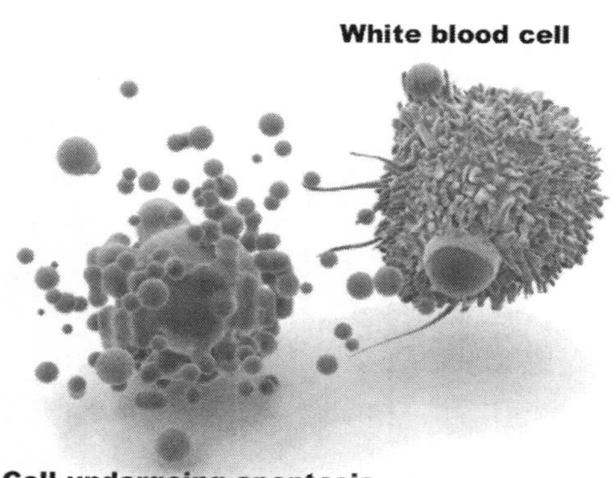

Figure 12.6. Cell undergoing apoptosis. After testosterone leads to apoptosis (cell death of a prostate cancer cell) a big white blood cell, also known as a macrophage, comes along and gobbles up the dead prostate cancer cell and eliminates it from the body. Image courtesy of US National Library of Medicine.

By increasing the rate of cell death, any remaining prostate cancer cells would be eliminated or they would grow so slowly that they would pose a minimal risk of causing death. The only prostate cancer cells that could thrive in this environment would be those with lots of intracellular androgen receptor. If there is any prostate cancer present and it's determined that the cancer population has mostly shifted to this makeup, then just teenage levels of testosterone plus some AI would eliminate most of these cells. Any cells that thrive with this treatment would either have lots of membrane androgen receptor and not that much intracellular androgen receptor or some nasty mutation on one of the androgen receptors that would result in some effect that strongly favors the survival of the cancer cell. In the latter case, testosterone supplementation would have to be discontinued. However, by alternating these treatment protocols, you are buying time—time to die from something *other* than prostate cancer. I know that dying from anything is not a pleasant prospect, but the reality is that if your local treatment fails and you're at risk of dying from prostate cancer, buying time in order to be able to die from something else that you probably would have died from eventually if you had never developed prostate cancer in the first place becomes a much more attractive prospect.

Since only localized treatment offers the chance of a cure, then the question becomes, Why would anyone not start with *that* treatment, followed by the systemic treatment outlined above? As mentioned before, angiogenesis is needed for distant metastases to grow large enough to become life-threatening. It turns out that, for most cancers, the primary tumor produces anti-angiogenic substances that interfere with the ability of distant metastases to obtain the blood vessels they need to grow larger. Studies have shown that in some cases, removal of the primary tumor allows distant metastases to grow much faster than before.[28] This means that if you have a treatment protocol that might increase the rate of cell death enough to kill prostate cancer cells throughout your body, then if you first destroy the primary tumor before administering this treatment when any distant metastases are already present, you may no longer be able to kill the cancer cells that make up these metastases that would have been vulnerable before the primary tumor was removed. This is a powerful reason for opting to use systemic treatment instead of surgery.

My own preference for treatment would be to stick to systemic treatments only. This avoids all the side effects associated with local treatment. Also, I like the concept of using treatment protocols to control the genetic makeup of cancer cells. Think of it like an hourglass full of sand. You allow two-thirds of the sand to empty from the top chamber to the bottom one, then you flip the hourglass over. At this point, you have two-thirds of the sand in the top chamber. You let the sand trickle to the bottom until it holds two-thirds, at which point you turn the hourglass over again. In theory, you could keep doing this forever or until a crack developed in one of the chambers and all the sand escaped through that crack.[29] The purpose of doing this is that each time you flip the hourglass, you succeed in killing the majority of cells in the top part, so with each flip (and each alteration in hormone therapy), you're significantly reducing the size of the cancer population or at least slowing down the rate of growth enough to hopefully avoid ending up dying of prostate cancer (see figure 12.7).

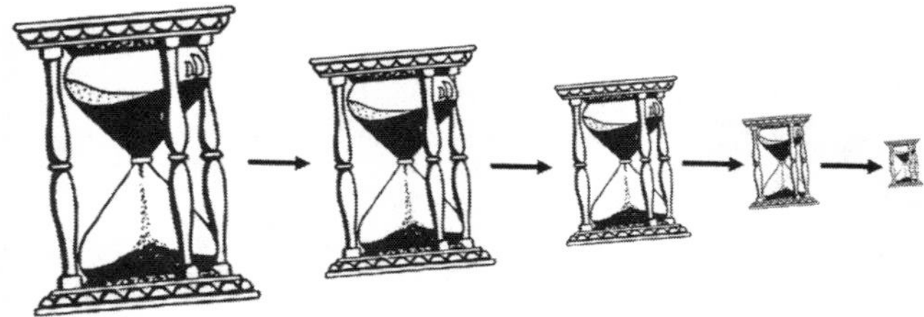

Figure 12.7. Hourglass analogy. Each time the hourglass is flipped, it gets smaller and there is less sand. In the same way, each time the Systemic Treatment Protocol is altered, the prostate cancer population gets smaller because there are fewer cancer cells.

THE SYSTEMIC TREATMENT PROTOCOL

The author's treatment plan manipulates hormone receptors to kill prostate cancer

The Systemic Treatment Protocol uses bioidentical hormone replacement therapy (BHRT), along with additional drugs, to destroy prostate cancer. In this way it totally avoids employing surgery or radiation. Even biopsies are avoided. There are no significant side effects, except that quite frequently during treatment patients feel like they're nineteen again.

The first thing to note about the Systemic Treatment Protocol is that it uses state-of-the-art knowledge about how hormone receptors work to kill prostate cancer cells. You might find it amazing that testosterone can, in many cases, kill prostate cancer cells. In light of the almost universal misunderstanding of testosterone's effect, you might even find it hard to believe that the hormone your family doctor is afraid to prescribe is actually the hormone that will save your life by destroying prostate cancer cells. The work of researcher Anastassia Hatzoglou and her colleagues confirms that testosterone can indeed kill prostate cancer. Testosterone does this killing of prostate cancer without side effects. In one important experiment, Dr. Hatzoglou gave testosterone to male mice that had been injected with human prostate cancer cells. These mice are specially bred not to reject human prostate cancer cells transplanted into their bodies so that we can test various drug therapies against the cancer without risking human lives. Dr. Hatzoglou reported that "one month of treatment with minimal doses of the agent [the testosterone] . . . caused a 60% reduction of [prostate] tumor size compared with that in control animals. . . . It is . . . possible that longer treatment periods would produce a more significant reduction of tumor size. The agent [that is, the testosterone] was nontoxic for the animals, even at concentrations 100 times higher than the effective ones. In this respect testosterone-BSA [the kind of testosterone administered] could represent a new antitumoral agent for prostate cancer." The researchers were naturally excited about their findings, and they went on to say, "*Our data provide the first evidence of an antitumoral effect of androgens in prostate cancer, acting through the activation of mAR both* in vitro *and* in vivo. The preferential expression of these sites in prostate cancer and the efficacy *in vitro* and *in vivo* of testosterone-BSA combined with its lack of toxicity point to a putative use of membrane testosterone activators as a new class of antitumoral agents in the treatment of prostate cancer"[30] (emphasis supplied). In other words, it has now been demonstrated that the membrane androgen receptor can be used to kill prostate cancer. Let's stop right here to emphasize this point. You are reading this book to learn how to fight prostate cancer, and you now have learned what a membrane androgen receptor is (it is described in chapters 2 and 4). You now see that this hormone receptor can start the process of apoptosis, that is, the process of instructing prostate cancer tumors to self-destruct. The way this happens, according to Dr. Hatzoglou, is that testosterone binds to the receptor on the cell surface. This binding triggers an almost instantaneous response. It doesn't take hours or days but mere minutes! In scientific language, the researchers said, "Recently, we identified in the LNCaP human prostate cancer cell line, an androgen-specific membrane receptor that modifies, upon activation, actin cytoskeleton dynamics *within minutes* through a specific signaling cascade. *This membrane receptor was also identified in human prostate tumors, showing a higher expression on cancer cells*"[31] (emphasis supplied). Put more simply, within minutes of binding to the membrane androgen receptor, testosterone sends a signal into the cell, beginning the process of killing the prostate cancer. Testosterone kills prostate cancer cells by causing the membrane androgen receptor to activate actin cytoskeleton dynamics. The actin cytoskeleton is a key factor in the initiation of apoptosis[32] (see figure 12.8).

Within minutes of binding to the membrane androgen receptor, testosterone sends a signal into the cell, beginning the process of killing the prostate cancer.

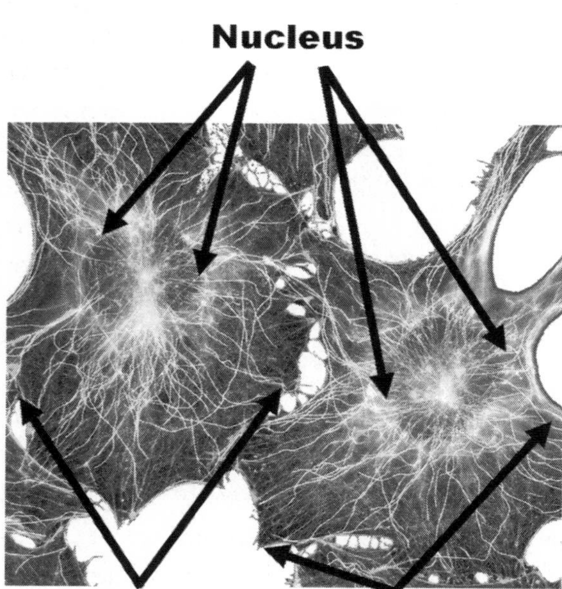

Figure 12.8. The irregularly shaped **actin cytoskeleton** of two cells is clearly visible in this 980 × micrograph. The nucleus and cytoplasm of cells are torn apart by actin cytoskeleton movement, killing the cells during the process of apoptosis. Testosterone can initiate this process of cell death within minutes of binding to membrane androgen receptors. The white lines are microtubules that contribute to the destruction of the dying cell by fragmenting it with spikes.[33] Image courtesy of NIGMS and Torsten Wittmann, Scripps Research Institute.

Applying the hourglass analogy to the Systemic Treatment Protocol, we begin with the fact that the prostate cancer population is initially made up mostly of cells with a high membrane androgen receptor-to-intracellular androgen receptor ratio. Treating these cells with a high testosterone, low DHT protocol will deliver a knockout punch to prostate cancer and at the same time will give a selective growth advantage to cells with a high intracellular androgen receptor-to-membrane androgen receptor ratio. As the population evolves, it will shift to contain more cells with a high intracellular androgen receptor-to-membrane androgen receptor ratio. It is not clear how long it will take for the appropriate genetic mutations to occur, but eventually it will occur in almost all the cells, so that switching the treatment to high testosterone, high DHT will prevent those cells from proliferating. However, cells with a high membrane androgen receptor-to-intracellular androgen receptor ratio will now have a selective growth advantage, and the population will evolve back closer to what it was before any treatment was started.[34] The whole point of switching the protocol is to encourage the destruction of prostate cancer cells, no matter what type of wild mutation they may develop.

Recent studies have shown that it is not necessary to wait for genetic mutations to occur. Using just finasteride greatly increases the amount of intracellular androgen receptor starting after one month and continuing through six months. Over 80 percent of both cancerous and noncancerous prostate cells show this increase in intracellular androgen receptor.[35] This means that our treatment can be repeated over and over again—each time with the same percentage of cells experiencing the increase in intracellular androgen receptor. This rapid increase in intracellular androgen receptor isn't due to a change in the genetic makeup of the cell; rather, it's a response of the cell adapting to its immediate environment. It remains to be seen whether high-dose testosterone plus finasteride will work in the same way as finasteride alone in increasing these receptors. Assuming that only finasteride will work in this way, then it may be better to maintain enough AI to keep estradiol levels at the low-normal level and to first use finasteride without additional testosterone and then alternate with high-dose testosterone (at least 2,000 ng/dL) without finasteride.[36] This treatment protocol may seem absurd to those still laboring under the misconception that testosterone is the worst thing that could be given to men with prostate cancer. They may find it inconceivable that the medical establishment would give this idea any credence. In fact, not only was this protocol published recently in the journal the *Prostate* but the editor wanted me to mention the fact that there were currently two clinical trials under way seeking to use testosterone plus additional drugs as therapeutic agents in treating prostate cancer. Although I wrote in that letter to the journal that the ideal length of time before switching treatments remains to be determined, my best guess would be about three months.[37]

If a man has early-stage prostate cancer with no metastases, then a choice must be made. Either thirteen months of androgen deprivation can be started or high testosterone-low dihydrotestosterone treatment can be started. I don't think testosterone ablation is best initially unless the patient has metastasized prostate cancer. It's not always easy to know when this happens, so I would say you definitely will want to start with androgen deprivation if your PSA is over 20, unless you have heart problems, in which case testosterone ablation would be too risky.[38] In either case, there will be a time period of three months during which no AI is given because we want to maximize the rate of cell death for prostate cancer cells that still have lots of ER-beta. After that point, the patient will be on an AI for the rest of his life because that reduces estradiol, the dangerous estrogen.[39] Just in case you forgot why too much estradiol is harmful, remember our discussion in chapter 4 about how it leads to excess epithelial prostate cell proliferation, which is a risk factor for prostate cancer.[40]

There are several reasons that we want to avoid androgen deprivation. First, the side effects tend to be pretty severe. Besides feeling worse physically and mentally, there's an increased risk of Alzheimer's disease, since androgen deprivation doubles the concentration of beta amyloid.[41] Also, if my hourglass treatment doesn't work, then androgen deprivation can always be implemented later. Of course, if distant metastases ever appear, then the multiple anti-angiogenic drugs espoused by Dr. Leibowitz need to be used. Finally, drugs presently available aren't as effective in blocking the intracellular androgen receptor as drugs that are currently under development. I expect that by 2022, androgen deprivation will be much more effective than it is today.[42]

THE RISKS OF TESTOSTERONE SUPPLEMENTATION

There is more risk for elderly men in *not* supplementing with testosterone than in supplementing, since low levels of testosterone are associated with increased coronary heart disease,[43] type 2 diabetes,[44] depression,[45] Alzheimer's,[46] and prostate cancer.[47] That being said, there are a few side effects to watch out for when using testosterone replacement therapy[48] The risks of testosterone replacement therapy are so minimal that even when using massive doses as athletes do, problems are so infrequent that they make headlines. When you use testosterone under the care of a physician, these risks are usually easy to manage. The side effects to watch for are the following:

Increase of red blood cells. Testosterone increases the production of red blood cells, which is usually a good thing because these cells carry oxygen to all parts of the body, giving you more energy. Too much of an increase of red blood cells (measured with a hematocrit blood test) is easily treated by reducing the dose of testosterone or by donating blood. If untreated, too many red blood cells increase the risk of blood clots.

Elevation of estrogen. Some men, especially those with a large amount of abdominal fat, experience a mild elevation in estrogen. This is due to aromatase converting testosterone to estradiol. This problem can be avoided by the use of an AI. It is important to note that in the presence of prostate cancer, testosterone will *always* increase *local* estradiol levels—even if it lowers *serum* estradiol levels. This is why it is so important to use AIs to minimize local estradiol. You can always supplement with estradiol or estriol if your serum estradiol level drops too low.

Increase of DHT. Dihydrotestosterone may increase when transdermal delivery is used. This is not necessarily bad, but if it gets too high, a 5-alpha-reductase inhibitor can be used to lower DHT.

As far as the delivery method, testosterone can be administered transdermally (with a gel or cream), through intramuscular or subcutaneous injection, with pellets, or with patches.[49] The only delivery requirement for all hormones is *not* to give them orally. Orally, they pass through the liver and get converted into other compounds. For example, estradiol given orally increases the risk of blood clots, but when not given orally, there is no such increase in risk.[50] So injection, pellet, cream, gel—all are fine as far as the Systemic Treatment Protocol is concerned.

WHY I RECOMMEND THE SYSTEMIC TREATMENT PROTOCOL

The Systemic Treatment Protocol is based on theory and logic, as well as on the clinical successes of Dr. Leibowitz and others.[51] Nevertheless, this treatment plan is experimental in the sense that it requires at least fifteen years before it can be adequately tested.[52] Unfortunately there are men who cannot wait fifteen years to see what the results will be. But I can tell you that if I were in their shoes, I would unhesitatingly opt for the Systemic Treatment Protocol. Overall, compared to surgery, it has less risk of side effects. Compared to radiation, it is much less risky. And compared to other hormone modulation protocols, it is state-of-the-art and superior in every way. For example, there are hormone modulation clinical trials now under way that don't even take into account the harmful effect of estradiol and that consequently fail to administer an AI to subjects. That is asking for trouble. As you will recall, whenever you give testosterone, you need to monitor estradiol levels carefully with periodic blood tests. Why? Because—as I have said numerous times—you don't want too much estradiol, which can lead to excess cell proliferation. In fact, if you take away only one message from this book, I suggest it be that estradiol, not testosterone, is the real culprit in causing prostate cancer, and you are justified in fearing too much estradiol, not too much testosterone.

There are hormone modulation clinical trials now under way that don't even take into account the harmful effect of estradiol and that consequently fail to administer an AI to subjects. That is asking for trouble.

Rumor has it that almost all men who decide to undergo watchful waiting and who opt for the treatment of high testosterone-low DHT, plus AI, have almost no rise in their PSA (at least in the initial first few years), whether or not they have first undergone thirteen months of enhanced androgen deprivation.

It is interesting to note that researchers at Johns Hopkins recently released some data regarding an experiment that is currently in progress. They are alternating two weeks of supraphysiological levels of testosterone plus the chemotherapeutic drug etoposide with two weeks of allowing the testosterone level to fall to near castrate levels. After three months, two of their four patients with castrate-resistant prostate cancer experienced a greater than 50 percent decrease in their PSA.[53] Treatment protocols for prostate cancer are generally not taken seriously unless they can achieve at least a 50 percent drop in PSA, and this protocol meets that criterion. It is not clear that etoposide is necessary to achieve these results. I doubt that the two-week cycle is the ideal time frame, and it would be interesting to see what would occur if AIs were incorporated as part of this protocol. The rationale behind this protocol is that during androgen deprivation those prostate cancer cells that survive tend to have more intracellular androgen receptor. As discussed earlier, testosterone prevents the proliferation of prostate cancer cells if they have lots of intracellular androgen receptors. This protocol is similar to what I have proposed, but it would be expected to have more side effects because of the near-castrate testosterone levels that are in place half of the time. I predict that this protocol will fail in the long run due to the lack of an AI.

One thing to keep in mind when discussing the effectiveness of various treatments is that besides the number of men who die from prostate cancer, the number who die from all other causes also needs to be taken into account. An early study from before the time that PSA was discovered found that after twenty-three years, there was no statistical difference in the overall survival rate of men who underwent surgery compared to men who chose watchful waiting.[54] A more recent Swedish study indicates that there's a slight but statistically significant survival benefit after fifteen years for men who undergo surgery as opposed to those who choose watchful waiting. While it may seem absurd that men who do nothing can survive roughly the same number of years as those who choose surgery, there are several possible explanations. One explanation is that the surgery somehow impairs men's health and contributes to an increased mortality rate. Personally, I don't think there's any convincing evidence of this. The explanation that I favor is that men with low testosterone are more likely to die earlier, either from prostate cancer or from some other cause. In statistics, this is referred to as competing risks in survival. In this case, it is known that men over forty with low levels of testosterone are much more likely to die each year from a host of causes than men with at least normal levels of testosterone.[55] So even if they're cured of prostate cancer but fail to eliminate the underlying problem—low testosterone—they won't show significantly longer overall survival rates. Of course, some men will die from prostate cancer even though they have higher levels of testosterone. However, Swedish researchers determined that men with lower levels of dihydrotestosterone at the time of diagnosis are more likely to die from prostate cancer than men with higher levels.[56] Since the only source of DHT is the conversion of testosterone, this indirectly demonstrates that low testosterone increases the risk of dying from prostate cancer.

Some anticancer nutritional supplements will interfere with the intracellular androgen receptor and therefore may interfere with the treatments described above. When using finasteride, mushrooms in the diet will be safe because they block the conversion of testosterone to DHT in a manner similar to what finasteride does. In fact, when undergoing androgen deprivation, all the anticancer supplements mentioned in the previous chapter will be safe to use. The only exception is resveratrol. It definitely has strong anticancer properties, but its promotion of angiogenesis is rather worrisome.[57] Even in early-stage prostate cancer, it can be fatal to assume that no metastases exist. More research is needed to determine exactly what levels of resveratrol lead to blood vessel growth. Ideally, a concentration will be discovered that still has anticancer properties without promoting angiogenesis.

PSA TESTING

Now let's go back to the traditional course of treatment mentioned at the beginning of this chapter. It makes no sense to do nothing following surgery when other options are available. "Teenage" levels of testosterone plus finasteride plus enough aromatase inhibitor to keep estradiol levels low is a logical step to try. If enough years go by with no indication that there are still any prostate cancer cells around, then eliminating finasteride becomes an option. Both of these systemic treatments will also lead to greatly improved quality of life.[58] If PSA tests indicate that there are still prostate cancer cells present, then cycling through finasteride followed by high testosterone (as described above) is in my opinion a better option than salvage radiation. If this procedure fails to stop the rise in PSA, then salvage radiation can always be employed later as a fallback treatment.

Currently doctors in some countries routinely administer PSA tests to men starting around age fifty, whereas doctors in other countries don't bother with PSA tests. In my opinion, it's ridiculous *not* to give PSA tests, especially in light of the fact that the prostate-specific death rate is higher in countries that don't give PSA tests. However, let's consider the ten-year study we discussed earlier. Before PSA testing, for every twenty men, sixteen men would not die whether or not they underwent surgery, two would die in either case, and two would avoid dying if they underwent surgery.[59] Now with PSA testing, prostate cancer is detected much earlier—some estimates are that the test detects the disease five years earlier than without testing. However, in addition to detecting the twenty men who would eventually have been diagnosed later, let's assume the test also catches twenty more men whose disease would never have progressed to the point where it would have been detected except for the fact that PSA testing triggered a biopsy that uncovered it. If all these men undergo surgery, then instead of two out of twenty dying, you have two out of forty dying. So without helping any more men, you've doubled the success rate of surgery. (In reality, earlier surgery would occasionally save the lives of some men, so a very small fraction of the additional men would actually be helped.) Of course, this will also improve the overall survival rate of men diagnosed with prostate cancer since those who were diagnosed as a result of PSA tests (and who otherwise would not have been diagnosed) would tend to be healthier and therefore would live longer. Another complicating factor is that some men being treated for prostate cancer will die from something related to their treatment but that won't show up in the statistics as dying due to prostate cancer. For example, some men undergoing androgen deprivation have an increased chance of dying from a heart attack, but for each man who does die that way, how can anyone be sure whether or not he would have died from a heart attack at that same time even if he had not undergone androgen deprivation? Because this is so messy, I don't see how anyone can state exactly to what extent PSA testing has improved the overall survival of men. If it is beneficial, then you would expect to see an improvement in the average life expectancy for men, but there are so many factors that potentially can affect the average life expectancy, it would be hard to attribute any improvement solely to PSA testing. Recently, the US Preventive Services Task Force recommended that routine administration of PSA tests be discontinued. I believe this was a mistake. In my opinion, men *should* get PSA tests but should *not* get biopsies no matter what their PSA results.[60] The value of getting a PSA test is that it enables you to monitor one important marker of prostate cancer. Then you can follow your PSA over time to see whether it goes up or down in response to your diet, lifestyle, or hormone protocol. Keep in mind that almost every man who is old enough to be given a routine PSA test will in fact have some prostate cancer within

Men *should* get PSA tests but should *not* get biopsies no matter what their PSA results.

him. The advantage of PSA testing is to monitor the velocity and see if by using hormones plus drugs you can get the velocity to go negative or at least to have so slow a rise that it's never life-threatening.

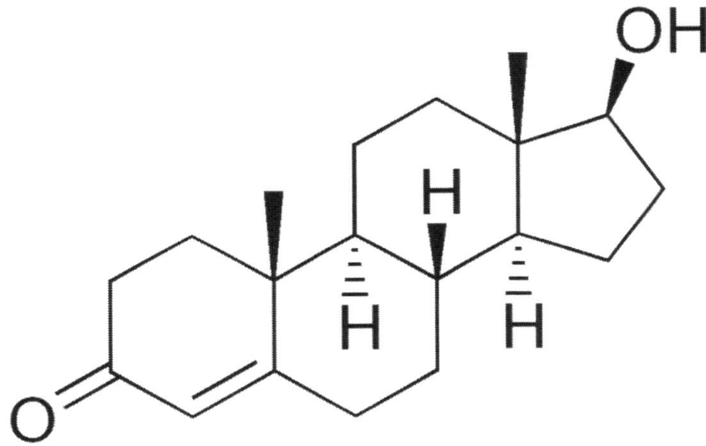

Figure 12.9. Testosterone. The chemical structure of testosterone is rather simple, but its effects are wide-ranging, multifaceted, and, when it comes to prostate cancer, literally lifesaving.

In the next few chapters, I'll show you how testosterone can also be used to fight breast cancer and Alzheimer's. That simple molecule in Figure 12.9 may start looking better to you the more you learn about its miraculous lifesaving potential. And the most remarkable thing is that testosterone—the primary male hormone—also has so much to offer women in terms of improved health, vitality, and longevity.

CHAPTER 13

THE STANDARD TREATMENT FOR BREAST CANCER AND HOW TO SIGNIFICANTLY IMPROVE UPON IT

Once a woman discovers that she has breast cancer,[1] she's usually given a choice of which type of surgery to undergo.[2] A mastectomy removes the entire breast, whereas a lumpectomy removes only the tumor and its surrounding tissue. Radiation is administered after a woman undergoes a lumpectomy.[3] In some cases chemotherapy is administered either before or after surgery. If a woman's breast cancer contains significant amounts of estrogen receptor (a condition doctors call estrogen receptor positive), then an aromatase inhibitor (AI) is prescribed for postmenopausal women, and the drug tamoxifen is prescribed for premenopausal women.[4]

Tamoxifen[5] is converted by enzymes in the liver into more potent compounds that block estrogen receptor-alpha[6] (ER-alpha) in breast tissue.[7] Five years of tamoxifen treatment reduces the recurrence rate from 28.7 to 16.4 percent, an improvement of 12.3 percent. Ten years of treatment yields an even more positive effect, reducing the recurrence rate from 40.1 to 25.9 percent, an improvement of 15.2 percent. There doesn't seem to be any further benefit after ten years or more of tamoxifen, with the reduction in the recurrence rate after fifteen years ranging from 46.2 to 33.0 percent, an improvement of 13.2 percent.[8] Between ten and fifteen years, 6.1 percent additional women who were not taking tamoxifen suffered recurrences as opposed to 7.1 percent for those women taking tamoxifen. Tamoxifen treatment is discontinued after five years because its use increases the risk of blood clots and endometrial cancer.[9]

Aromatase inhibitors have proven superior to tamoxifen in preventing recurrences in postmenopausal women. The AI anastrozole is 2.8 percent better than tamoxifen in preventing recurrences after five years and 4.8 percent better after nine years.[10] Doctors don't use AIs for premenopausal women except in combination with drugs to suppress ovarian function because the resulting decrease in circulating estrogen results in an increase in the hormone gonadotropin, which increases the production of hormones by the ovaries.[11]

Recurrences are removed surgically, if possible. If this isn't possible because the cancer has become metastatic, then the prognosis is especially poor. The five-year survival rate in the 1920s was 5 percent. It increased to 25 percent in the 1960s but has not improved significantly since then. Treatment is typically chemotherapy, but even the introduction of combination drug protocols has done little to improve the survival rate.[12]

Breast cancer possessing the HER2 membrane receptor is particularly aggressive. The drug trastuzumab, commonly known as Herceptin®, has been shown to be beneficial in treating this type of cancer. Herceptin treatment typically lasts one year, although studies are being done to determine the optimal duration of treatment. Women with HER2-positive breast cancer who are treated with Herceptin following surgery have a three-year recurrence rate of 26.0 percent, compared to 35.5 percent for those who don't receive Herceptin. There have been rare cardiac side effects for women using Herceptin, with one recent study reporting a 2.1 percent increase in heart problems either during or after Herceptin treatment.[13] Herceptin has also been added to chemotherapy in treating women with metastatic HER2-positive breast cancer, resulting in an improved average survival time of 25.1 months as opposed to 20.3 months for women who don't take Herceptin.[14]

TESTOSTERONE FIGHTS BREAST CANCER

Testosterone has been used to treat metastatic breast cancer since 1939. In some cases, dramatic improvement is achieved, but in general, the response has been unpredictable and transient.[15] Unfortunately, when testosterone was first employed to combat breast cancer, AIs hadn't yet been discovered. In addition, testosterone dosages were quite large, typically large enough to prevent the ovaries from producing hormones, leading to masculinizing side effects, such as growth of facial hair. We now know that it's a mistake to use testosterone to shut off the ovaries because aromatase converts too much of that testosterone, resulting in an unacceptably high local level of estradiol. What is remarkable is that any of the tumors responded positively to such a treatment. Presumably, those cancers that showed regression were unable to take advantage of the higher local levels of estradiol, possibly due to a lack of ER-alpha.

The truly interesting question is, "What happens when an AI is administered along with testosterone?" According to the Hormone Receptor Model, this would be an especially effective protocol because both androgen receptors (membrane and intracellular) would act to reduce the production of Bcl-2, and excess estradiol would not be produced.

The truly interesting question is, "What happens when an AI is administered along with testosterone?" According to the Hormone Receptor Model, this would be an especially effective protocol because both androgen receptors (membrane and intracellular) would act to reduce the production of Bcl-2, and excess estradiol would not be produced.

Dr. Rebecca Glaser reported in the 2010 ASCO Breast Cancer Symposium that implanting testosterone pellets plus the AI anastrozole improved the quality of life for fifty-five breast cancer survivors. No recurrences were reported in any of these women for up to three years of treatment. In addition, two women with metastatic breast cancer were treated with pellets and had no progression of disease.[16] On the surface, these results seem fantastic, but it's too early to get excited. The lack of recurrences is definitely encouraging, but the abstract did not indicate how many years had gone by since their surgery before these women started pellet therapy.

I believe that if started immediately after surgery, this pellet protocol will come close to achieving zero recurrences after five years, but I still expect that there will be some recurrences. This is because decreasing Bcl-2 will increase the rate of cell death, thus killing some cells and slowing down the rate of the rest. Because of the heterogeneous nature of breast cancer, I expect that some cancer cells will survive, with some fast-growing cancer cells now becoming slow-growing cancer cells. I also expect that in some cases, what would have been slow-growing breast cancer cells will now die out. Similarly, the lack of progression in metastatic breast cancer is encouraging, but again we're dealing with a heterogeneous population. I expect that while overall there is no progression of the disease, in reality some of the cancer cells are dying while others are still growing—but at a slower rate. It's definitely too soon to say that Dr. Glaser's work represents the end of breast cancer, but in my opinion, it represents the beginning of the end of breast cancer.

THEORETICAL TREATMENTS FOR BREAST CANCER

There are additional theoretical treatments to try in addition to what Dr. Glaser is doing. One obvious improvement is to add RU-486 plus progesterone. RU-486 has been shown to inhibit the growth of breast cancer cells whether they're progesterone receptor positive or negative.[17] The authors of this study suggested that RU-486 might be acting on membrane progesterone receptors, and I agree with that conclusion. If RU-486 blocks membrane progesterone receptors that bind to "bad progesterone,"[18] that would explain why it inhibits cancer growth. It has also been discovered that the combination of progesterone plus RU-486 works better than either one alone in inhibiting breast cancer growth.[19] Researchers believe there is a synergistic interaction between RU-486 and progesterone. They also believe that 400–600 mg. of RU-486 will produce therapeutic blood plasma concentrations.

Another possible improvement is to make use of the pro-apoptotic proteins produced by the membrane androgen receptor.[20] According to the Hormone Receptor Model, this can be accomplished by decreasing binding to the intracellular androgen receptor while increasing binding to the membrane androgen receptor. There are two ways to accomplish this—either use a drug to block the intracellular androgen receptor or use a drug such as finasteride to decrease the conversion of testosterone to dihydrotestosterone (DHT). Even if you're using a drug to block the intracellular androgen receptor, you'll still want to use finasteride because then you gain the advantage of reducing the amount of "bad progesterone" present. This protocol has not yet been tried, so there's no data available today on exactly how much extra testosterone needs to be administered.

NEW DRUGS FOR BREAST CANCER

There are several promising new drugs that will hopefully be approved for treating breast cancer in humans. The first, MDX-12C, is a combination of testosterone conjugated with human serum albumin. It binds to the membrane androgen receptor but not to the intracellular androgen receptor. So far, it has been effective against prostate cancer cell lines,[21] and it is also expected to be effective against breast cancer.[22]

Another promising new drug that may play a role in the war against breast cancer is Rexin-G®.[23] Rexin-G is a nanoparticle that targets metastases. It has almost no side effects and has been shown to be effective in some women with metastatic breast cancer.[24] Currently, this drug seems to work well for some women and not at all for others. However, it appears that it's worth trying if nothing else proves effective.[25]

PERSONAL CHOICES FOR BREAST CANCER

There are a number of personal choices to be made in treating breast cancer, not only whether to have a lumpectomy or a mastectomy. It's not always clear what the best choice is—in some cases, you're balancing quality of life with a chance of increased survival. Each individual has to decide with her doctor which path to take. The following describes what I would personally do if I were a woman diagnosed with breast cancer. Philosophically, I don't want to sacrifice my quality of life or undergo unduly invasive procedures in the hopes of a marginally improved chance of success.

At this point, most women would be considering whether to undergo a lumpectomy or a mastectomy. Personally, I would be considering whether or not to have surgery at all! It appears that a number of breast cancers regress on their own if left untreated. Because of this regression, some researchers have recommended using tamoxifen or an AI for women with estrogen receptor–positive breast cancers and monitoring them to see if surgery is even necessary.[26] However, I would improve upon their suggestion and start with the anastrozole-testosterone pellets used by Dr. Glaser.[27] I would also adopt an aggressive vitamin, mineral, herb, and cofactor regimen, taking nutritional supplements known to fight breast cancer. Besides vitamin D, calcium, vitamin K2, walnuts, mushrooms, and green tea, I would also start taking curcumin,[28] pomegranate,[29] resveratrol,[30] oil of oregano,[31] indole-3-carbinol (I3C),[32] diindolylmethane (DIM),[33] inositol hexaphosphate (IP6),[34] broccoli sprouts,[35] and a tocotrienol complex.[36] There are plenty of other nutrients that fight breast cancer, but these are some of the most effective. If you search the Web, you'll find that almost every fruit and vegetable contains anticancer constituents. Although we might not know the optimal dosage for some of these supplements, I would avoid taking massive amounts, since that might cause unintended consequences if they interfered with your hormone receptors. The safest thing for now is to follow the directions given with each supplement or by your health care provider.[37] Needless to say, I would continue taking these supplements for the rest of my life, no matter what subsequent treatments I received.

Assuming that this protocol fails to stop the growth, I would then proceed to a lumpectomy. Personally, I would forego radiation. Even though it might be helpful in the short run, I'm reluctant to expose myself to possible secondary cancers years later.[38] After surgery, I would continue with anastrozole-testosterone pellets. If premenopausal, I would also add tamoxifen, but only for two years instead of five in order to minimize the risk of side effects.

Assuming that in spite of this treatment there is a recurrence of breast cancer, I would undergo another lumpectomy, if feasible. However, if the cancer had spread and was now metastatic, I would turn to more aggressive measures. First, I would implement Dr. Leibowitz's anti-angiogenic protocol. If I lived in a country where it was legal to use RU-486 to treat breast cancer, I would take that plus progesterone. In addition I would take finasteride to minimize the amount of "bad progesterone" produced. To compensate for the lack of dihydrotestosterone, I would increase the amount of testosterone to aim for a free testosterone level five times higher than the normal maximum.[39] I would aim for five times more testosterone because DHT binds five times more strongly to the intracellular androgen receptor than testosterone.[40] This protocol can also be expected to result in much more binding to the membrane androgen receptor than to the intracellular androgen receptor, which will increase the amount of pro-apoptotic proteins produced. This protocol will additionally provide sufficient testosterone to bind to the intracellular androgen receptor, effectively preventing side effects due to testosterone deficiency. In addition, I would maximize the amount of aromatase inhibitor taken to try to prevent the conversion of testosterone to estradiol as much as possible. I would also add estriol to make sure that the estriol level is greater than the combined levels of estrone and estradiol.[41] Estriol improves hormonal health by binding to estrogen receptor-beta and by interfering with estradiol's and estrone's binding to estrogen receptor-alpha. If I were in the United States, I would follow the above procedure but without using RU-486 or progesterone.[42] Without RU-486, progesterone is too dangerous because it increases Bcl-2 in cancer cells that possess plenty of progesterone receptor A.

Finally, if after all of this the cancer was still growing too fast, and if I had the money, I would go to a country where Rexin-G was legal and try that.[43] In theory, Rexin-G increases the rate of cell death, and testosterone with an AI decreases the amount of Bcl-2. Combining these protocols will in theory lead to more effective killing of cancer, as well as less protection for cancer against this killing; however, nobody has tried this combination yet. If nothing else works and my cancer is HER2 positive, then I would use Herceptin. I'm wary about the short-term cardiac problems that have been observed with Herceptin. Even though the percentage is small, it causes me concern that something this obvious is happening shortly after treatment. It makes me wonder whether something bad that is not obvious is happening to other women receiving Herceptin.

I hope the preceding discussion has helped you appreciate why I would make the personal choices I have described, and I trust that my reasoning has enabled you to understand the powerful role that hormones play in causing, and also fighting, breast cancer. It's only natural that radiologists and surgeons might fail to take the time to educate their patients about successful hormonal treatment options, but once you see how effective testosterone can be as a weapon in the war on cancer, I'm sure you'll feel more open to discussing with your doctor the possibility of trying these state-of-the-art methods of treating the disease. If my approach is right, and I have every reason to believe that it is, then the future will see much less cutting and radiating, and much more bioidentical hormone replacement therapy being employed to improve women's health.

CHAPTER 14

A NEW PROTOCOL FOR CURING EARLY-STAGE ALZHEIMER'S AND FOR HALTING LATE-STAGE ALZHEIMER'S

With all the overwhelming evidence pointing to hormones as the solution, it will come as no surprise that I advocate the use of hormones for treating Alzheimer's disease. The real question is, why am I the only scientist to support this treatment protocol? The answer is quite simple. *I am* not *the first scientist to realize that hormones are the answer to Alzheimer's!* Let me call your attention to an excerpt from a 2002 article in the *Proceedings of the National Academy of Sciences,* one of the most prestigious journals in the world: "Testosterone given alone to aging men and given with estradiol to postmenopausal women would probably prove beneficial in preventing and/or treating Alzheimer's disease."[1]

"Testosterone given alone to aging men and given with estradiol to postmenopausal women would probably prove beneficial in preventing and/or treating Alzheimer's disease."

Clearly, other researchers have seen the value in using testosterone to fight Alzheimer's. I am, however, the first scientist to realize that using aromatase inhibitors (AIs) when administering testosterone prevents breast and prostate cancer as well as enhances the effect of testosterone in fighting Alzheimer's.[2] I'm also the first one to recognize that because estrogen receptor-beta (ER-beta) is protective against Alzheimer's (meaning that when this receptor is activated by something binding to it, Alzheimer's diminishes), estriol should be more effective than estradiol.[3]

This is because, unlike estradiol, estriol binds preferentially to ER-beta.[4] While most doctors, even anti-aging doctors, have a philosophy of using as little of a hormone as possible and for as short a time as possible to address a problem, my philosophy is that, within limits, *it is safer to have higher levels of hormones than lower levels of hormones, with the exception of estrone and estradiol.*

Since a number of scientists already know that hormones are the answer to Alzheimer's, why haven't doctors done clinical trials to test this approach to treating this disease? For women, doctors have always thought that the 2002 WHI (Women's Health Initiative) study was the definitive clinical trial that showed that hormone replacement increased the risk of both breast cancer and Alzheimer's. They had no way of knowing at the time that all the bad results could be explained by the fact that synthetic progestins almost totally block the intracellular androgen receptor (as discussed in chapter 3). Even to this day, very few doctors are aware of this fact, in large part because the article revealing the problem with progestins was published in a biological journal, not a medical journal.[5]

However, it's a different story for men. There's no question that doctors were taught in medical school that testosterone was dangerous. While writing this book, I had an interesting conversation with a retired cardiologist. He seemed to be interested in my work on Alzheimer's. However, when he realized that my treatment involved administering large amounts of testosterone, he said, "You can't do that. It will cause these men to develop prostate cancer." At that point, I explained my work on prostate cancer and how testosterone can cause prostate cancer only when it is converted to estradiol. His response was, "Let me know when your book comes out." This fear of prostate cancer also often makes its way into scientific literature. Here are two excerpts from a 2000 article in the *Proceedings of the National Academy of Sciences* that discuss the possibility of using testosterone to prevent Alzheimer's in men: "Our results . . . suggest that androgen supplementation for aging men . . . may be protective against the development of Alzheimer's disease." "These possible benefits must be weighed against potential deleterious effects of testosterone, including the development of prostate cancer in men . . ."[6]

For both men and women, it is clear that brain cells are dying as Alzheimer's progresses. No treatment is going to resurrect dead cells. This means that the most any treatment can do is to stop more brain cells from dying. However, people with Alzheimer's and other forms of dementia have some days that are better than others. As I envision it, the best-case scenario would be to restore the mind to what it is on a "good" day and to allow new memories to be retained so that the person can relearn much of what was forgotten. Whether in fact this can be achieved remains to be determined.

TREATING ALZHEIMER'S IN MEN

In spite of their fear, doctors actually explored giving testosterone to men with Alzheimer's. They did a double-blind study with men who had mild Alzheimer's and treated half with testosterone gel and half with a placebo. After twenty-four weeks, the men given testosterone had their free testosterone increase from an average of 5.1 ng/dL to 9.4 ng/dL. Objective tests showed no decline in cognitive functions in the treated group, whereas there was some statistically significant decline in the placebo group. The caregivers also reported a noticeable improvement in the quality of life in the treated group.[7]

This study is worthy of discussion. Since there was no decline in objective test scores and a subjective improvement, the results suggest that not only did testosterone stop the progression of Alzheimer's but that the men were also slowly improving. The increase in free testosterone in the treated group was over 80 percent, which sounds like a lot. However, as was previously discussed (in chapter 11), the Mayo Clinic reference range for free testosterone in men is 9–30 ng/dL. So this experiment raised free testosterone to just above the lowest level of normal. I look at these facts, and two questions pop into my mind. First, if we continue the experiment for years, will Alzheimer's progress in any of these men? Second, what would happen if higher levels of testosterone were given, say, 12, or 20, or perhaps even 30 ng/dL?

While this seems obvious to me, it did not seem to be obvious to this article's authors. I was surprised to learn that in the discussion section of this paper, the authors were giving credence to the WHI studies involving hormones and women. They cited a WHI study in which both horse estrogen by itself and in conjunction with synthetic progestins increased the risk of Alzheimer's.[8] As I have mentioned before, synthetic progestins will increase the risk of Alzheimer's by blocking intracellular androgen receptor. However, to understand why horse estrogen increases the risk of Alzheimer's, you simply have to realize that estrone makes up half of horse estrogen.[9] The Hormone Receptor Model posits that estrogen receptor-alpha (ER-alpha) increases the risk of Alzheimer's, while ER-beta decreases the risk. Therefore, the only way administering estrogen can result in an increase in Alzheimer's is if it increases binding to ER-alpha. Since, as was mentioned in chapter 2, estrone binds to ER-alpha five times more strongly than to ER-beta, we need look no further to explain why horse estrogen would increase the risk of Alzheimer's.

Another experiment is currently under way in Australia to test the effect of testosterone on men with Alzheimer's. Specific details of the study have not yet been published, but the study's website claims that after four months, most of the men showed a reduction in their beta amyloid.[10] The fact that they said "most" and not "all" is a red flag to me. This sounds like another study where the target testosterone level will be at the low end of normal rather than the high end.

These two experiments are the only ones I could uncover on treating Alzheimer's with testosterone, and in my opinion, this second experiment will fail to achieve a cure just as the first one failed. Speaking as a theoretical biologist, there is a logical way to treat Alzheimer's to try to achieve a cure, and while it is possible that testosterone alone might be sufficient, I suspect that a multi-pronged approach is essential and certainly much safer.

If I were a doctor treating a male patient with Alzheimer's, these are the steps I would follow. First, if he smokes, he would be instructed to stop[11] and stay away from other people's smoke, since air pollution increases beta amyloid. I would attempt to keep his serum vitamin D3 level very high at 70–90 ng/mL to facilitate the transport of beta amyloid out of the brain.

Of course, I would keep free testosterone high, shooting for the maximum of 30 ng/dL in order to counteract the biochemical reactions associated with Alzheimer's. In addition, I would try to get serum estradiol as low as possible by using an AI to allow testosterone to work even more efficiently. I would then add estriol to try to maximize the binding to ER-beta. This is a little tricky because once ER-beta is saturated, any further estriol would make things worse by binding to ER-alpha. If a sufficiently high enough amount of estriol is administered, it is even possible to saturate both estrogen receptors—the same result that would occur if very high amounts of estradiol were administered. While further research is needed to determine optimal levels of estriol, I believe that it would be higher than the levels of estrone and estradiol combined.

I would be very surprised if all this fails to halt Alzheimer's in its tracks, but clinical trials are needed to verify my prediction. This is one of the reasons I'm writing this book—without it, nobody would dream of taking such a multi-pronged approach. However, if in fact Alzheimer's still progresses even after applying the above treatment, then I would add all the nutritional supplements mentioned in the following section on treating women. If all this still isn't sufficient, then I would consider raising free testosterone to higher than physiological levels, but that has to be done carefully because nobody has studied the potential side effects of such a protocol.

TREATING ALZHEIMER'S IN WOMEN

There is some question about whether there is any point in using testosterone to treat women with Alzheimer's. The maximum physiological level of free testosterone in women is over fifteen times less than it is in men. However, I'm convinced that it needs to be taken into account. A postmenopausal female relative of mine who was taking bioidentical hormone replacement had some testosterone added to her regimen. She informed me that it felt like all the cobwebs had been cleared out of her brain—except she had no idea that there were any cobwebs there until they were cleared out! Of course, a single anecdotal case is "at the very bottom" of "the hierarchy of evidence-based medicine," but "they can be the vehicle for novel observations" and they "can generate hypotheses for subsequent systematic research."[12] As one researcher noted, "Individual case reports can also be educational and thus illustrative of what may be already well known but often forgotten."[13] In fact, there is already enough evidence to support using testosterone in women, and I was going to suggest it even without this anecdote. However, hearing it gave me more confidence that I was on the right track.

For that reason, I would treat a woman similarly to how I suggested treating a man: no smoking, a very high level of vitamin D3 (70–90 ng/mL), the maximum level of free testosterone (for women, 1.9 ng/dL), and enough AI to minimize the amount of estradiol present. Just as with men, I would use estriol to try to maximize the binding to ER-beta. I would maximize progesterone for ten days every thirty days at the teenage level of 27 ng/mL.[14] There is a chance this might work by itself, but because testosterone levels are so much lower in women than in men, I would suggest adding the following nutritional supplements: niacinamide,[15] curcumin,[16] sage,[17] and rosemary. While 750 mg per day of rosemary is helpful, higher dosages actually make things worse.[18] The optimal dosages for the other supplements I listed above still have yet to be determined. Also, I recommend that the equivalent of three cups of coffee worth of caffeine be ingested each day.[19]

One final thing to try is to counter the lowered glucose uptake to brain cells associated with Alzheimer's disease by using ketones to fuel the brain in place of glucose. Ketones can be produced by fasting or by a ketogenic diet, which consists of very low levels of carbohydrates along with very high levels of saturated fat. Ketogenic diets have been shown to reduce the amount of beta amyloid in mouse brains by 25 percent.[20] However, it is a difficult diet to follow and risks other health problems.[21] Therefore, researchers have tried using medium-chain triglycerides (such as coconut oil), which are converted to ketone bodies following their ingestion. One such experiment demonstrated that medium-chain triglycerides could help some people with Alzheimer's or mild cognitive impairment.[22]

An inexpensive way of producing ketone bodies is by eating coconut oil.[23] Some people with Alzheimer's have reported being helped by coconut oil, but no clinical tests have been done, and at this point there is no evidence that it is effective.[24]

CONCLUSIONS

My own research and visits to support websites for Alzheimer's patients indicate that a number of people are taking the nutritional supplements listed above, as well as coconut oil. Unfortunately, nobody is reporting being cured, although some people believe that their dietary regimen might be slowing down the progression of the disease. I'm not surprised that nobody is being cured by these supplements, since hormone levels decline as people age and declining hormone levels will increase all the biochemical markers associated with Alzheimer's. So even if some relief of symptoms occurs with supplements and diet changes, the only way to stop progression of the disease is to prevent the decline in hormone levels.

To summarize: for men, no smoking, high levels of vitamin D3 and free testosterone, and an AI and estriol can be expected to be enough to put an end to Alzheimer's. If not, then the nutritional supplements listed for women should be added. Finally, if none of these things work, then serious consideration needs to be given to raising free testosterone above the maximum physiological level as well as raising estriol levels.

For women, no smoking, high levels of vitamin D3 and free testosterone, an AI and estriol, ten days of high progesterone each month, plus all the nutritional supplements mentioned in this chapter need to be employed. If that plan doesn't work, then higher levels of free testosterone, progesterone, and estriol all need to be considered.

CHAPTER 15

QUESTIONS AND ANSWERS

The following are questions I'm often asked by people familiar with my work, as well as questions that might be occurring to readers of this book. In each case, I've replied to the question with some additional context to orient those of you who are learning about the Hormone Receptor Model for the first time. In this way, you'll get a better idea of some of the major issues involved with my approach to the prevention and treatment of disease.

You mention that increased levels of testosterone will reduce body fat and increase muscle mass. Does that mean that we will all end up looking like body builders?

No, not at all. There are still many teenagers who are overweight or obese in spite of having plentiful hormones. What testosterone does is make exercise more effective in reducing body fat and increasing muscle mass. But you can't just sit on your couch watching television and expect to end up with a great physique. Without hormone replacement therapy, most people discover that, as they age, their muscles become weaker, and they accumulate more fat even if they're working out regularly. Teenage levels of testosterone will change all that.

I have heard that aromatase inhibitors can cause some side effects. Is there any way to prevent this?

Yes, some women experience pain and fatigue when taking aromatase inhibitors (AIs). Although the causal mechanism is not well understood, the discomfort is most often felt in the joints of the wrists and ankles and is probably related to reduced estrogen levels.[1] A recent study discovered that increasing serum vitamin D3 reduces the number of women who experience these side effects. This study raised serum vitamin D3 to 57 ng/mL,[2] which is less than the 70–90 ng/mL that I recommend. I suspect that higher levels of vitamin D3 will be even more effective than what was tried in this study.

Another study tried to determine whether there was any relationship between serum hormone levels and aromatase inhibitor side effects. They discovered that women who had no side effects had higher levels of dehydroepiandrosterone-sulfate (DHEA-S) than those who experienced joint discomfort.[3] Unfortunately, nobody has yet tried administering DHEA-S to women who suffer side effects to see what happens.

Finally, I always recommend the use of estriol whenever AIs drop estradiol levels too low. Estriol will reduce inflammation and, in conjunction with high serum levels of vitamin D3, eliminate the side effects of AIs. If anyone still suffers from side effects, then I believe increasing serum DHEA-S levels will remedy that.

For some hormones and supplements, you're very specific about dosage. Why are you vague on others?

I wish I could be specific about everything. The problem is that I would only be guessing. Even when I mention specific values, such as the optimal level of free testosterone, it is a bit of a guess. Basically, I'm picking the top of the normal range for hormones that are beneficial, since, by definition, the normal range is the range that is seen in the majority of people, that is, people not in a disease state. It would be irresponsible for me to advocate higher-than-normal levels of a hormone without evidence to demonstrate its safety. It is entirely possible that higher-than-normal levels would be beneficial for some people, just as it is possible that the top of the normal range might be too high for other people. This is one of the reasons that I wrote this book. I hope to encourage researchers to explore what happens when senior citizens receive teenage or even higher levels of hormones. I would not be surprised if the optimal hormone levels for some people turn out to be even higher than teenage levels. Also, this is why I repeatedly emphasize that you need to seek a knowledgeable anti-aging doctor to work with you to modify your hormone levels.

I'm confused about the concept of binding affinity. How can estriol increase the activity of estrogen receptor-beta by interfering with estradiol?

I find this concept a bit confusing myself. Estriol will interfere with estradiol binding to estrogen receptor-beta (ER-beta) and to estrogen receptor-alpha (ER-alpha). Because estriol's binding affinity is much *lower* for ER-alpha than for ER-beta, it will almost never successfully allow ER-alpha to bind to its estrogen response element (meaning it will rarely activate the receptor), since estriol will dissociate from ER-alpha first. Estriol will occasionally successfully allow ER-beta (because of its higher binding affinity) to bind to its estrogen response element. However, irrespective of binding affinity, massive amounts of estriol would obviously saturate both estrogen receptors. This is because if enough estriol is around, then even when it dissociates from an estrogen receptor, there will be plenty more estriol waiting to take its place.

Ideally, when using estriol, you want just barely enough to saturate ER-beta. This will produce the best ratio of ER-beta to ER-alpha activity. If no ER-beta is present, then you want just enough estriol to generate maximum *interference* with the binding of estradiol to ER-alpha. You might think of estriol like a good football player who is doing his best to make sure that the other team doesn't get the ball. Unfortunately, we have to wait for researchers to discover exactly what the ideal amount of estriol is in each of these cases. However, even without such studies having been completed, it's almost certainly beneficial to have more estriol present than the combined amount of estradiol and estrone.

Once I start taking hormones, how long do I have to keep taking them?

You can stop taking hormones any time you choose; you just have to be prepared to accept the consequences for doing so. Remember, decreasing your hormone levels as you age is one of the ways that nature ensures that the older generation will die out and make room for the young. If you stop taking hormones, you can expect your hormone levels to drop to what they would have been at that age if you had never taken hormone supplements, and they will continue to drop as you age.

Isn't it dangerous to give very high levels of hormones to somebody who has lived for years with very low levels?
It may be dangerous in some cases. However, there is no need to go directly to the highest levels of hormones. A competent anti-aging doctor can monitor what happens as your hormone levels gradually increase and can determine how high a level can safely be administered.[4]

You keep referring to estriol in the book, but my doctor says that he can't prescribe estriol for me because of FDA restrictions. So how are we supposed to get estriol?
Actually, the FDA has not restricted the use of estriol but has added an extra layer of paperwork for doctors who wish to use it. Doctors must fill out an Investigational New Drug Application form, and each patient must fill out an informed consent form. In theory, this shouldn't interfere with doctors being able to prescribe estriol, but in practice it's time-consuming and therefore is a definite roadblock. In my opinion, it's absurd to set up such roadblocks for any hormone that so strongly fights breast cancer, prostate cancer, and Alzheimer's disease.

Why do you keep recommending estriol when no clinical trials have been done to study its effect on breast cancer, prostate cancer, or Alzheimer's? Also, why do you always recommend an aromatase inhibitor when you recommend estriol?
I base my recommendations on the properties of the hormone receptors as determined by the Hormone Receptor Model. To give you an absurd hypothetical scenario, assume that doctors someday discover that ER-alpha helps eliminate bunions, while ER-beta promotes them. In this case, I would recommend the use of estrone plus an aromatase inhibitor (AI) to eliminate bunions, even if no clinical studies had yet been done. My reasoning is that this combination would maximize ER-alpha activity while minimizing ER-beta activity. In other words, it gets the job done.

The reason I recommend AIs when using estriol is to maximize the binding of the hormone to ER-beta while minimizing what binds to ER-alpha. Aromatase produces estradiol, which strongly binds to ER-alpha. An AI reduces the amount of estradiol present, in the process helping estriol, the more beneficial estrogen, to act. In order to create the greatest imbalance in favor of ER-beta, you always want to use an AI. Although this seems obvious to me, unfortunately, the medical profession typically ignores this combination. Estriol has been found to be useful in the treatment of multiple sclerosis, but as far as I know, no researcher has tried using an AI and increasing the level of estriol in order to maximize the imbalance in favor of ER-beta. This can be expected to minimize inflammation of the brain even more than estriol by itself does and may be an even more effective treatment of multiple sclerosis.

You claim that it's not possible to prescribe RU-486 in the United States, but isn't it true that any doctor can prescribe it if they get approval from an Institutional Review Board (IRB)?
In theory, yes, but in practice, not a chance. There are several problems with getting such approval. I personally was called in as an expert in a vain attempt by a physician to try to get an IRB to grant permission for him to use RU-486 on a patient who had progesterone-dependent prostate cancer. The head of the IRB was not pleased to learn that RU-486 was a generic, for which the amount of profit to be made was limited. Also, while he may have considered RU-486 as a sole treatment option (which should have very limited clinical value), there was no way he was going to even consider approving a multi-pronged approach, which in my opinion is the *only* sensible way to use RU-486 in attacking cancer.

BREAST CANCER

Do you agree with the US Preventive Services Task Force recommendation that mammograms be given every other year for women between the ages of fifty and seventy-four?
In part I do agree. I'm concerned about the potential cancers that may be caused by too-frequent mammograms, especially for women with BRCA1 or BRCA2 mutations.[5] Eventually, I would love to see the day when mammograms are no longer needed, because the preventive protocols detailed

in this book are shown to be 100 percent effective. However, for now, the task force recommendations make sense.

Why do you recommend the anastrozole-testosterone pellets of Dr. Glaser for women with metastatic breast cancer, when she has published data on only two patients?

From the point of view of a clinical trial, her numbers are too low to draw any conclusions. However, I base my recommendations on the Hormone Receptor Model. There's no way that using testosterone with an aromatase inhibitor can increase the rate of growth of breast cancer, but it will increase the rate of cell *death* in virtually every breast cancer cell. The fact that Dr. Glaser published data on only two patients with metastatic breast cancer with no progression of the disease is something I use to verify what my model already predicts. I would be recommending that combination even if nobody had published anything about it. It's important to note that the results reported by Dr. Glaser are different from what doctors observe when using chemotherapy. Chemotherapy might kill 90 percent of a cancer population. However, after four doublings, you'll have more cancer cells than you had before you started chemotherapy. After that point, the cancer would grow even *faster* than before, because chemotherapy effectively performed a thinning of the herd.

With testosterone and an aromatase inhibitor, you don't see an initial big drop in a cancer population. However, the lack of progression of disease indicates that almost all the cancer cells have an increased rate of cell death, so some tumors will gradually disappear while others are still growing, albeit at a slower rate than they did before treatment. This protocol isn't going to be curative, but if the doubling time of a cancer population becomes slow enough, then a patient may be able to eventually die with the cancer cells instead of because of them. My personal prediction is that no patient with early-stage metastatic breast cancer who follows this treatment will die within five years, although the best that other doctors are doing for such women is a 25 percent five-year survival rate.

I read a book claiming that iodine deficiency causes breast cancer and that iodine cures breast cancer. Why don't you emphasize iodine more?

There's no question that having an iodine deficiency increases the risk of breast cancer. Iodine can also be helpful in the treatment of breast cancer, but it's not a cure. There is also at least one breast cancer cell line that is immune to the effects of iodine.[6] Therefore, iodine will perform a thinning of the herd but will not be curative. Still, there's no reason not to raise iodine to high-normal levels.

You mentioned that some breast cancers vanish on their own. How can that possibly happen?

If you recall, estrone causes breast tumors, but they vanish after estrone is removed. This is because estrone is not mutagenic, so the mutations necessary for cancer to occur never happen. On the other hand, a high local level of estradiol *does* result in mutations. However, there is no guarantee that those mutations will include the ability of the cell to undergo cell division in the absence of high local levels of estradiol. So, once a breast cell starts producing factors that result in high aromatase activity—leading to more local estradiol—a tumor forms around it. But that tumor will vanish if the right mutations are not present to allow the tumor cells to divide in the absence of high levels of estradiol. All that's needed for the tumor to vanish is for the rate of cell death to be greater than the rate of cell growth in all the cells producing the factors that cause high aromatase activity. Think of it this way—high local levels of estradiol are equivalent to high local levels of estrone unless the estradiol causes just the right mutation. In both cases, tumors will vanish once the high local levels of hormones binding to ER-alpha ceases.

How do you explain the results of the WHI study that showed horse estrogen by itself reduced the incidence of breast cancer?

It's true that the WHI study with horse estrogen alone showed a reduction in the incidence of breast cancer. However, because of the relatively small sample size, there was a 91 percent chance that horse estrogen reduced the incidence of breast cancer and a 9 percent chance that it didn't.[7] The much larger Million Women Study showed that *there was a greater than 99.99 percent chance that horse estrogen increased the incidence of breast cancer.*[8] It seems obvious to me that the explanation of this WHI study conclusion is that, unfortunately, its results were just a statistical anomaly—something that was expected to happen 9 percent of the time.

Why can't you use the cycling trick in breast cancer to increase, then decrease, the amount of intracellular androgen receptor—just the same as is done in prostate cancer?
It may be possible that you can; however, nobody has done any research on this. Because women have much lower testosterone levels than men, it's unlikely that finasteride alone will change the amount of intracellular androgen receptor present. However, a combination of high testosterone plus finasteride just might do the trick. This combination would increase the amount of pro-apoptotic proteins being produced, except for those cancer cells that increase their production of intracellular androgen receptor. If this works, then a cycle of much higher-than-teenage levels of testosterone plus finasteride followed by a cycle of teenage levels of testosterone without finasteride might be a powerful treatment protocol.

PROSTATE CANCER

Since low Gleason score prostate cancer divides on average every sixty-five days and dies on average every seventy days, how does the tumor grow? Shouldn't the cancer cells be dying five days after they divide?
This is another concept that is hard to visualize. If you think of a woman giving birth to a girl, then you can tell who the parent is and who the daughter is. But cancer growth is more like that of an amoeba—there's no way to tell who the parent is and who the daughter is after a cell divides. In addition, cancer cells are not all individually dividing every sixty-five days. What happens is that there is a statistical chance that any cell will be dividing or dying every day. If, for example, you have a low Gleason score prostate cancer tumor that contains one million cells, then on average there will be 15,400 cells dividing and 14,200 cells dying on that day,[9] for a net gain of 1,200 cells.

Do you agree with the US Preventive Services Task Force recommendation to no longer routinely use PSA testing to screen for prostate cancer?

The task force's arguments make sense if you look at the way prostate cancer is currently being treated—with surgery and radiation. There is only a very small reduction in the rate of death from prostate cancer and no reduction in the overall rate of death for men who receive PSA screenings as compared with men who do not.[10]

However, if men follow my recommended protocol for prevention, raising testosterone to teenage levels and taking aromatase inhibitors, then PSA screening becomes essential. This is because there will be some men who already have prostate cancer cells within them before they start this protocol. Some of those men will have their cancer cells die off because of the treatment, but others will have cancer that continues to grow. For men who experience too high a rise in PSA velocity, the existence of prostate cancer must be assumed, and they are advised to start the treatment protocols described in chapter 12.

Do you believe that biopsies should be done to detect prostate cancer?

The problem with prostate biopsies is that some men experience serious complications, with more than one in twenty-five requiring hospitalization within thirty days who wouldn't have needed hospitalization without the biopsy.[11] Biopsied men with complications involving an infection have an increased risk of dying within thirty days. I strongly doubt that any man who died as a result of a biopsy ever thought beforehand that such a thing was possible.

Personally, I suspect that almost all men have some prostate cancer cells within them by the age of forty. Therefore, I strongly encourage men to start with the preventive protocols outlined in chapter 11, and if their PSA happens to rise too rapidly, then they can switch to the more aggressive treatment protocols outlined in chapter 12. The standard approach of most urologists today is to perform biopsies in order to verify the existence of cancer cells and to justify the use of surgery and radiation, both of which worsen a man's quality of life. Raising a man's testosterone level will improve his quality of life, so there is no reason to wait until being sure that prostate cancer is present before starting on testosterone replacement therapy, as detailed in chapters 11 and 12.

Why is the rate of prostate cancer for African Americans in the United States so much higher than for other races, and why is it more deadly?

Dr. Rick Kittles answered this question during a recent talk, and I believe that his reasoning is absolutely correct. Basically, there are some mutations found in people from Western Africa that increase the likelihood of prostate cancer being more aggressive when it develops, and these mutations have been identified in many African Americans. More important, though, is the fact that the darker your skin pigmentation, the less efficiently your skin can make vitamin D3 from sunlight. Also, the farther north from the equator you live, the less vitamin D3 is being made from sunlight.[12] In general, the less vitamin D3, the more aggressive the prostate cancer (the population increases more rapidly due to a lower rate of cell death). Men with more aggressive forms of prostate cancer are more likely to die of the disease than men with less aggressive forms. So the high prostate cancer death rate in African Americans can be explained by a combination of unfortunate genetic mutations plus low serum levels of vitamin D3. The decreased rate of cell death associated with these genes and with low levels of vitamin D3 explain why people with dark skin have a higher overall rate of prostate cancer—the rate of cell death becomes lower than the rate of cell growth at an earlier age.

Shouldn't I avoid sun exposure to prevent deadly skin cancer?

No. This is a common misconception.[13] There are basically two types of skin cancer, melanoma and non-melanoma. Melanoma is the more serious kind. But you're *less* likely to develop melanoma if you receive adequate sun exposure.[14] Michael Holick, professor of medicine at Boston University Medical Center and a pioneer in vitamin D research, recently observed that "you have about a 30 to 50 percent decreased risk of developing colon, prostate, and breast cancer if you maintain adequate vitamin D levels throughout your life."[15]

A large multinational study concluded that "Vitamin D production in the skin seems to decrease the risk of several solid cancers (especially stomach, colorectal, liver and gallbladder, pancreas, lung, female breast, prostate, bladder and kidney cancers)."[16] The key to healthy sun exposure is to be out when the sun is at least "30 degrees above the horizon or whenever the temperature is warm enough to expose large amounts of skin."[17]

Why is the rate of prostate cancer so high in the United States compared to the rest of the world?
I believe that there are two factors that account for our high rate of prostate cancer. First, since the United States is not near the equator, there are many men with too little vitamin D3. Second, the diet of people in the United States is typically high in junk food (nobody has yet identified any anticancer properties associated with angel food cake or French fries) and low in natural foods known to prevent prostate cancer. If Americans consumed more broccoli, mushrooms, walnuts, and green tea, then our prostate cancer rate would drop enormously.

Why are so many mutations found on the intracellular androgen receptor as prostate cancer progresses?
Because doctors are so convinced that the intracellular androgen receptor is the key to understanding prostate cancer, intracellular androgen receptor is the hormone receptor most commonly studied. As cancer progresses, all sorts of mutations will arise throughout the DNA that ultimately benefit the cancer population. But if you focus your attention on only one specific area, then that's where you'll see (and categorize) lots of mutations. There are so many other mutations that benefit cancer growth, that in theory, anywhere you focus your attention you will see more and more mutations as cancer progresses.

I heard that Dr. John Lee claimed that one of his patients with metastatic prostate cancer had his metastases vanish when treated with progesterone. On the other hand, Dr. Robert Leibowitz claims that his patients who take progesterone have rapidly rising PSA. Who is telling the truth here?
Actually, I believe that both doctors are telling the truth. If a patient has

naturally low progesterone levels, then there's no selective advantage for the prostate cancer to have lots of progesterone receptor A. If progesterone is given to such a man, it will almost certainly lower the amount of Bcl-2 produced and increase the rate of cell death, quite possibly eliminating metastases. However, for men with normal amounts of progesterone, some of their prostate cancer cells will have enough progesterone receptor A to thrive in the presence of progesterone. I suspect that the patients Dr. Leibowitz saw first experienced a drop in their PSA as those prostate cancer cells with a lot of progesterone receptor B died off. Then there was a pronounced increase in PSA because the thinning of the herd left only prostate cancer with a lot of progesterone receptor A.

I've read about something called the Saturation Model that seems to explain the behavior of testosterone and prostate cancer. How is that different from your model?

The Saturation Model was developed by Dr. Abraham Morgentaler of Harvard University. Dr. Morgentaler is one of the real pioneers in determining the truth about testosterone and prostate cancer. He went through medical school at a time when doctors were taught that testosterone fueled prostate cancer. His genius is exemplified by a question that one of his students posed and that Dr. Morgentaler quoted in one of his papers: "If testosterone is so bad for prostate cancer, then why is it so hard to prove?"[18] While untold thousands of doctors have shrugged off similar questions in the past, Dr. Morgentaler took this question to heart and came up with what he called the Saturation Model. Basically, this model claims that testosterone is necessary for prostate cancer growth, but that above a certain point, the intracellular androgen receptor becomes saturated, and there's no more growth benefit from additional testosterone.[19] Besides coming up with a model, Dr. Morgentaler had the courage to actually use testosterone in treating men who had early-stage prostate cancer, which caused an average *drop* of their PSA by one-third after an average of two and a half years of treatment.[20]

The Saturation Model offers an explanation as to why reducing testosterone to castrate level or below kills most prostate cancer cells—these cells have insufficient testosterone to live. This model also explains why no increase in the rate of prostate cancer is seen in men undergoing testosterone replacement therapy; even if they have prostate cancer, their testosterone level is already high enough for maximal growth of their prostate cancer cells. Increasing their testosterone level is not capable of increasing the rate of growth of their prostate cancer cells.

The problem with the Saturation Model is that it is too simplistic, specifically because it takes no account of the conversion of testosterone to estradiol or of the presence of membrane androgen receptor. It has no explanation for how testosterone can prevent prostate cancer cell division in certain cell lines, such as LNCaP 104-R2, which has an overabundance of intracellular androgen receptor.[21] Also, it has no explanation for how testosterone can kill a prostate cancer cell line that has no intracellular androgen receptor.[22]

While I applaud Dr. Morgentaler for using testosterone to treat men with prostate cancer, I'm extremely concerned about the long-range consequences of allowing testosterone to be converted to estradiol. I pointed this out in a letter to the editor of the *Journal of Urology*, urging the use of AIs, but Dr. Morgentaler dismissed my concerns[23] by citing an article that showed no correlation between the serum level of estradiol and the rate of prostate cancer.[24] I have to assume that he was unaware of a different article that showed a strong correlation between the serum level of estrone and prostate cancer.[25] This strong correlation means that either (1) estrone is causing prostate cancer or (2) that prostate cancer is increasing the level of estrone. Since work with breast cancer has already demonstrated that estrone *lacks* the mutagenic properties necessary to cause cancer, it seems obvious that prostate cancer is increasing estrone levels. There must be a selective growth advantage for prostate cancer to be doing this, and obviously it must be the increased activity of ER-alpha that results from increased levels of estrone. Since aromatase is required to produce estrone in men,[26] I am steadfast in my opinion that administering testosterone to prostate cancer patients without accompanying it with AIs is going to be disastrous in the long run.

I am steadfast in my opinion that administering testosterone to prostate cancer patients without accompanying it with AIs is going to be disastrous in the long run.

Why does taking finasteride or dutasteride to prevent prostate cancer actually increase the rate of aggressive prostate cancer? Both of these drugs block the conversion of testosterone to DHT. For finasteride and dutasteride, studies have shown a decrease of approximately 25 percent in the overall rate of prostate cancer but an increase of 0.5–0.7 percent in the rate of high Gleason score prostate cancers.[27] High Gleason scores are correlated with more aggressive cancers, which are more likely to be fatal. The medical profession currently has no explanation for this increase in aggressive cancers.

One suggestion has been made that the more aggressive cancers were caused by less DHT, which caused less 3beta-Adiol, which caused less ER-beta activity.[28] This explanation has one fatal flaw. Reducing ER-beta activity would increase Bcl-2 and decrease the rate of cell death, consequently making the cancer more aggressive. However, all the cancers detected in these studies existed before the drugs were administered. In other words, these studies were showing what effect the drugs had on being able to detect prostate cancers that were already growing, not brand-new prostate cancers. Therefore, increasing Bcl-2 would make it easier to detect all the prostate cancers, and there is no way that there would be an overall 25 percent decrease in the amount of prostate cancer detected if this explanation had been correct.

The Hormone Receptor Model supplies a logical explanation for these results. All that's needed is one vital piece of missing information. Dr. Robert Leibowitz has observed that a number of men he treated who were taking finasteride had their PSA rise faster than expected. He determined that those men were very often consuming phytoestrogens, such as soy products or flaxseed. When he instructed them to discontinue those products, their PSA usually declined.[29] Ordinarily, phytoestrogens increase ER-beta activity, since normal prostate cells don't tase activity. However, in the presence of high local levels of estradiol, phytoestrogens interfere with estradiol's binding to ER-beta and thus increase Bcl-2. Most phytoestrogens have anticancer properties independent of their interaction with the estrogen receptors. This is a situation where low DHT increases the rate of cancer cell death but also increases Bcl-2, and phytoestrogens increase the rate of cancer cell death and increase Bcl-2 as well. The way both low DHT and phytoestrogens kill prostate cancer cells is not additive—each acts independently. However, the increase in Bcl-2 due to low DHT and phytoestrogens *is* additive. Having lots of Bcl-2 is extremely protective for cancer cells—high-enough levels even prevent cell death when exposed to radiation![30]

So now we have a straightforward explanation for these experimental results, which so far have confounded the medical profession. Finasteride and dutasteride reduce the percentage of men diagnosed with prostate cancer because of the increased level of cell death caused by having more pro-apoptotic proteins. Both drugs block the formation of "bad progesterone," which will increase the rate of cell death even more. This slows down the growth of existing prostate cancer cells and prevents them from being detected. Unfortunately, men who ingest large amounts of phytoestrogens experience an increase in Bcl-2 that is great enough to decrease the rate of cell death and therefore make their cancers more aggressive.[31]

If I'm right, then there should be a higher percentage of men who ingested significant amounts of soy, flaxseed, and other phytoestrogens in the group that took finasteride or dutasteride and ended up with an aggressive prostate cancer than in the group that ended up with a less aggressive cancer. This is a readily testable prediction.

ALZHEIMER'S DISEASE

You claim that air pollution causes an increase in beta amyloid production. How do you know that other pollutants in our food and water don't cause this increase too?

The answer to this one is simple—I don't. In my opinion, it's quite likely that there are chemicals in our food and water that act to increase beta amyloid production, but I have no idea what they might be. For that matter, nobody seems to have identified exactly which pollutants in the air cause an increase in beta amyloid. Ideally, researchers could use animal studies to identify exactly which chemicals in our air, food, and water increase beta amyloid production.

If air pollution increases Alzheimer's, shouldn't people who live in rural areas, like the Amish, have lower rates of Alzheimer's?

Actually, the Amish *do* have much lower rates of Alzheimer's and dementia than the general population.[32] In fact, it seems that rural communities have statistically lower rates of dementia than other communities.[33]

Since beta amyloid seems to cause Alzheimer's, why not just develop a drug to totally block its production?

While an *excess* of beta amyloid appears to be responsible for Alzheimer's and other forms of dementia, beta amyloid is actually an essential protein for the proper functioning of the brain.[34] Drugs have been developed to reduce beta amyloid formation, but so far none have demonstrated the ability to slow down Alzheimer's.[35] My opinion is that there may already be too much beta amyloid present in people with Alzheimer's, so preventing further production of beta amyloid is not enough to help them. You also want to increase the breakdown of existing beta amyloid and stop the formation of hyperphosphorylated tau protein, all of which can be accomplished by increasing hormone levels.

One other reason that I prefer hormones to drugs is that the body tends to have feedback loops with regard to natural substances. I can't imagine testosterone ever totally shutting down the production of beta amyloid, whereas a drug might well shut down beta amyloid so much that normal brain cells would be deprived of the minimal amount needed to function properly. Also, as discussed in chapter 6, all the biochemical reactions associated with Alzheimer's increase as hormone levels decrease. Therefore, even if a drug were to succeed initially, I doubt that it could permanently stave off the development of Alzheimer's unless the continued decrease in hormone levels associated with aging were to be stopped as well.

Even if a drug were to succeed initially, I doubt that it could permanently stave off the development of Alzheimer's unless the continued decrease in hormone levels associated with aging were to be stopped as well.

How long will it take for your treatment protocols to have a noticeable effect on Alzheimer's patients?

This is a question that has to be answered by clinicians and researchers, but I suspect that noticeable improvement would occur within weeks for men and months for women. The different prognosis for men and women stems from the fact that the level of testosterone that can safely be administered to men is much higher than the amount that can be given safely to women, and testosterone is the most powerful hormone for combating Alzheimer's.

CHAPTER 16

A BETTER TOMORROW: HOW THEORETICAL BIOLOGY CAN HELP CURE DISEASE

One thing that amazed me while I was conducting research for this book was how much the Internet has changed the process of solving problems using theoretical biology. When I received my PhD, there were no articles available online. I had to spend untold hours in the library stacks searching for articles that were relevant to my investigations. In some cases, this involved following the work of researchers I knew were publishing in the field and then trying to locate articles that cited those authors. This was incredibly time-consuming, and I have no idea how many important papers I may have missed. But today all that has changed, and the Internet has allowed me to complete the research that led to this book in just a few years instead of decades.[1]

Because of the speed with which the Internet makes communication possible, if someone created a clearinghouse that listed ideas from experts for important new experiments and made those ideas available to researchers around the world capable of doing such experiments, then enormous medical breakthroughs would be possible. A few examples will illustrate my point. Imagine that there was a theoretical biologist suggesting that research be done to determine the effect of estriol on the biochemical reactions associated with Alzheimer's. Or imagine that a researcher suggested trying RU-486 in combination with progesterone in treating breast cancer.[2] Once these proposals were online, researchers could then perform the experiments and find the answers to important questions. To succeed, such a clearinghouse would need to be open to everyone, meaning it would be run by a nonprofit organization or government agency. It's frustrating to look at diseases that are known to be affected by hormones, such as ovarian cancer and colon cancer, and not be able to produce a useful model because researchers haven't yet categorized the effects of each hormone receptor on the production of pro-apoptotic and anti-apoptotic proteins. I suspect that teenage levels of hormones will protect against many cancers, but if the right research were done, then it might be possible to change that guess into a certainty.

In the past seven years, I've made a number of suggestions that have literally changed the lives of two families. I'm including these stories here—even though a single anecdotal case is irrelevant scientifically—because I find the theory behind the treatments quite credible and the results of these two cases close to being miraculous. I received enormous personal gratification from the good that resulted in these two cases, and I feel morally obligated to share this information in case other people might also benefit. These anecdotal stories are true, but I've changed the names of the people involved to protect their privacy. These examples vividly illustrate how a theoretical biologist can make suggestions based on theory that prove to be life-changing when put into practice.

AUTISM

As I was doing my research, it became apparent that testosterone confers many health benefits for both men and women, in addition to fighting breast cancer, prostate cancer, and Alzheimer's. Therefore, I was a bit taken aback by some scientists suggesting that testosterone might be the cause of autism. Admittedly, four times more males than females develop autism, and there's some evidence that higher levels of testosterone in the womb lead to some similarity in psychological tests to what is observed in autism.[3] However, the most convincing study I've seen shows that 499 out of 503 autistic children exhibit evidence of an abnormal metabolism of metals, with 428 having an abnormally high copper-to-zinc ratio.[4] This strongly suggests a problem with the functioning of **metallothioneins**, a class of proteins that protect against metal toxicity. Metallothionein levels are higher in women than in men[5] (which might explain why females are less likely to develop autism). A study on the concentration of metallothioneins in blood serum showed that there was no difference between autistic and non-autistic children.[6] However, no measurement of the functionality of the metallothioneins was done in this study, nor was any measurement made of the amount of metallothionein-III present. Metallothionein-III acts to eliminate excess neurons during early infancy, so if it's not functioning properly you would expect to see increased brain volume and head diameter,[7] which is in fact what is observed in autistic children.[8]

The nonprofit Pfeiffer Institute has been treating autistic children since 2001 with protocols designed to improve the functioning of metallothioneins. Their protocol involves some nutritional supplements, which all the children receive along with customized supplements for each individual child. When I learned that a woman I knew, Jane, had an autistic son, Tommy, I suggested that she look into getting him treated by the Pfeiffer Institute.

Jane discovered that her son was autistic when he was two years old. Her daycare provider expressed concern about the boy's screaming and his practice of keeping away from other children. Tommy was two when he had his first evaluation, and there was no question that he was autistic.

The boy showed almost no improvement as the months went by, and experts told Jane to accept that this was how Tommy was always going to be. When he was three and a half, he started preschool. His vocabulary consisted of just a few words, and he wasn't toilet trained. His first school experience was very negative, with frequent bouts of screaming and not paying attention in class. Jane was forced to remove him after a few weeks and transfer him to the district's special-education preschool.

Shortly after that, Jane started her son on a protocol under the supervision of the Pfeiffer Institute. This involved urine, blood, and hair analysis to determine which nutritional supplements to administer. A new supplement was added every few weeks. If it improved behavior, it was continued—otherwise it was discarded.

The Pfeiffer Institute also ordered X-rays that revealed a blockage in Tommy's intestines. They cleaned it out and had him take cod liver oil daily. Soon Tommy (and Jane) was sleeping through the night for the first time since Tommy had been born. The Pfeiffer Institute had Tommy follow a year-long treatment to train his bowels, and he has never had another problem with them since.

Jane also observed other improvements as soon as her son started taking his supplements and cod liver oil. Tommy had never spoken more than one or two words previously. However, while walking outside just one week after starting this treatment, Jane was astonished to hear him say, "It look moon the mom." While Tommy's words were out of order, Jane clearly understood their meaning.

A few months later, after more supplements had been added, one of Tommy's teachers said hello to him, then did a double-take when he replied by saying hello. The teacher explained to Jane that she greeted Tommy each morning, but that this was the first time he had responded.

That spring, Tommy began pulling a chair into the circle at school instead of sitting on the floor. Jane realized that he was trying to imitate students in his class who were in wheelchairs. She decided that if he was starting to imitate the students around him, then she wanted him in a preschool with typical children in the fall. His current school informed Jane that he had outgrown the level that this school functioned on, and they could no longer meet his needs. Tommy had experienced significant academic, social, and physical improvements while at this school, but there is no way to determine to what extent his improvement was due to the school as opposed to the supplements.

Before starting treatments, Tommy would almost always have what Jane called "meltdowns," where he would scream and flail about on the floor no matter where they were. Jane hated the dirty looks and inappropriate advice that strangers gave her, assuming that she must have done something wrong to cause her son to misbehave like that.

The whole family's social life changed as Tommy kept improving. Before his treatment, Jane couldn't take her family to church because of Tommy's meltdowns. Now she discovered that they could all go to church, and Tommy would spend most of his time running around with other children in the kid's area. Previously, Jane had to turn down invitations to parties, but now her entire family could go, although they couldn't stay until the end because Tommy would get tired and bored after a while.

That summer, Jane decided to take a road trip to visit relatives, even though they lived five hundred miles away. She was pleased when her instincts turned out to be right, and Tommy was fine during the trip.

Later that summer, Jane took Tommy to visit a farm that allowed people to feed their animals. Jane had taken him there the previous year, but he had stayed in his own world, showing no interest in the animals. Now, not only was he interested in the goats and pigs, he said things to Jane that made it clear he remembered their prior visit. This time, instead of ignoring the animals, Tommy gently fed the goats. I found this story remarkable because it strongly suggests that even when some autistic children seem to be in their own world and oblivious to what is around them, at some level of consciousness, they're actually aware of what is happening.

That fall, Jane enrolled Tommy in the same preschool that had asked him to leave the previous year. Jane had successfully managed to toilet train him, which was a requirement for this class. Tommy proceeded to test his boundaries to see what he could get away with, and he only did well with his main teacher. One day he ran out of the classroom to the outside playground. But he had stood with his hand on the doorknob, waiting until he was sure his teacher was watching him before he ran out. Because of this and similar incidents, and since Tommy wouldn't respond to the teacher's assistants, the school hired an aide for him because he showed potential and, according to his teacher, was a good fit for the program.

Tommy thrived in that preschool. He ignored all attempts the other students made at teasing him. Many of the girls in his class were especially protective of him. He loved to run around at recess time, and he found a number of other children who ran with him and who pulled him into other games. His social skills continued to improve, and he started to catch up developmentally.

Several months after school started, Jane was walking Tommy to school one morning, holding his hand. They approached the school building and spotted Sue, a little girl in Tommy's class, who was walking toward them, holding her mother's hand. Tommy let go of his mother's hand and started running toward Sue. At the same time, Sue got her hand free and ran to meet Tommy. Jane was fearful of what might happen, but to her amazement, the two children gave each other a hug and walked hand in hand to the school building. There were tears in Jane's eyes as she told me this story, and it brought tears to my eyes as well.

That winter, Tommy developed an interest in drawing. Before that time, he had been unable to do anything with pencils or crayons. One Sunday he spent hours on end trying to draw. Eventually, he succeeded in drawing stick figures—essentially improving to the level of his peers. He went to school the next day, full of enthusiasm about his accomplishment. His enthusiasm was infectious, and his classmates started to do extra drawing too. Prior to this, Tommy had followed a ritual each day, taking off his coat and putting it in his locker, ignoring everyone and everything until this action was completed. But once he started getting interested in drawing, things changed. One morning, shortly after Tommy started drawing, a classmate named Will came up to him to show him *his* picture as Tommy was taking off his winter coat. Jane was amazed when Tommy stopped taking off his coat, looked at Will's picture, and said, "Will, that is a wonderful picture."

Tommy continued improving throughout preschool, especially with vocabulary. One day he told his mother that his ear hurt, and his parents were able to have him treated by his doctor for an ear infection. In the past, he would have screamed from the pain, making it very difficult for anyone to determine exactly what was wrong.

Jane took Tommy on a road trip that summer to visit her relatives. They stayed in the same motel as they had the previous year. Jane was surprised when Tommy said that he knew where their room was and led the way. It turned out that he took them to the same room they had stayed in the year before. He also interacted more with his grandparents and extended family during the visit.

Tommy went to kindergarten in the fall, again with an aide. He had a little trouble adjusting to the new routines, especially to unstructured time. One day Jane had a meeting with Tommy's teacher, who explained that there was a big improvement in her son that had started two weeks earlier. That was when Jane had changed the formulation of his supplements. Every six months, he was tested and his formulation changed to take into account new test results. Lab work revealed that he had abnormally high levels of copper, tin, and arsenic. His symptoms lessened as these levels dropped closer to normal.

One day that winter, Tommy came up behind his mother, gave her a hug and said, "Mommy, I love you. You're my best friend." Hearing this brought tears to her eyes. Months earlier, the evening news had featured the story of a woman who had killed her autistic child, apparently out of frustration. The local newspaper carried letters to the editor from mothers who said how difficult it was to raise an autistic child. One letter in particular stood out in my mind. In it, a mother said that she would give anything in the world just to hear her child say, "I love you."

On Tommy's sixth birthday, he asked whether he could have a birthday party and named a few classmates he wanted to invite. Before starting treatment, he had sat passively during birthday parties, ignoring his presents. He had seemed to be in another world as his mother opened presents for him. Now, after just a few years of treatment, he was looking forward to the party and to the gifts he might receive.

Shortly after this, Tommy took his annual test with a psychologist who specialized in autism. Although the results indicated that he was still autistic, they also revealed that he had improved by leaps and bounds developmentally. Before starting treatment, he had been about two years behind on all scores. Now he was testing low normal for his age in almost all categories. He was actually slightly above normal in mechanical aptitude.

Jane had to move, and the next year Tommy ended up in a new school in which the first-grade teacher set no boundaries for him and failed to communicate with Jane. Tommy made it clear that he hated school and didn't want to continue. He finished up that year mostly in a special-education classroom. In the following year, he was also in special education, making good progress. Health problems forced him to attend alternative schools for the next two years. He is now in fifth grade and extremely happy with school. His reading and writing are three years behind his peers, but he's slowly being mainstreamed into normal classes. Now that he enjoys school again, Jane is hopeful that he can start to catch up on his schoolwork and possibly be totally mainstreamed by the time he enters high school.

As Jane kept telling me how well Tommy was doing, I was always hoping that he would test out of the autistic range spectrum. However, although he keeps improving, he's still considered autistic. When Jane asked her doctor at the Pfeiffer Institute about the possibility of her son becoming non-autistic, he explained that a little over 1 percent of the children they treat eventually test out of range. While this may seem like a small percentage, it's much higher than the approximately 0 percent achieved by mainstream medicine. Although Tommy hasn't yet tested out of range, he has gone from being in his own world and almost totally unresponsive to living in the real world and interacting with others. Jane certainly has no regrets about choosing this path for her son.

What amazes me is that even after the Pfeiffer Institute findings, which clearly show metal metabolism disorders in almost all autistic children, mainstream medicine continues to ignore their work. Doctors don't hesitate to treat children if their blood sugar or cholesterol is too high. However, it's unheard of for a mainstream doctor to check metal levels in autistic children. I can't understand why a doctor would think that having abnormally high levels of cholesterol is unacceptable, but somehow an autistic child's having abnormally high levels of copper is acceptable.

STOMACH ACID

You might think that stomach acid has nothing to do with breast cancer, prostate cancer, or Alzheimer's disease, but you would be wrong. Just think of all the anticancer chemicals inside mushrooms or the anti-Alzheimer's chemicals inside the rosemary or sage that you eat. How do these chemicals get into your bloodstream? It's clear that the food you eat goes to your stomach, where stomach acid breaks it down and allows those helpful chemicals to enter your bloodstream. However, if you don't have sufficient stomach acid, then food will pass through your body with little or no benefit to you.

But surely low stomach acid must be a rare thing. We've all seen commercials that show *too much* stomach acid present after a meal, and this acid is then neutralized by the antacid brand being advertised. Since acid indigestion is so common, then too much stomach acid must be the norm, not too little, right? Well, actually, the opposite is the case. Stomach acid production *decreases* with age, and the average forty-year-old produces *half* as much stomach acid as the average twenty-year-old.[9]

Dr. Jonathan Wright has pioneered research in this field and has written a book about the benefits of stomach acid.[10] According to Dr. Wright, acid reflux occurs when the lower esophageal sphincter muscle loosens inappropriately. He presents evidence that high levels of stomach acid force this muscle to stay closed, whereas low levels allow it to open. When open, acid escapes from the stomach and burns the esophagus, causing heartburn. He also explains that stomach acid is essential for proper digestion, especially for the release of water-soluble vitamins and minerals. Dr. Wright has had significant success treating heartburn patients with *increased* levels of stomach acid. While there are medical conditions that cause too much stomach acid, they are rare, and when someone develops acid reflux in middle age, the culprit is almost always too *little* stomach acid.

My second story is about a young man who started taking daily acid blockers at the age of twenty-nine after being diagnosed with GERD (gastroesophageal reflux disease). John initially thought these drugs were terrific because the burning disappeared. He soon discovered, however, that this drug wasn't a cure-all. There were many foods he still couldn't eat without the burning coming back. Even with the foods he could eat, he would have to be careful not to consume too much at one time. He experimented with various ways to avoid GERD and discovered that lying on his left side and raising his head three inches helped before going to bed.[11]

When John told me about his condition, he had been taking acid blockers daily for approximately ten years. His health had been steadily deteriorating, with increased tiredness, depression, constipation, and heart palpitations. He thought this was a natural consequence of aging, even though he was under forty. I suggested that he read Dr. Wright's book about stomach acid. After he had done so, I suggested that he speak with his doctor about discontinuing the acid blockers and instead *increase* stomach acid production.[12] In his book, Dr. Wright discussed the fact that anything that tasted bitter seemed to stimulate the production of stomach acid,[13] and so he recommending eating something bitter around fifteen minutes before each meal. Once John had obtained his doctor's blessing for this experiment, he discontinued his medication and put a few drops of bitters on his tongue before each meal. He used alcohol-free liquid bitters with ginger—an inexpensive product readily available in health food stores.

At first, John tried switching from acid blockers to bitters, but he had to give up after a few days because the pain was too intense. He tried again but this time using antacids when the pain became intolerable. As the days went by and his stomach started to produce more acid, he gradually decreased the amount of antacid until, after a few weeks, he wasn't using any at all. Thrilled that he could now eat all the foods he had been denying himself for the past ten years, he started keeping a record of what he ate, how many drops of bitters he used, and how he felt. This journal was extremely helpful in allowing him to adjust exactly how many drops of bitters to take before each meal. He even discovered nuances that weren't mentioned in Dr. Wright's book. For example, he experienced discomfort whenever he ate hot foods, but when he let the food cool down to close to room temperature, there was no problem.[14] He also discovered that putting a few drops of bitters on his palm and licking it off with lips and tongue seemed more effective than putting drops directly on his tongue. In addition, when he ate a big meal, it often helped to take bitters in the middle of the meal as well as before the meal. At this point, he was able to eat everything without discomfort except very spicy food.

All of John's previous health problems have vanished since switching to bitters. He used to feel exhausted at work around four p.m. When he came home after work, he used to be totally exhausted and had no energy to play with his children. Now he has energy throughout the day, and he is handling with ease multiple difficult problems that would have been overwhelming before he started using bitters. John is experiencing no more depression,[15] constipation, or heart palpitations. He feels at least ten years younger, and his doctor has noted on his medical record that his GERD is gone after being treated "holistically." In my opinion, there are no medicinal properties of bitters that alleviated John's problems. Instead, I'm convinced that his problems were due to a chronic vitamin and mineral deficiency while he was taking acid blockers. If this is in fact the case, then all the bitters did was allow his food to be properly digested so that he was able to receive sufficient nutrients.

While bitters worked for John, this is only a single anecdotal case, and it doesn't mean it will work for everyone. However, a number of his friends and relatives (some of whom used to make fun of him when they saw him taking bitters) have also tried using bitters, and all are now experiencing similar benefits.

These anecdotes about autism and stomach acid illustrate the way a theory can lead to a breakthrough in therapeutic outcome. In the same way, the theories we have been discussing in this book about hormone receptors can be put into practical use today. In fact, the Hormone Receptor Model, which is based on a theory about how hormones affect their receptors, has the potential to change your life. It may take mainstream medicine decades before it catches up with the notion that teenage hormone levels can fight breast cancer, prostate cancer, and Alzheimer's. Luckily, you won't have to wait that long. There are anti-aging doctors doing cutting-edge work, and finding one will enable you to reap the rewards of theoretical biology today.

CHANGING THE WORLD

My overriding purpose in writing *The New Testosterone Treatment* has been to demonstrate that it's possible for one person to change the world for the better, armed only with logic and the truth. I'm confident that the facts revealed in this book will eventually lead to beneficial change for anyone interested in better health. Even if some of my predictions turn out to be wrong, the only way to prove that is to conduct experiments demonstrating what is right, and *that* will result in the advance of science, too.

I think by now my message is clear: *You* are in charge of your own health. And you don't need a medical degree to understand the logic in a sound argument. You've seen throughout this book that a strong argument can be made that teenage hormone levels are associated with good health. You've also learned that, contrary to popular misconception, testosterone doesn't cause prostate cancer; excess local estradiol does. Estradiol is also a risk factor for breast cancer because of the way it binds to estrogen receptors and increases cell proliferation.[16] Finally, you've seen that high hormone levels are powerfully protective against cognitive decline and Alzheimer's. In the end, logic is all you need to see the strength of these lines of reasoning—and to see the wisdom in acting on the advice to bring your hormones into the optimal range.

Last but not least, as a theoretical biologist, I've written this book to provide practical applications for my research findings. After all, what good is the Hormone Receptor Model unless it can help people?

I sometimes joke with my friends that my research will end up *saving* Medicare while putting a *strain* on Social Security—because people will live longer, healthier lives. However, there may be more truth than humor in my statement. There's no doubt that when people take hormones and blood tests to monitor them, it costs more each year than simply getting an annual physical. However, just balance this modest cost with the enormous savings that would result if there were no more breast cancer, prostate cancer, Alzheimer's, type 2 diabetes, colon cancer, ovarian cancer, depression, acid reflux, and GERD. Imagine all that money not being spent on drugs, doctors, and hospitals! I suspect that additional health benefits and savings would be realized as people optimize their hormones—just think of all the medical problems that teenagers *never* have.

In chapter 7, I talked about teenage levels of hormones being essential if a real fountain of youth is ever discovered. We now have to add sufficient levels of stomach acid as well. I predict that eventually almost every biochemical feature of the teen years is going to have to be incorporated into any effective fountain of youth. While teenage levels of hormones may make you feel young, there are many other biochemical activities occurring inside your body during your teenage years that don't affect how you feel but that do affect your overall health. Hopefully, this book will dispel the irrational fear that doctors have of teenage hormone levels and will encourage researchers to find new ways to return other biochemical reactions to teenage levels as well. And, as I've said all along, I sincerely hope that this book will inspire you to take control of your health and enjoy all the emotional and physical advantages of the new testosterone treatment.

LIST OF ILLUSTRATIONS

ACKNOWLEDGMENTS

In preparing this volume, I've benefited from the guidance of many scholars. Special thanks, however, must go to Dr. Robert Leibowitz. I have only spoken with him on one occasion, but he related inexplicable and paradoxical facts about prostate cancer. This is what launched my research—I couldn't get those paradoxes out of my head until I finally developed a model that explained them all.

I'm infinitely obliged to numerous scholars who prefer to remain nameless and to receive their accolades in the bylines of scientific journals. Without the fact that they took up their pens and transmitted to the scientific community so much of their findings, I would have been left in the dark and unaware of the breakthroughs that have lighted our way to a better understanding of how to prevent and fight three of the biggest scourges of the modern age.

I'm confident that the book you're reading will demonstrate that our subject is worthy of attention from scientists, physicians, and laypersons alike. I trust that while I have done an acceptable service to science and to the public, I have at the same time to some degree contributed to the advancement of the renown of the countless clinical researchers, epidemiologists, and physicians toiling in the corridors of institutions of higher education and in hospitals and investigative centers around the world in their attempts to push back the ravages of disease and usher us all into a more benign and healthful state of being.

When the idea for this book first crossed my mind, it was with some trepidation that I ventured to imagine its organization. Now that it is completed, I wish to thank my literary agent, Steve Harris at CSG Literary Partners, for his astute guidance in helping my ideas find a home. There were many nights when he was out and about in the New York literary scene, assisting other authors with their book parties, but always in the back of his mind was this volume, of which he said on numerous occasions, "It *must* be published. It's an important book." He believed in this project from the start and helped me validate my own belief. For that insight, he deserves a round of applause from all whom this book will touch in a beneficial way, both today and in the far future, when the ideas contained herein become mainstream medicine, as they surely must. How a man who has so many other books on his desk could find time to understand my work and believe in it is a miracle in my life.

I'm very aware of the fact that a work of this nature might have appeared to much greater advantage had it been undertaken by an abler hand, but I am not without hope that what I have now brought to a conclusion will meet with a favorable reception, and notwithstanding its deficiencies, may have its use in helping many see the true nature of the value of natural hormones for contemporary men and women. All that I have aimed at is by faithfully interpreting the current state of research to convey to my readers a true sense of what is now known—and admittedly much still remains unknown—about the safety and the benefit of using hormones to alleviate distress both psychological and physical. I must own that I take some degree of pride in the opportunity to share with you the fruits, such as they are, of a long and arduous journey of discovery in this often thankless area of research.

Words could never express sufficient appreciation for my coauthor, William Cane. A marvel of dexterity with ideas, a redoubtable companion in challenging the status quo, and a tireless researcher in his own right, he jumped into this project with a true love of the adventure it posed and a realization of the uphill battle that we would fight to express scientific ideas in straightforward language. True, he tended to require me to explain complex concepts repeatedly until I had reduced the most perplexing philosophies to the likes of "This will kill you!" . . . "This will keep you alive!" but when finally he had grasped my theories and concepts, he was full of unbridled enthusiasm for them and eager to put the argument together in a way that I know will be understood by all. He was kind enough, too, to let me keep in all the mind-numbing references to drugs, enzymes, and hormones that are such an integral part of this story, including the tongue-twister designations of some of the hormone receptors . . . such as estrogen receptor-alpha-alpha homodimer. If after reading this book you have even a passing understanding of what these beasts do, you can join me in thanking *him*.

At Prometheus Books, I wish to acknowledge the conscientious copy editing of Julia DeGraf, whose careful reading and editing helped clarify many of my ideas. A special thanks to editor in chief Steven L. Mitchell for having the vision to see that this book broke important new ground, and for encouraging me to make my technical writing accessible to the general reader.

I wish to express my gratitude to Dr. Paul Savage for answering questions about bioidentical hormone replacement therapy and for taking the time to discuss my model with me. He helped me understand that doctors were being taught almost the exact opposite of what my research was showing to be true. I especially want to thank Dr. Rebecca Glaser for answering my questions about breast cancer. Her encyclopedic knowledge of the literature enabled her not just to answer my questions but also to supply multiple references to back up her answers.

Upon reviewing current scientific and medical opinion, I found so much inaccuracy and uncertainty that I soon resolved to take nothing on trust but to consider the subject as wholly new, and I have had abundant reason to be satisfied with my determination on that head; for by inquiries and researches in every quarter where information was likely to be obtained—especially the 2007 *FASEB* article showing that progesterone is categorically different from synthetic progestin, the former free from untoward risks and adverse effects, the latter fraught with unacceptable cancer risk—I have procured more materials than my most optimistic expectations had promised. These academic and intellectual endeavors, though not without their intermittent rewards, were also followed by the most sustained sense of gratification when I realized that they had cleared away much confusion and error, and enabled me to ascertain several key facts, which I can assure readers appear underscored in the previous pages with a degree of certainty hitherto impossible to achieve, all tending toward the inescapable conclusion that the use of bioidentical hormones, especially testosterone, can help men *and* women achieve unprecedented levels of health and happiness.

I wish to thank the many professors at the University of Chicago who taught me the importance of objectivity in science. I especially wish to thank Professor Jon Alperin. Although he is a mathematician and not a biologist, he took the time to look for logical inconsistencies in my work, and in the end he understood my model well enough to discuss it intelligently with me. Special thanks are due to Paulina Glozman at the College of Staten Island for feedback on numerous technical and editorial aspects of the manuscript. For his creativity in developing the modern citation style used in this book, I wish to thank Frank J. Sulloway.

Before I conclude, I should think myself guilty of the highest ingratitude did I not make all due acknowledgments to those praiseworthy persons who have greatly obliged me in their favorable opinions and heartily recommended this work as appears from several letters and communications I have received to that effect from Dr. Terry Grossman, a distinguished author and physician who has done much to bring cutting-edge research to the general reader. I hope I may be excused for making this public mention in particular of the many great favors I have received from the prestigious urologist Dr. George W. Yu, an expert in prostate cancer and the coauthor of the classic *Critical Operative Maneuvers in Urologic Surgery*. The fact that such an eminent person as Dr. Yu respected my work gave me immense confidence that I was on the right track.

Final thanks must go to my sister-in-law, Anne York, who acted as a sounding board and a devil's advocate. Her insights were especially helpful when I was first starting to publish my articles. Last but not least, I would like to thank my wife, Shelly, who was unbelievably supportive during the many hours I put in to this project, and my sons, Daniel and David, who listened patiently and pretended to understand what I was saying while I talked to them enthusiastically about my research.

GLOSSARY

adipose tissue. Fat cells, including cells in the breast.

agonist. A synthetic molecule that binds to a hormone receptor and mimics the action of the hormone. It may have a slightly greater or lesser effect compared to the actual hormone.

AI. See aromatase inhibitor.

androgen. A hormone that binds to the androgen receptor. The primary androgens are testosterone and dihydrotestosterone.

antagonist. A chemical that opposes a hormone, binding the hormone's receptor to prevent the hormone from acting.

antimicrobial peptides. Proteins that kill bacteria and viruses. Exposure to the UVB rays in sunlight increases these highly beneficial peptides.

apoptosis. The process by which a cell destroys itself. Apoptosis is needed to get rid of defective cells. It is also the chief way that cancer cells are destroyed by hormonal treatment.

aromatase. An enzyme that converts testosterone to estradiol. Excess aromatase activity, especially in breast and prostate tissue, is harmful because it leads to higher local levels of estradiol, which can cause cancer.

aromatase inhibitor (AI). A drug or an herbal compound that inhibits the action of the aromatase enzyme. The chief function of an aromatase inhibitor is to reduce local and systemic levels of estradiol. The main reason for reducing estradiol is because it can lead to the initiation and development of prostate and breast cancer.

AS3. A helpful protein that stunts cancer growth by preventing cancer cells from undergoing cell division and multiplying.

bad progesterone. Metabolites of progesterone, such as 5alpha-pregnanes, that increase cancer's rate of growth.

basal epithelial cells. In the prostate, a layer of small, often inconspicuous epithelial cells adjacent to the basement membrane and subjacent to the luminal/secretory epithelial cells. The basal cells are the presumed progenitor cells of the prostate epithelium (SCGAP Urologic Epithelial Stem Cells Project).

Bcl-2. An anti-apoptotic protein that protects cells from programmed cell death. Its presence is generally bad for you when cancer is present because it prevents cancer cells from dying.

bicalutamide. An anti-androgen used to fight prostate cancer by blocking the intracellular androgen receptor (brand name Casodex®).

binding affinity. A measure of how likely it is that a particular ligand will stay in a hormone receptor until it causes an effect.

bioidentical hormone. A hormone identical to one produced by the human body.

BPH. Benign prostatic hyperplasia, a noncancerous enlargement of the prostate.

BRCA1 and **BRCA2.** Tumor suppressor genes that are good for you because they repair DNA and prevent cancer. Mutations (defects) in these genes make women more likely to develop breast cancer. Women with BCRA1 and BCRA2 mutations have a lot of progesterone receptor A (which is bad for them because this receptor increases Bcl-2), and they also have no progesterone receptor B (which is also bad because this receptor decreases Bcl-2).

calreticulin. A protein that protects prostate cancer from calcium ion overload.

Casodex®. See bicalutamide.

DHT. Dihydrotestosterone. An androgen produced from testosterone that binds to the intracellular androgen receptor five times more strongly than testosterone does.

dimers. Two hormone receptors attaching to each other to create a new sort of receptor, in which both receptors need the appropriate hormone attached before it does anything.

DNA binding domain. An area on p53 that attaches to DNA.

epithelium. Cells covering body organs, including the inside of arteries and veins.

estrogen receptor. A hormone receptor that binds to estrogen.

estrogen receptor-alpha. Increases Bcl-2, which is a harmful effect that causes cancer to grow.

estrogen receptor-beta. Decreases Bcl-2, which is a positive effect that causes tumors to die.

5alpha-pregnanes. See bad progesterone.

4-pregnenes. See good progesterone.

Gleason score. A way for pathologists to tell how aggressive prostate cancer is likely to be based on its appearance. Higher Gleason scores indicate cells that are more misshapen and that should correspond to more aggressive cancer.

good progesterone. Metabolites of progesterone, such as 4-pregnenes, that fight cancer.

G protein. A messenger protein that detaches from a membrane hormone receptor (the G protein–coupled receptor) and sends an amplified signal into the cytoplasm and nucleus.

G protein–coupled receptor. A membrane hormone receptor with a G protein connected to it in the interior part of the cell. The G protein is waiting to be activated by the appropriate hormone binding to the part of the receptor that sticks up from the outer layer of the cell membrane.

heterodimer. A double hormone receptor (dimer) in which the two receptors are of different types. Example: estrogen receptor-alpha-beta, which needs two molecules of estradiol to function.

homodimer. A double hormone receptor (dimer) in which the two receptors are of the same type. Example: estrogen receptor-alpha-alpha, which needs two molecules of estradiol to function.

hormone receptor. A protein complex located in a cell membrane or in the interior of a cell that captures passing hormones and then produces specific effects in the cell, such as stimulating replication, apoptosis, or protein manufacture.

HRT. Hormone replacement therapy, the process of using exogenous hormones for anti-aging and disease prevention.

intracellular androgen receptor. Decreases Bcl-2 (which is a good effect), decreases pro-apoptotic proteins (a bad effect), increases AS3 (a good effect), and increases calreticulin (a bad effect).

ligand. Any substance (such as a hormone, a SERM, or a drug) that binds to a hormone receptor and causes an effect.

LNCaP. The most common line of prostate cancer cells used for research. (Pronounced "Lynn cap.") It is considered androgen dependent but will grow in the presence of estrogen.

local levels. Levels of various hormones in prostate or breast tissue. Not to be confused with serum blood levels. Serum estradiol may be normal, for example, but local levels of estradiol may be high enough to initiate cancer.

membrane androgen receptor. Resides on the cell surface. Increases the production of pro-apoptotic proteins for both breast and prostate cancer.

non-genomic. This term refers to the action of hormones on membrane receptors causing effects that do not involve transcription or modification of genes.

progesterone receptor A. This receptor is bad for you because it increases Bcl-2. Women with BRCA1 and BRCA2 mutations have a lot of this harmful receptor in their breasts and none of the good progesterone receptor B.

progesterone receptor B. This receptor is good for you because it decreases Bcl-2. Women with BRCA1 and BRCA2 mutations have very little of this good receptor.

progestin. A synthetic molecule based on (but not identical to) the hormone progesterone.

RU-486. A synthetic steroid patterned after progesterone that works as a progesterone antagonist. It binds to progesterone receptor A and prevents progesterone from binding there.

SERMs. Selective estrogen receptor modulators are substances that can attach (with various levels of affinity) to estrogen receptors. Examples are soy and flaxseed. SERMs are important because in some situations they *increase* receptor activity, mimicking estrogen. In other cases, they *reduce* receptor activity because they are like bad keys and do not work, or do not work as well as estrogen would. Because they have attached to the hormone receptor, they can *prevent* estrogen from attaching and thereby reduce the activity of an estrogen receptor.

SHBG. Sex hormone binding globulin. A protein in the blood that binds to testosterone, DHT, and estradiol, effectively inhibiting the effect of these hormones by taking a significant percentage of them out of circulation.

signal transduction. The process by which a hormone binds to a membrane receptor and transmits a signal (which can be amplified) down into the cell.

Src. A cancer-promoting gene. Pronounced *sarc*, and short for *sarcoma* (tumor), it is also known as p60src.

supraphysiological. An amount or dose of a hormone that is greater than one found naturally in the body of a healthy young person.

tipping point. In the development of prostate cancer and breast cancer, this is the point at which the rate of cell growth becomes greater than the rate of cell death. Hormones and their interaction with hormone receptors affect this tipping point because hormone receptors control many proteins and other factors that either retard or accelerate the rate of cell growth and the rate of apoptosis.

transcription. The first step in a process in which the genetic information in DNA is read and eventually ends up with the production of proteins.

transduction. See signal transduction.

WHI study. The Women's Health Initiative, a large study that examined the effect of hormone supplementation on women's health and found an increased risk of breast cancer when synthetic progestin was used by women. The study is widely misused to support the claim that hormones cause cancer. In reality, the study only supports the proposition that synthetic hormones can increase cancer risk. The study says nothing about bioidentical hormones.

NOTES

CHAPTER 1. WHY HORMONES HAVE GOTTEN A BAD RAP

1. Safe hormone replacement therapy uses bioidentical hormones and is monitored by an anti-aging physician. The proper procedure is described in detail in this book.
2. Rossouw et al. 2002.
3. Million Women Study Collaborators 2003.
4. See, e.g., "FDA Approved 'HRT' IS Risky," http://tahomaclinicblog.com/fda-approved-hrt-is-risky/ (accessed May 26, 2012), where Jonathan V. Wright, MD, describes the dangers of using synthetic hormones and recommends instead the use of natural bioidentical hormones.
5. Fournier, Berrino, and Clavel-Chapelon 2008.
6. Fournier, Berrino, and Clavel-Chapelon 2008.
7. Parker-Pope 2011.
8. Fournier, Berrino, and Clavel-Chapelon 2011.
9. Huggins, Stevens Jr., and Hodges 1941.
10. Noble 1977.
11. Fowler Jr. and Whitmore Jr. 1981.
12. The thirty-day mark is significant because cancer will evolve to try to foil any treatment given (often through cells with just the right mutations surviving), but the early effect of a treatment gives a better understanding of the worth of a treatment. If something good happens right away, then it might be possible to build on that treatment to make it more effective. If something bad happens right away, then the treatment is almost certainly doing more harm than good.
13. However, there always seem to be some prostate cancer cells that are able to survive and grow in the absence of testosterone. The modern terminology for those cells is castration-resistant prostate cancer (CRPC).
14. Morgentaler and Rhoden 2006.
15. Morgentaler et al. 2011.
16. Szmulewitz et al. 2009; Morris et al. 2009.
17. Isaacs et al. 2012.

18. Friedman 2005.

19. Friedman 2007.

20. Bonkhoff and Berges 2009.

21. Friedman 2007.

22. Bonkhoff and Berges 2009.

23. Bonkhoff et al. 1999.

24. Fowler Jr. and Whitmore Jr. 1981.

25. Some of these men, however, may have had enough estrogen receptor-alpha to greatly increase their cancer's rate of growth if they were exposed to high enough levels of estradiol, which would occur if enough testosterone were administered and converted to estradiol.

Because this is an important point about a classic study, I would like to clarify what I'm saying. What is going on in the study is that there is a group of men with metastatic prostate cancer, but they are in stable condition. That is, they are experiencing a slow, not rapid, worsening of their condition. Some of these men saw a rapid worsening of their condition when given testosterone, others noticed an improvement. The point I'm making is that if you have a moderate amount of estrogen receptor-alpha (ER-alpha), then small amounts of estradiol aren't going to rapidly make you get worse. But a moderate amount of ER-alpha along with very high amounts of estradiol is disastrous. The reason that the men have very high amounts of estradiol is because they were given very high amounts of testosterone, enough of which gets converted to estradiol to cause this problem.

On the other hand, some of these men with stable conditions were lucky enough to still have a very small amount of ER-alpha. For these men, the high level of testosterone would be beneficial, and even the high level of estradiol might have helped if their cancer still had plenty of estrogen receptor-beta (ER-beta).

26. This is a highly unlikely claim in light of the observation that as men age and testosterone levels drop, this "testosterone starvation" does not reduce prostate cancer; on the contrary, it increases the incidence of prostate cancer. See, e.g., Morgentaler and Rhoden 2006.

27. Martikainen and Isaacs 1990.

28. Bcl-2 was the anti-apoptotic protein used in this study (Raffo et al. 1995).

29. Bosland, Ford, and Horton 1995.

30. Hu et al. 2011.

31. Yu et al. 2011.

32. Ricke et al. 2008.

CHAPTER 2. HORMONE RECEPTORS

1. Matthews and Gustafsson 2003.

2. Receptors in the cytoplasm enter the nucleus once they bind to the appropriate hormone. Receptors in the nucleus are sometimes called nuclear receptors, which is a subcategory of intracellular receptors.

3. This seven-loop structure of membrane receptors is known as a 7-transmembrane domain motif (TMD).

4. Friedman 2007.

5. Another way to envision hormone receptors is to imagine a mouse pad representing a cell with tens of thousands of wispy thin hairs protruding from the surface of the mouse pad, each hair representing a hormone receptor. There are between two thousand and one hundred thousand receptors for a particular hormone in each cell (Holt and Hanley 2012:29). When a hormone is in plentiful supply, the number of hormone receptors is reduced (downregulated); when a hormone is in short supply, the number of hormone receptors is increased (upregulated) to increase the likelihood of the hormone being captured by that cell.

6. Narvaez and Walsh 2001.

7. Guzey, Kitada, and Reed 2002.

8. Stambolsky et al. 2010.

9. Whenever Bcl-2 is mentioned in this book, keep in mind that I am almost always referring to Bcl-2 plus many other anti-apoptotic proteins.

10. Risbridger, Ellem, and McPherson 2007.

11. Bonkhoff and Berges 2009.

12. Shaaban et al. 2003.

13. Researchers are starting to talk about progesterone receptor B neutralizing the effects of progesterone receptor A, but I look at it differently. I believe that most of the effects of these two receptors are in direct opposition to each other. For all the other hormone receptor pairs, there are hormones that bind with different affinities to each member of that pair. However, no hormone has yet been identified that binds differentially to progesterone receptors A and B, although I predict that someday such a hormone will be discovered.

14. Friedman 2007.

15. Dimers are present in both the cytoplasm and in the cell membrane (Razandi et al. 2004). Unfortunately, no one has yet done an experiment to find out whether it is membrane dimers or intracellular dimers that are the receptors responsible for producing telomerase activity.

16. Nanni et al. 2002.

17. Malet et al. 1988.

18. Chieffi et al. 2003.

19. Nanni et al. 2002.

20. Ricke et al. 2008.

21. Bonkhoff and Berges 2009.

22. Friedman 2007.
23. Risbridger, Ellem, and McPherson 2007.
24. Bonkhoff and Berges 2009.
25. Fernö et al. 1990.
26. Friedman 2007.
27. Unfortunately, prostate and breast cancer research money is not always spent wisely. There is altogether too much busywork being done investigating synthetic drugs and woefully little being spent on natural ways of defeating prostate and breast cancer and Alzheimer's through manipulating hormone receptors.
28. Friedman 2007.
29. Wiebe 2006.
30. Zhu et al. 2006.
31. Löfgren et al. 2006.
32. Friedman 2007.
33. Until a way to kill breast cancer cells with calcium overload is discovered, the presence of calreticulin in breast cancer cells is irrelevant.
34. Friedman 2007.
35. Szelei et al. 1997.
36. Hatzoglou et al. 2005.

CHAPTER 3. BIOIDENTICAL HORMONES

1. There are exceptions to this general rule about achieving hormone levels equivalent to a teenager for optimum health. When treating some disease states, it is at times valuable to achieve either supraphysiological levels or abnormally low levels of specific hormones.
2. Prystupa et al. 2012. Most NSAID deaths are due to deadly stomach complications.
3. FDA 2008:13. In an embarrassing display of disingenuous naïveté, the FDA has campaigned long and hard against the use of bioidentical hormones, clearly as a result of pressure from pharmaceutical companies like Wyeth. See, e.g., FDA 2008:3. In this connection, it is ironic to note that the FDA has admitted that it is incompetent and that it cannot do the job it was mandated to do (Faloon 2008).
4. Holtorf 2009.
5. Moskowitz 2006.
6. See Somers 2012, in which she argues for the use of testosterone to fight prostate cancer; Somers 2009 and Somers 2006.
7. Beck 2012.
8. Beck 2012.
9. Pharmaceutical company marketing departments are oriented toward maximizing

income. After all, they're being paid to sell a product, and spin sometimes sells better than full disclosure. Spin occurs when PR firms pay researchers to cherry-pick data and publish only favorable articles about their products. Pharmaceutical companies also hire press agents, and somehow Wikipedia and scholarly articles are skewed to their viewpoint. This misinformation eventually trickles down to the popular press, which (as we pointed out in chapter 1) is the primary reason why most people mistakenly fear hormones. In other words, the good news about the safety of bioidentical hormones has not yet reached the public or the doctors who need to hear it most.

10. Testosterone binds to the intracellular androgen receptor in a breast cancer cell. It results in less protection against apoptosis. This binding is blocked by the synthetic "hormone" Provera®, which results in more protection against apoptosis, or, in other words, a slower rate of cell death.

11. Pizzorno 2012.

12. To be fair, we have no long-term studies on the safety of bioidentical hormones (the longest is eight years), but all the studies to date (2013) have confirmed the hypothesis that bioidentical hormones are safe when used as directed.

13. "Progesterone . . . down-regulates Bcl-2 and up-regulates p53, thereby stopping cancer growth" (Lee, Zava, and Hopkins 2002:60). See also Lee, Zava, and Hopkins 2002:58 and 174. This assumes normal genetics in which there is more progesterone receptor B than progesterone receptor A.

14. Birrell et al. 2007. This groundbreaking *FASEB Journal* article explains how progestin interferes with proper hormone receptor functioning (androgen signaling), contributing to an increased risk of breast cancer.

15. National Cancer Institute conclusion at "Oral Contraceptives and Cancer Risk," http://www.cancer.gov/cancertopics/factsheet/Risk/oral-contraceptives (accessed July 15, 2012).

16. Do not waste your time asking your family doctor for testosterone. He will not prescribe it, and even if he does, he is unlikely to administer it in the safest manner. With rare exceptions, only anti-aging doctors understand the value of prescribing testosterone for andropause.

17. Morgentaler and Rhoden 2006.

18. Powers and Florini 1975.

19. Morgentaler 2006. There are two exceptions to the statement that testosterone doesn't make the prostate grow. If testosterone is converted into excess local estradiol by the aromatase enzyme, it can result in cell proliferation and cancer. And if testosterone is converted into high local levels of DHT by the 5-alpha-reductase enzyme, it can lead to BPH. Luckily, both scenarios are preventable.

20. Testosterone kills prostate cancer by binding to the membrane androgen receptor, which sends a signal within minutes into the cancer cell, instructing it to eventually self-destruct. This programmed cancer cell death is facilitated by actin cytoskeleton dynamics, a crucial part of apoptosis (Hatzoglou et al. 2005). See also Kampa et al. 2006 and Papadopoulou et al. 2008, which elucidate the method by which testosterone effectively initiates apoptosis in prostate cancer cells.

21. The anti-tumorigenic role of membrane androgen receptors for colon cancer cells is fully outlined in Gu et al. 2009. See also Gu et al. 2011.

22. Gu et al. 2009.

23. Gu et al. 2009. The implication, since mice and humans are so close genetically, is that similar or better results would obtain in humans.

24. Unfortunately, almost all general practitioners are still in the Dark Ages when it comes to the use of hormones to prevent and fight disease, so it really is a good idea to seek a physician from alternative health organizations, such as the American Academy of Anti-Aging Medicine (http://www.a4m.com) and the American Board of Integrative Holistic Medicine (http://www.abihm.org). A particularly effective way to find a doctor in your area is to call a local **compounding pharmacy** (not to be confused with a regular pharmacy) and ask which physicians send their patients to that pharmacy. Compounding pharmacies mix generic bioidentical hormones individually for each patient.

25. Davis 2009.

26. Tambi and Imran 2010.

27. Neychev and Mitev 2005.

28. Saad and Gooren 2011.

29. Kelly et al. 2001:6.

30. Kapoor et al. 2006.

31. Saad and Gooren 2011.

32. Li, C. et al. 2010.

33. Salam, Kshetrimayum, and Keisam 2012. Type 2 diabetes is caused by overconsumption of carbohydrates and, according to Joseph Mercola, DO, is totally curable with exercise and diet. Says Mercola, "You will want to eliminate ALL sugars and grains—even 'healthful' grains such as whole, organic or sprouted ones" (Mercola 2010).

34. A series of informative videos on the connection between low testosterone and type 2 diabetes can be found on the website of Barry Gordon, MD, at the Hidden Disease, http://www.thehiddendisease.com/blog/educational-videos (accessed July 10, 2012).

35. Key et al. 2002.

36. Dimitrakakis et al. 2004.

37. Glaser 2010.

38. Birrell et al. 2007.

39. Dimitrakakis et al. 2003.

40. Dimitrakakis et al. 2003.

41. Birrell et al. 2007.

42. Chlebowski et al. 2003.
43. Dimitrakakis et al. 2004.
44. Rossouw et al. 2002.
45. Million Women Study Collaborators 2003.
46. Davison et al. 2005.
47. Shumaker et al. 2003.
48. Davison et al. 2011.
49. Paoletti et al. 2004.

CHAPTER 4. A *NEW* MODEL OF PROSTATE CANCER

1. Men who experience twenty-one or more ejaculations per month over the course of their lifetime have a reduced risk of prostate cancer (Leitzmann et al. 2004).
2. Endocrine glands include the pituitary, thyroid, and pancreas.
3. Incidentally, chemicals and radiation are less likely to initiate prostate cancer than are high local levels of estradiol.
4. Anderson and Appella 2005:97.
5. Klein 2007:431.
6. Defective p53 causes harm independent of hormone levels; a recent study found that it is "associated with earlier onset prostate cancer" (Sun et al. 2010).
7. Kamradt et al. 2003. Telomerase activity is needed initially, but as prostate cancer (PCa) advances, other mechanisms can take its place, so you actually see less telomerase activity in advanced PCa, not more. Tumor suppressor p53 kills cells that try dividing without telomeres, but mutated p53 allows PCa to grow without telomeres, although the DNA tends to become very scrambled. There is also a process called alternative lengthening of telomeres (ALT), which somehow lengthens telomeres without using telomerase. The exact mechanism of ALT has not yet been worked out.
8. Chieffi et al. 2003.
9. Nanni et al. 2002.
10. Abate-Shen and Shen 2000.
11. Approximately 90 percent of prostate cancers have been observed to have telomerase activity. There are alternative mechanisms to increase cell division without requiring telomerase, but it's not clear whether the 10 percent of cells without telomerase activity are using such alternative mechanisms or whether they already have a great enough telomere length so that telomerase activity is no longer essential.
12. For most men, the first prostate cancer cell starts up when they're in their twenties (Berges et al. 1995). Although autopsy studies show that 0–2 percent of men have prostate cancer between the ages of 20–29, 27–29 percent of men have prostate cancer between the

ages of 30–39, and 32–34 percent of men have prostate cancer between the ages of 40–49. The reason I give a range of percentages is that there are two different studies (Sakr et al. 1993 and Sakr et al. 1994) with slightly different numbers. One study stops at age 49; the other shows 55 percent of men having prostate cancer between the ages of 50–59 and 64 percent of men having prostate cancer between the ages of 60–69. The actual incidence of prostate cancer is certainly even higher than what has been uncovered in autopsy studies since it's nearly impossible for an autopsy to spot a single cancer cell or even just a few cells.

13. Lung cancer is number one.

14. Brawley 2012.

15. Autopsy studies show that for men under thirty, 0–2 percent prostate cancer has been detected.

16. John R. Lee, MD, calls this altered ratio **estrogen dominance**, and he argues that it's the cause of many ills in men. We now know that prostate cancer is caused by high levels of estradiol within epithelial cells, but BPH may be caused by high levels of estradiol binding to SHBG, which is attached to the membrane surface of stroma cells (Farnsworth 1996).

17. Risbridger et al. 2003.

18. This excess proliferation is not the same as benign prostatic hyperplasia (BPH), a condition that affects most aging men. BPH typically only occurs later in life, with frequency increasing with age, so it may well be due to a decrease in the rate of apoptosis (which, as I discussed earlier in this chapter, is also a problem occurring during the formation of prostate cancer). Normal prostate cells are supposed to die after about five hundred days, and testosterone binding to the membrane androgen receptor (mAR) induces the proteins that cause apoptosis (programmed cell death). This necessary apoptosis is prevented by DHT binding to intracellular androgen receptor (iAR). As cells age and iAR loses its functionality, apoptosis is supposed to occur to let those cells die. (A separate mechanism kicks in when mAR loses functionality.) But as men age, their levels of testosterone decrease, and this reduces their ability to produce favorable apoptotic proteins from mAR. The result is that it is easier for prostate cancer to thrive if it starts up.

19. In women, ovarian cancer and uterine cancer probably are associated with high levels of estradiol, but more research must be done to definitively prove this.

20. High Gleason score localized prostate cancer divides on average every 68 days and dies on average every 76 days for an average population doubling time of 495 days. Low Gleason score localized prostate cancer divides on average every 65 days and dies on average every 70 days for an average population doubling time of 577 days. Late high grade prostate intraepithelial neoplasia (HGPIN) divides on average every 56 days and dies on average every 56 days for an average of no growth (Berges et al. 1995).

21. In plain English, a **model** is a scientific description of something; in this case, of prostate cancer.

22. My model predicts that it is impossible for prostate cancer to develop without a properly functioning membrane androgen receptor since this receptor is needed to decrease AS3. However, no known case of a mutated membrane androgen receptor has yet been reported (probably because nobody has ever looked for any).

23. Ricke et al. 2008.

24. I believe Professor Risbridger deserves a Nobel Prize for her research involving estrogen and prostate cancer. Her work in this field has been profound and prolific—she has reported that the aromatase activity in prostate cancer is just as high as in breast cancer, that it's impossible to get prostate cancer without properly functioning aromatase (unless you add external estrogen), and—most important of all—that it's impossible to develop prostate cancer if there's no estrogen receptor-alpha.

25. Taylor et al. 2012.

26. This is unfortunate because if you're a male, your family doctor is unlikely to prescribe testosterone for you. He will be afraid that it will cause cancer. And yet the evidence is clearly against him. This means that you'll need to find an anti-aging doctor to prescribe testosterone. Anti-aging doctors understand that testosterone is good for your health, and they generally understand the importance of controlling excess estrogen.

27. Nakai and Nonomura 2012.

28. Risbridger, Ellem, and McPherson 2007.

29. Inflammation definitely increases the chance of developing breast or prostate cancer. Basically, inflammation is associated with increased levels of nuclear factor kappa B (NFKB), and NFKB prevents apoptosis (similar to Bcl-2 preventing apoptosis but by different chemical pathways). But that doesn't mean that inflammation *causes* prostate cancer.

30. There is, however, one known gene fusion that's associated with more aggressive cancer. And there's no question that, all things being equal, men with prostate cancer containing the gene fusion TMPRSS2:ERG are worse off than men whose cancer doesn't contain that gene fusion. However, no study has been done on men with that gene fusion to show whether more testosterone is beneficial (since higher levels of testosterone reduce Bcl-2) or harmful (since higher levels of testosterone result in more TMPRSS2:ERG gene product). Of course, any time testosterone is given, an aromatase inhibitor must also be administered, otherwise the effects of estradiol on the estrogen receptors may overwhelm the effects of testosterone on the androgen receptors.

31. Gorlov et al. 2009.

32. Berges et al. 1995.

33. Gat, Joshua, and Gornish 2009.

34. Risbridger et al. 2003.

35. There are two known ways that a gene is inactivated. One is by the methylation of the section of DNA that codes that gene, and the other is by RNA interference specific for that gene. Since a mutation is required for RNA interference to fail, my model proposes that it is the failure to methylate the aromatase gene that ultimately causes the first prostate cancer cell to arise. DNA methylation involves the addition of a methyl group (which is composed of one carbon and three hydrogens) to DNA. It's a fundamental biological process that is crucial for life.

36. For cancers in most other tissues, a random mutation has to occur in just the right gene in order for them to become immortal. Of course, the same mechanism that causes cancer in other tissues may be responsible for some of the cancers in the prostate, but if so, they would be expected to be found at a low rate similar to what is observed in other tissues.

37. Chieffi et al. 2003.

38. As we have seen, one of the mutations necessary for cancer is in proto-oncogenes, which become oncogenes upon mutation and cause cells to divide in an uncontrolled manner. Another mutation that is necessary is the ability to invade other cells—one of the hallmarks of cancer.

39. As men age, the intracellular level of dihydrotestosterone decreases in prostate epithelial cells but stays constant in prostate stroma cells. In addition, as men age, the level of estradiol remains constant in prostate epithelial cells but increases in prostate stroma cells (Krieg, Nass, and Tunn 1993).

40. Almost all the estradiol produced in men is due to the enzyme aromatase acting on testosterone. So having no testosterone means having no estradiol, and consequently there would be no initiation of prostate cancer. In chapter 9 I will provide detailed information on exactly how a lack of testosterone, a lack of DHT, or a defective intracellular androgen receptor can lead to potential cancer cells acquiring a rate of cell death greater than the rate of cell growth, and I'll also describe in detail exactly what role ER-alpha plays in the immortalization of prostate cells.

41. It's possible that cells that are just neighbors of cells that have aromatase activity can thrive in the absence of estradiol because, after the fusion, they might be able to activate the needed estradiol genes simply by androgens binding to the intracellular androgen receptor. This is speculation on my part.

42. In some rats, super-high levels of just testosterone can cause prostate cancer almost 20 percent of the time (Noble 1977). This cancer, however, is caused by testosterone converting to estradiol.

43. The Internal Spermatic Vein Model reported that repairing the damage to the veins was beneficial to patients. The authors' explanation was that the resulting decrease in intracellular androgen receptor activity killed the cancer cells. The explanation of the Hormone Receptor Model would be that the benefit was due to the reduction in local estradiol levels. This is a testable prediction.

44. Fowler Jr. and Whitmore Jr. 1981.

45. Ricke et al. 2008.

46. Hu et al. 2011.
47. Yu et al. 2011.
48. Elements of the treatment protocol I advise (which is described in chapter 12) are being used today with remarkable results by Dr. Robert Leibowitz.

CHAPTER 5. HOW BREAST CANCER ARISES FROM ESTROGEN

1. An overview of the types of breast cancer and how they are traditionally classified into estrogen-positive and estrogen-negative can be found in Rakha, Reis-Filho, and Ellis 2008, which also discusses how a more sophisticated classification into gene expression patterns and DNA copy number alterations may lead to improved therapy.
2. There had been speculation that estradiol might cause breast cancer either directly or through its metabolites, but this study concluded that the specific metabolites of estradiol tested do not cause breast cancer; instead, it is estradiol itself that is the causative factor (Turan et al. 2004).
3. Cutts and Noble 1964.
4. Estriol, another estrogen, appears to protect against breast cancer (Dimitrakakis et al. 2010).
5. "Breast Cancer Statistics," MEDTV, http://breast-cancer.emedtv.com/breast-cancer/breast-cancer-statistics.html (accessed May 20, 2012).
6. "Breast Cancer Risk in American Women," National Cancer Institute, http://www.cancer.gov/cancertopics/factsheet/detection/probability-breast-cancer (accessed May 20, 2012).
7. "Breast Cancer Risk by Age," Centers for Disease Control, http://www.cdc.gov/cancer/breast/statistics/age.htm (accessed May 20, 2012).
8. Feigelson and Henderson 1996.
9. Nanni et al. 2002.
10. Liehr 2000 (emphasis supplied).
11. However, there is still some effect from the serum, since breast tissue estradiol levels in postmenopausal women are approximately 25 percent less than those of premenopausal women (van Landeghem et al. 1985).
12. Zhou et al. 2001.
13. It is also possible that the metabolites of estradiol might increase the rate of mutations (Liehr 2000), which would increase the likelihood that breast cancer would succeed in starting up.
14. Santen, Yue, and Heitan 2012.
15. Spratt Jr., Kaltenbach, and Spratt 1977.

16. Santen, Yue, and Heitan 2012.
17. The Surveillance Epidemiology and End Results data showed a 9.1 percent reduction for the same time frame. The computer model did not take into account that increasing the rate of cell death would prevent a small number of women from developing breast cancer—a group for whom the rate of cell death would now be greater than the rate of cell growth. This could explain the observed extra 2.1 percent reduction in the breast cancer rate that was not predicted when using the occult tumor model.
18. Other mutations that raise the risk of breast cancer include mistakes in p53 and PTEN/MMAC1 genes, although these are more rare than BRCA mutations.
19. Nathanson 2001.
20. Mercola 2009a. Certain ethnic groups are more likely to have these mutations. Most notably, women in the Ashkenazi Jewish population are five times more likely to possess BRCA1 and BRCA2 mutations (National Cancer Institute n.d.).
21. Grann et al. 1998.
22. Poole et al. 2006.
23. Sartorius et al. 1994.
24. Mote et al. 2004.
25. Sabourin et al. 1994.
26. Ma et al. 2006.
27. Veronesi et al. 2005.

CHAPTER 6. CAN ALZHEIMER'S BE CURED?

1. The leading health organization in Alzheimer's care openly admits that "current medications cannot cure Alzheimer's or stop it from progressing" (Alzheimer's Association, n.d.).
2. Jonsson et al. 2012.
3. Actually, this is not strictly true. Bioidentical hormone replacement therapy brings back so many of the healthy conditions associated with youth that this probably explains why testosterone, estrogen, and progesterone replacement reduce all the causal factors associated with Alzheimer's.
4. Bachmeier et al. 2013.
5. Ito et al. 2011.
6. Gouras et al. 2000.
7. Carroll et al. 2010.
8. Spies et al. 2010.
9. McAllister et al. 2010.
10. Tyler et al. 2002.

11. Vincent and Govitrapong 2011.
12. Cole and Vassar 2007.
13. Nixon 2000.
14. "Gamma Secretase Activating Protein, A Role in Alzheimer's Disease?" Pharmacology, December 5, 2011, http://www.pharmacology.org/news/gamma-secretase/ (accessed May 25, 2012).
15. McAllister et al. 2010.
16. Amtul et al. 2010.
17. Miners et al. 2006.
18. McAllister et al. 2010.
19. Liang et al. 2010.
20. Papasozomenos and Shanavas 2002.
21. Carroll et al. 2010.
22. Gong et al. 2006.
23. Zitmann et al. 2001.
24. Lannert et al. 1998.
25. Syed et al. 1992.
26. Driscoll and Resnick 2007.
27. Salom et al. 2001.
28. Not surprisingly, a nineteen-year study involving 574 men found that the average amount of free testosterone in men who developed Alzheimer's was roughly half the amount found in men who didn't (Moffat et al. 2004).
29. Calderón-Garcidueñas et al. 2004.

CHAPTER 7. THE MIRACLE OF TEENAGE HORMONE LEVELS

1. Rice et al. 2008.
2. Yeap 2009. Vasopressin affects memory, and testosterone restores depleted vasopressin in senescent rat brains. Researchers speculate that sex steroids may do the same in humans. Estrogen, which is known to boost cognitive capability in females with Alzheimer's, may operate, in part, through the restoration of vasopressin innervation. Therefore, the administration of testosterone replacement therapy may play an important role in cognitive improvement via its effect on the vasopressin system (Goudsmit, Fliers, and Swaab 1988). Testosterone reverses vasopressin depletion in aging rat brains and may have a similar effect in humans suffering from Alzheimer's, contributing to a reversal of cognitive impairment (Goudsmit, Fliers, and Swaab 1989).
3. Schutter et al. 2005.

4. Schutter et al. 2005.

5. Yeap 2009; testosterone (testosterone undecanoate 160 mg/day) and carnitines (propionyl-L-carnitine 2 g/day plus acetyl-L-carnitine 2 g/day) both contribute to improved peak systolic velocity, end-diastolic velocity, and resistive index (Cavallini et al. 2004); testosterone reduces inflammation and heart problems and may play a role in the fight against arthritis. Sex hormones have "immune-modulating effects; testosterone in particular appears to suppress activation of pro-inflammatory cytokines. Men with low testosterone levels are at increased risk of coronary artery disease" (Malkin et al. 2003); short-term administration of testosterone induces a beneficial dilation effect on exercise-induced myocardial ischemia in men with coronary artery disease (Rosano et al. 1999; Morgentaler 2008:90).

6. Orshal and Khalil 2004; sex steroid hormones bind to membrane receptors in the blood vessels and cause rapid non-genomic relaxation (Khalil 2005).

7. Ready et al. 2004.

8. Torkler et al. 2011; Walker 1942.

9. Isidori et al. 2005.

10. For example, testosterone replacement improves elderly men's spatial cognition (Janowsky, Oviatt, and Orwoll 1994).

11. Yeap 2009.

12. Ready et al. 2004 describes the low energy and apathy as men report that they have less "get up and go" or that they feel "out of gas."

13. Tamimi et al. 2001. See also Yeap 2009.

14. Unfortunately, most doctors never check testosterone levels. Those who do almost never test bioavailable testosterone. Men can request such tests when routine blood draws are ordered by their general practitioner. Insurance may not cover the cost of such tests, but if a man complains of low libido, insurance may be more likely to cover the cost.

15. Yeap 2009.

16. Axell et al. 2006.

17. Rabkin, Wagner, and Rabkin 1999.

18. Wagner, Rabkin, and Rabkin 1998.

19. Ready et al. 2004.

20. In addition to the beneficial effects of testosterone, this study also found that carnitines (propionyl-L-carnitine and acetyl-L-carnitine) had a similar effect in reducing fatigue in elderly men. The study concluded that because testosterone could increase prostate size, it might be preferable to use only carnitines (Cavallini et al. 2004).

21. Bachmann et al. 2002.

22. Bachmann et al. 2002.

23. Davis and Tran 2001.

24. Davis et al. 2008.

25. Guay and Jacobson 2002.

26. Burger et al. 1987:937.

27. Travison et al. 2006.

28. This study defined low testosterone as a level below 300 ng/dL along with clinical symptoms such as low libido, erectile dysfunction, osteoporosis or bone fracture, lethargy, sleep disturbances, depression, and low physical performance. A correlation was found between low testosterone and low sex drive (Araujo et al. 2007).

29. Morgentaler 2008.

30. van Wingen et al. 2009.

31. van Honk, Peper, and Schutter 2005.

32. Perman 2012.

33. Hall 1979, and Hall 1984. See also Ambady 1995.

34. van Honk, Peper, and Schutter. 2005.

35. van Wingen et al. 2009.

36. Delville et al. 1996. Vasopressin, a hormone that regulates the way water is retained in tissue, also increases sexual pleasure. According to Thierry Hertoghe, it is an important hormone to supplement with as we age since it can keep skin smooth and youthful by retaining water in tissue (Hertoghe 2002:185). Dr. Hertoghe, who John Crisler regards as the finest mind in hormone research today, recently spoke about the value of vasopressin replacement therapy in an engaging video (Hertoghe 2010).

37. Testosterone also boosts libido in postmenopausal women (Davis et al. 2008, APHRODITE study).

38. Barrett-Connor et al. 1999.

39. Barrett-Connor et al. 1999.

40. Schutter et al. 2005.

41. The term *low testosterone* is usually defined by blood labs as the levels of 90 percent of the men tested. They cut off the top 5 percent and the bottom 5 percent and lump everyone else into what they call a normal range. But as Barry Gordon, MD, and others have pointed out, this is a fiction, since most men over age forty have lost their ability to make sufficient testosterone; therefore the lab reference range is not optimal. According to anti-aging doctors, optimal ranges for total testosterone are 800 to 1,000 for men. While I agree that testosterone should be maintained in the higher ranges, I believe that it is preferable to measure free testosterone instead of total testosterone.

"Mainstream medicine's ignorance regarding the need to maintain free testosterone in the higher ranges is a significant cause of premature disability and death in aging men" (Faloon 2012a).

42. Wang et al. 2000. Similar results were obtained by Wang et al. 2004.

43. Wang et al. 1996.

44. Researchers found short-term (six-week) supraphysiological doses had little or no

negative psychological effect on most men, saying, "Testosterone administration, 600 mg/wk increased ratings of manic symptoms in normal men. This effect, however, was not uniform across individuals; most showed little psychological change, whereas a few developed prominent effects" (Pope et al. 2000).

45. Ebinger et al. 2009. On the dopamine boosting power of testosterone, see also Simpson 2001.

46. Simpson 2001.

47. Simpson 2001.

48. Simpson 2001. See also Urban et al. 1998. In hamster brains, testosterone upregulates vasopressin receptors (Young et al. 2000).

49. Sahay et al. 2002.

50. Bachner-Melman et al. 2005.

51. Seidman et al. 2001.

52. Giovannucci et al. 1997.

53. Adolescent males exhibit more or less androgen-influenced traits (including aggression, risk taking, dominance, and self-esteem) based on free testosterone *and* sensitivity to androgen as calculated by CAG repeat lengths (Vermeersch et al. 2010). Another factor in how men respond to androgen is the coactivators that are present near the receptors.

54. Wingfield et al. 2006.

55. Aikey et al. 2002.

56. Hermans, Ramsey, and van Honk 2008. See also Hermans et al. 2006; van Honk, Peper, and Schutter 2005.

57. Greenwell 2002. See also Kryger 2007:143.

58. Nielsen, Pelsen, and Sørensen, et al. 1988.

59. Terburga, Morgan, and van Honk et al. 2009.

60. Coccaro et al. 1998.

61. Liening and Josephs 2010.

62. Delville, Mansour, and Ferris 1996.

63. Hermans, Ramsey, and van Honk 2008.

64. Trainor et al. 2006.

65. Trainor et al. 2006.

66. Trainor et al. 2006.

67. Nathan, Cahill, and Gardner 1963.

68. Rolf et al. 2002.

69. Isidori et al. 2005.

70. Lee et al. 2003.

71. Jaminet and Jaminet 2010; Sisson 2012.

72. Bhasin et al. 2007.

CHAPTER 8. HOW TO USE HORMONES SAFELY

1. I recommend you see the anti-aging doctor primarily for hormones and keep your family doctor for all other general health issues and referrals to specialists.

2. Both documents are widely available online, including at All Things Male, http://www.allthingsmale.com/publications.html (accessed September 2, 2012).

3. The underarm testosterone "Teddy" received was Axiron®, which costs around $300 per bottle after a free trial.

4. Crisler 2009:2.

5. Shibayama et al. 2009.

6. Worthman and Stallings 1997.

7. The bioavailable testosterone blood test has been called "the gold standard for serum androgen evaluation" (Crisler 2009:3).

8. Crisler 2004:16–17.

9. Crisler 2004:16–17. See also Shogo, Forchielli, and Dorfman 1963. Gonadotropins significantly increase side-chain cleavage of cholesterol, boosting levels of downstream hormones (Scott et al. 1990).

10. Sahelian 1997. Those who have experimented with hallucinogens have compared pregnenolone to a much milder form of LSD in the way it sharpens the enjoyment of sensory input, including taste, vision, and touch (Sahelian 1997). One of the reasons young people gradually awaken to a love of music in their teen years is undoubtedly because hormones, including pregnenolone and DHEA, are at a maximum level. Pregnenolone levels peak at age sixteen through seventeen, and 17a-Hydroxypregnenolone levels peak between eighteen through twenty (Hill et al. 2005).

11. Lee, Zava, and Hopkins 2002. See also Hopkins n.d.a.

12. Lee, Zava, and Hopkins 2002:163.

13. Lee, Zava, and Hopkins 2002:153–71. Estriol may even be efficacious in the fight against existing metastatic breast cancer (Lee et al. 2002:164).

14. In this article, the terminology is a bit strange—the term *low potency estrogen* is used to refer to estriol, and *local estrogen* is used to refer to estriol cream. In any case, no increase in breast cancer for "local estrogen" use is found (Rosenberg et al. 2006).

15. Holtorf 2009:78.

16. Brinton, Hoover, and Fraumeni Jr. 1983. Other studies suggest that a woman's age at first birth is not as important as number of children in conferring protection against breast cancer (Layde et al. 1989).

17. Hermsmeyer et al. 2008.

18. Canonico et al. 2007.

19. Is it possible to explain the rest of the adverse effects of the 2002 WHI study simply as a case of depriving women of the testosterone they need to maintain their health? The

2002 WHI study reported that there was also a significant increase in coronary heart disease, stroke, and blood clots in the women receiving HRT. The blood clots can be explained by the fact that horse estrogen was being taken orally. There doesn't appear to be any correlation between testosterone and heart disease or strokes, meaning there's no difference whether women have normal, slightly below-normal, or above-normal levels of testosterone. Put more simply, a woman taking testosterone would not lower her risk of heart disease or stroke if she started with normal or slightly below-normal levels of testosterone. The only exception is for women who have the lowest 20 percent of endogenous testosterone (Sievers et al. 2010), who had significantly more heart disease and strokes, and who would presumably benefit most from testosterone replacement therapy.

20. There is a synthetic form of testosterone called methyltestosterone that used to be administered to men. It was given in an oral form, and eventually it was determined that it was too dangerous—longtime usage caused liver damage in some men (Nieschlag 1998). Methyltestosterone was even combined with horse estrogen to treat some menopausal women. However, this combination roughly doubled the chances of a woman developing breast cancer (Tamimi et al. 2006).

21. One exception to this recommendation against oral delivery is the observation that pregnenolone is probably best administered with tablets under the tongue (Sahelian 1997). Oral administration is also safe for DHEA (Panjari et al. 2009). With oral delivery, a patient swallows a product; with sublingual, he puts it under his tongue, where it's absorbed into the venous circulation, largely bypassing the liver. Inevitably, however, some sublingual product is ingested and processed through the digestive tract, reaching the liver, which is why hormones that aren't suitable for oral use are also not recommended for sublingual delivery. Pregnenolone and DHEA, however, can be taken orally, sublingually, and topically.

22. On the other hand, John Crisler, DO, is of the opinion that transdermal is the best way to deliver hormones. "The constant variability of serum androgens provided by T gels mimic the hormones of a young man; the stable daily level provided by T injections mimic the hormones of an old man; those of implantable pellets mimic the hormones of no one" (Crisler 2004:7). On October 31, 2012, he posted a YouTube® video advocating the subcutaneous injection of testosterone (http://www.youtube.com/watch?v=n98LOFQwUGA).

23. There is some evidence, however, that estriol can be used to fight existing breast cancer (Lee, Zava, and Hopkins 2002. See also Hopkins n.d.a, and Holtorf 2009).

24. Holtorf 2009.

25. Holtorf 2009. That one study is Lippman, Monaco, and Bolan 1977. This result is totally expected. When only estriol is administered to a breast cancer tissue culture, sufficiently high levels of estriol can take the place of estradiol and bind to ER-alpha. However, when both estradiol and estriol are present, estriol will interfere with the binding of estradiol to ER-alpha, which is why all the studies not using tissue cultures demonstrated that estriol exhibited anticancer properties.

26. "Acting alone, estriol is a weak estrogen, but when given with estradiol, it functions as an antiestrogen. Interestingly, estriol competitively inhibits estradiol binding and also inhibits activated receptor binding to estrogen response elements, which limits transcription" (Holtorf 2009).

27. Men with estradiol significantly above or below this optimal range experienced much higher mortality rates, emphasizing the need for neither too high nor too low levels of estradiol, and again underscoring the necessity of periodic blood tests during HRT (Jankowska et al. 2009).

28. van Landeghem et al. 1985.

29. Balunas et al. 2008.

30. It is important to measure estradiol with a sensitive assay for males. As Dr. Crisler observes, "Unless you specify a 'sensitive' assay for your male patients, the lab will default to the standard estradiol designed for females, which is useless for our purposes here. I have run the standard assay and the sensitive assay concurrently on a number of my patients, and the two results may be as night and day. However, patient symptomology is best described by the sensitive assay" (Crisler 2009:4).

31. For an answer to the question "If local levels of estradiol in the prostate are not dependent on serum levels of estradiol, then why would an aromatase inhibitor help the prostate?" see chapter 9.

32. Chen et al. 2006.

33. The DO degree (Doctor of Osteopathic Medicine) is in every essential way equivalent to an MD (Medical Doctor) degree.

34. Hoyos et al. 2012.

35. Bixler et al. 2001.

36. Morgentaler 2006.

37. Basaria et al. 2010.

38. Basaria et al. 2010. This study was criticized for its failure to include aromatase inhibitors in a transdermal protocol administered to elderly men, a puzzling error, especially in light of the fact that it's now common knowledge that men convert transdermal testosterone into estrogen and that this estrogen needs to be controlled with aromatase inhibitors (Joyal 2010).

39. Liu, Death, and Handelsman 2003.

40. Phillips et al. 1983.

41. Basaria et al. 2012.

42. Basaria et al. 2010.

43. Not all men experience increased estradiol when using testosterone; some see estradiol decrease. "I do not use an AI [aromatase inhibitor] initially, even when E2 [estradiol] is elevated, because some patients will actually see a drop in estrogen over baseline on follow-up. We would have otherwise added an unnecessary (and relatively expensive) medication" (Crisler 2009:13). Men with abdominal body fat produce more estradiol

(Cohen 1999). In addition, local levels of estradiol in certain tissue, such as prostate cancer tissue, can be higher than serum levels because certain tissue has significant aromatase, an enzyme that converts testosterone to estradiol (Simpson et al. 2002). Aromatase within the prostate is normally present "in the stroma of benign tissue, while in malignancy there is an [increase in] epithelial [aromatase]" (Ellem and Risbridger 2006).

CHAPTER 9. THE BIG PICTURE

1. Prostate epithelial cells will be referred to as **normal prostate cells** in the rest of this book.
2. Litvinov, De Marzo, and Isaacs 2003.
3. Geck et al. 2000.
4. Src is a tyrosine kinase enzyme associated with tumors (Chieffi et al. 2003).
5. Nanni et al. 2002.
6. Singh et al. 2006.
7. Taylor, Tolvanen, and Risbridger 2010.
8. Taylor et al. 2012.
9. Garber 2010.
10. Martikainen and Isaacs 1990.
11. In the former case, all the cancer cells have to do to survive is have a high enough level of anti-apoptotic proteins or other mutations that prevent apoptosis due to calcium ion overload. On the other hand, if testosterone is essential for cell division, then really major mutations must occur for it to cause prostate cancer in cells that cannot bind to androgen. In fact, when Bcl-2 is added to a prostate cancer cell line (LNCaP) that needs testosterone to grow, it can now grow in the absence of testosterone (Raffo et al. 1995). Chalk one up for my point of view.
12. Cell division stops at the same point in all these cells (Bai et al. 2005).
13. Castagnetta et al. 1995.
14. Even if apoptosis never finishes (LNCaP is more resistant to apoptosis from low levels of testosterone than normal prostate cells).
15. Friedman 2007.
16. This natural decline in performance is one reason why many athletes look to steroids for help. Although it is against the rules of Major League Baseball to use performance-enhancing drugs, a better option would be to let players bring their hormone levels into the high-normal range as they age so that they can perform at their optimal ability. I fully realize that some athletes, and some young people, abuse steroids by taking more than are needed, and as a result they suffer negative consequences. But under an anti-aging doctor's supervision, such problems would be unlikely to occur, which is why it is

so important to encourage adults to consult a trained physician who has experience with bioidentical hormones.

17. Friedman 2007.

18. Good progesterone also plays a role in fighting breast cancer (Wiebe et al. 2000). See also Wiebe 2006. I suspect that men with BRCA1 or BRCA2 mutations may have a situation similar to breast tissue in women, in which there is almost all progesterone receptor A and no receptor B so that progesterone should increase Bcl-2 levels. In any case, the presence of either of these BRCA mutations increases the lifetime risk of prostate cancer being diagnosed in men (Liede et al. 2004).

19. Even autopsy studies fail to find prostate cancer in young men.

20. Wilbert, Griffin, and Wilson 1983.

21. Kuiper et al. 1997.

22. Risbridger et al. 2003.

23. Kjellman et al. 2008.

24. Berges et al. 1995.

25. Assuming that none of those cells have a mutation that decreases the rate of cell death enough for them to survive even though the tipping point has not been reached.

26. Even though the cell population will not be increasing, with the rate of cell growth and the rate of cell death both being around two months.

27. Stathopoulos et al. 2003.

28. Dambaki et al. 2005.

29. Takeda et al. 1996.

30. Hatzoglou et al. 2005.

31. There is a minimum amount of pro-apoptotic proteins needed to kill a cancer cell. One reason that high testosterone will be worse for cancer is that it lowers the threshold of membrane androgen receptor necessary to produce this amount of pro-apoptotic proteins.

32. Bonkhoff and Berges 2009.

33. Demichelis et al. 2007.

34. Sekine et al. 2007.

35. Krieg, Nassi, and Tunn 1993.

36. The male teen range for *total* testosterone is 300 to 1,200 ng/dL; the range for *free* testosterone is 9 to 30 ng/dL.; the top of the normal range for adult men is around 950 ng/dL (Mayo Medical Clinic).

37. Isbarn et al. 2009. See also Morgentaler and Rhoden 2006.

38. Parsons et al. 2005.

39. In theory, elderly men with very low testosterone levels who have not yet been diagnosed with prostate cancer should have less biopsy-detected prostate cancer than similar men with higher levels of testosterone. This has recently been shown to be true (Muller et al. 2012).

40. Berges et al. 1995.
41. Gray et al. 1991.
42. Hyde et al. 2012.
43. Kapoor et al. 2006.
44. Cherrier et al. 2004.
45. McAllister et al. 2010.
46. Jonsson et al. 2012.
47. Shores et al. 2006.
48. López-Otín and Diamandis 1998.
49. Löfgren et al. 2006.
50. Sabourin et al. 1994.
51. Dimitrakakis and Bondy 2009.
52. Nanni et al. 2002.
53. Löfgren et al. 2006; Shaaban et al. 2003.
54. Gonzalez et al. 2008.
55. Pich et al. 1999.
56. This is the primary reason why women are at a greater risk of developing Alzheimer's than men.
57. Davison et al. 2005.
58. Carroll et al. 2010.
59. See, e.g., Kurzweil and Grossman 2004.
60. Follingstad 1978.
61. Sieri et al. 2009. The fact that testosterone is converted into estradiol doesn't mean that women should avoid supplementing with testosterone. Testosterone replacement can provide many unique positive effects in aging women, including boosting libido. But when using testosterone, it's important to use an aromatase inhibitor and/or measure hormone levels before and after supplementation to protect against excessive amounts of estradiol, one of the chief culprits in carcinogenesis.
62. "Woody Allen," The Quotations Page, http://www.quotationspage.com/quote/52.html (accessed February 15, 2013).

CHAPTER 10. PREVENTION THEORY

1. Santen, Yue, and Heitan 2012.
2. Krishnan, Swami, and Feldman 2012.
3. Korach 1994.
4. You may be wondering why I'm recommending taking an aromatase inhibitor (the chief function of which is to *reduce* local levels of estradiol) *and* also recommending *raising*

serum estradiol. The answer is that the level of estradiol inside breast cancer cells is not directly correlated to the serum level of estradiol but rather depends on local aromatase activity (van Landeghem et al. 1985).

CHAPTER 11. PREVENTION PRACTICE

1. Lachman and Firth 2004:328.

2. Before we get into the specifics for men and women, it may be useful to note that people with breast cancer or prostate cancer should avoid refined sugar and products that contain refined sugar. High sugar intake has been linked to increased IGF-1 levels, and high IGF-1 levels have been linked to an increased growth rate of almost all cancers, not just breast and prostate cancer.

3. In this study, the male mice lacking aromatase but containing a mutation that caused Alzheimer's-like symptoms ended up with twice the normal level of testosterone. *These mice demonstrated a better memory than normal mice* (McAllister et al. 2010).

4. Michael F. Holick, a vitamin D pioneer at Boston University, makes a convincing case for obtaining vitamin D preferentially through appropriate exposure to sunlight (or UVB tanning beds in winter months in northern latitudes), with oral supplementation as a backup strategy (Holick 2010).

5. Faloon 2012b.

6. A reference range is generally defined as the level found in 90 percent of test subjects, excluding the lowest and highest 5 percent. "Test ID: TTFB," Mayo Clinic, http://www.mayomedicallaboratories.com/test-catalog/Clinical+and+Interpretive/83686 (accessed August 7, 2012).

7. Prescriptions for supplementation will not be written by most general practitioners, who mistakenly believe that the normal range is adequate for health. If you wish to get your testosterone into optimal range, you will usually have success only by visiting an anti-aging doctor who understands the value of bioidentical hormone replacement therapy.

8. "Testosterone Replacement Therapy," Cleveland Clinic, http://my.clevelandclinic.org/services/testosterone_replacement_therapy/hic_testosterone_replacement_therapy.aspx (accessed June 14, 2012).

9. Donating blood is an effective way for men to reduce excess iron. Since menstruating women lose iron every month, they usually don't have this problem. The best test for iron is serum ferritin. Aim for levels between 40–60 ng/mL (Mercola 2009b).

10. "Adding HCG to Testosterone Replacement Therapy," Steroidology.com, March 31, 2010, http://www.steroidology.com/adding-hcg-to-testosterone-replacement-therapy/ (accessed October 17, 2012).

11. Jankowska et al. 2009.

12. When testing for estradiol, men need to use the sensitive assay for males (Crisler 2009:4).

13. Landau et al. 2012. However, no convincing explanation for how mental activity protects against Alzheimer's has been advanced. It is entirely possible that geriatric mental activity is not protective but is rather a result or side effect of having high-normal hormone levels. In other words, while there is admittedly an association between mental activity and lack of dementia, there is no evidence that mental activity *causes* lack of dementia (Zamosky n.d.). It is entirely possible that some third variable—such as high hormone levels—causes both geriatric mental activity and an absence of dementia.

14. Cao et al. 2012. An even stronger link has been found between caffeine consumption and protection against Parkinson's (Palacios et al. 2012).

15. Venkateswaran et al. 2007.

16. Davis et al. 2012.

17. Davis 2011:96.

18. Kristal and Lampe 2002.

19. Chen et al. 2005.

20. Luk et al. 2011.

21. Lakshman et al. 2008.

22. White et al. 2010.

23. Chau et al. 2007.

24. Price et al. 2006.

25. Price et al. 2006.

26. Bettuzzi et al. 2006.

27. Bettuzzi et al. 2006.

28. Luk et al. 2010.

29. Yang et al. 2012.

30. Vucenik and Shamsuddin 2003.

31. Paoletti et al. 2004.

32. Shankle and Amen 2005:110–11.

33. Hopkins n.d.b.

34. Pirskanen et al. 2005.

35. Calderón-Garcidueñas 2004.

36. Morinaga et al. 2007.

37. Takahashi et al. 2000.

38. Goss et al. 2011.

39. The real dilemma would be if progesterone receptor A turned out to protect against Alzheimer's (which I suspect it doesn't). In that case, progesterone would be more protective against Alzheimer's for women with BRCA1 and BRCA2 mutations, but it would increase the risk of breast cancer for those women because they have lots of progesterone receptor A in their breasts, which increases harmful Bcl-2.

40. Poole et al. 2006.
41. Song, Coghlan, and Gelmann 2004.
42. Basina et al. 2012.
43. Bouker and Hilakavi-Clarke 2000.
44. Bosetti et al. 2012.
45. Zhang et al. 2009.
46. Green tea fights cancer "through multiple mechanisms such as anti-oxidation, induction of apoptosis, inhibition of angiogenesis and metastasis" (Li, Yu. et al. 2010). In addition, "EGCG can prevent and inhibit breast tumorigenesis independently of ER status" (Li, Yu. et al. 2010). One of the newly discovered ways that green tea fights hormone-resistant (estrogen receptor alpha-negative) breast cancer—a more aggressive cancer—is that EGCG (a main component of green tea) reactivates estrogen receptor-alpha expression, making cells more sensitive to chemotherapy with tamoxifen and other drugs (Li, Yu. et al. 2010).
47. Petrova et al. 2005.
48. Smith-Warner et al. 1998.
49. A number of mechanisms have been proposed to explain the association between alcohol consumption and breast cancer, including "alcohol's interaction and effect on oestrogen secretion; number of oestrogen receptors; the generation of acetaldehyde and hydroxyl free radicals; cells migration and metastasis; secretion of IGF1 and interaction with HRT and folate metabolism" (Al-Sader et al. 2009).
50. Kumle et al. 2002.
51. Kim et al. 2012
52. For example, a novel approach to prevention involves extract of eggplant that has anticancer properties for breast cancer and may also confer immunity. Researchers reported that their approach can be injected or applied topically and that it may be superior to other forms of therapy in that it induces apoptosis of cancer cells while sparing normal cells (Cham and Chase 2012).

CHAPTER 12. A NEW TREATMENT PROTOCOL

1. Numerous clinical trials are currently being conducted to test the best way to use testosterone to fight prostate cancer. To date, the most successful physician who uses testosterone as one of his primary tools to fight prostate cancer is Dr. Robert Leibowitz, MD, the director of Compassionate Oncology. Although he has had great success, my protocol, described in this chapter, will suggest ways to improve on his already phenomenal results.
2. "Prostate Cancer Treatment: Treatment Option Overview," National Cancer Institute, http://www.cancer.gov/cancertopics/pdq/treatment/prostate/HealthProfessional/page4 (accessed September 2, 2012).

3. Although taking vitamin D3 is almost always very beneficial, in a small fraction of cases, advanced cancers might mutate to the point where even this treatment would speed up cancer growth (Stambolsky et al. 2010). If this happens, stopping vitamin D3 supplementation would slow down the rate of cancer growth.

4. Numerous drugs and supplements reduce dihydrotestosterone (DHT) by interfering with 5-alpha-reductase (5AR), reducing the conversion of testosterone to DHT, including mushrooms, saw palmetto (Serenoa repens), nettle root extract, *Epilobium*, progesterone, beta-sitosterol, enterolactones, ECG, EgCG, and finasteride. Enterolactones also provide another useful function, inhibiting the enzymes 17-beta hydroxysteroid dehydrogenases (HSDs), which convert estrone to the most harmful estrogen, estradiol.

5. The reason you should avoid strong SERMs like soy and flaxseed when taking 5-alpha-reductase (5AR) inhibitors (which prevent the conversion of testosterone to DHT) is that 5AR inhibitors (like finasteride) reduce DHT too much. True, DHT is essential for initial prostate cancer growth because it protects cancer from membrane androgen receptor-induced apoptosis, but DHT plays even more of a role in *fighting* prostate cancer. If you reduce DHT too much, you'll increase Bcl-2, and you don't want to increase Bcl-2, since it helps prostate cancer grow. (Note: DHT has a contradictory action: it reduces Bcl-2 a lot by binding to intracellular androgen receptor (iAR) at the same time it increases Bcl-2 a little by binding to mAR. Experiments show that its binding to iAR has more of an effect than its binding to mAR, so DHT results in a net reduction in Bcl-2.) Remember that Bcl-2 is a harmful anti-apoptotic protein that protects prostate cancer by preventing it from dying. Reducing DHT increases harmful Bcl-2, and SERMs increase harmful Bcl-2 (by interfering with the binding of estradiol to ER-beta), and the combination of the two can be extremely detrimental. Dr. Leibowitz observed rapidly increasing PSAs in his patients who used this combination, which usually dropped back down after the SERMs were discontinued (http://www.compassionateoncology.org/pdfs/RECOMMENDEDVITAMINLIST.050305.pdf [accessed October 16, 2012]).

6. Lu-Yao and Yao 1997.

7. In my opinion for surgery to be curative, all the cancer cells must be removed, which means that biochemical failures do not qualify (Boorjian et al. 2011).

8. Karakiewicz et al. 1998.

9. Potosky et al. 2004.

10. "PSA Rising after Prostate Cancer Therapy—Now What?" *PCRI Insights* 14 no. 3 (August 2011), http://prostate-cancer.org/PDFs/Is14-3_p10-14.pdf (accessed November 3, 2012).

11. Zietman 1999.

12. Doctors from Sweden published a paper comparing surgical removal of the prostate with watchful waiting for men with localized prostate cancer and an average PSA of 13.5. During the ten years after the men received surgery, 8.6 percent died from prostate cancer and 15.3 percent died from other causes (Bill-Axelson et al. 2005).

13. Roundy, Turner, and Leibowitz 2011.

14. Bill-Axelson et al. 2005.

15. Hatzoglou et al. 2005.

16. This patient was still alive, according to the last posting about him on Dr. Leibowitz's website in 2007 ("TRT Case Reports," http://www.compassionateoncology.org/pdfs/TRTcase_reports-05-09.pdf [accessed November 3, 2012]).

17. Phytochemicals sometimes kill cancer via mechanisms other than binding to hormone receptors and upregulating pro-apoptotic proteins. Like mercenary soldiers, they have ingenious cancer-killing techniques. EGCG in green tea, for instance, is an effective killer that fights cancer through multiple modalities.

18. "Bad progesterone" refers to 5alpha-pregnanes (Wiebe 2006).

19. It should be noted that there are class-action lawsuits against Merck, the maker of Propecia® (finasteride to prevent hair loss), claiming it permanently reduces sexual function. Dr. John Crisler is critical of finasteride and has vowed never to use it in his practice. It is my opinion, however, that these claims stem from the fact that users of the drug are mostly elderly and were suffering from sexual dysfunction even before using finasteride.

20. Finasteride inhibits type II 5-alpha-reductase, whereas dutasteride inhibits type I and type II 5-alpha-reductase. Type II is the dominant type within the prostate.

21. Leibowitz et al. 2010.

22. Umekita et al. 1996.

23. Keep in mind that even if the PSA doesn't drop, the protocol is still successful if it results in enough of a decrease in PSA velocity. For example, if your PSA still rises, but the PSA doubling time is fifteen years, it would typically take about 150 years for prostate cancer to kill you—so that treatment protocol can be considered a success.

24. Less than one year after Dr. Leibowitz's patient had his PSA below 2, the PSA rose to almost 4. Dr. Leibowitz then discontinued testosterone supplementation and the patient's testosterone level dropped to below castrate level and the PSA became undetectable. However, this patient never received an aromatase inhibitor (AI), and the increase in PSA may well have been due to increased estradiol. The flaw in giving testosterone without an AI is that there's no way to know whether the results (good or bad) are due to the effects of the androgen receptors or the effects of the estrogen receptors. In the long run, testosterone supplementation without AIs will always turn out badly, since prostate cancer cells with lots of ER-alpha will receive a huge survival benefit over other prostate cancer cells and will eventually dominate the population. Modern AIs are either anastrozole or exemestane.

25. "Antiangiogenic Cocktail," Compassionate Oncology Medical Group, http://www.compassionateoncology.org/pdfs/AntiangiogenicCocktail082508.pdf (accessed November 13, 2012). Related articles are available at http://www.compassionateoncology.org/publications.php.

26. It bears repeating that whenever a drug such as finasteride is used that results in low dihydrotestosterone, strong SERMs (such as soy and flaxseed) should be eliminated from your diet.

27. These pro-apoptotic cancer killers include proteins such as BAD and Fas. Here's one case where "bad" is good.

28. Coffey et al. 2003.

29. In this analogy, the crack in the hourglass signifies an unlikely mutation that can't be successfully treated with this alternating hormone therapy.

30. Hatzoglou et al. 2005.

31. Hatzoglou et al. 2005.

32. Gourlay and Ayscough 2005; White et al. 2001.

33. Moss et al. 2006.

34. At some point, a mutation might arise that grows at maximum speed independent of androgen receptors, or a mutation might arise that causes testosterone to increase the growth rate to maximum independent of the amount of DHT present. This is the equivalent of a crack in the hourglass. This kind of mutation would be rare, and if it occurred, would be random. So while it is possible that the very first cancer cell might have such a mutation, it almost certainly would take many, many years before such a devastatingly harmful mutation occurred.

35. Because the genetics are identical in noncancerous prostate cells, there must be a random process involved that determines which cells will show this increase and which will not. To expand on this, if 80 percent of cancer cells show this increase, whereas 100 percent of normal cells show this increase, then the logical conclusion would be that those cancer cells—cells we know contain a heterogeneous makeup—whose genetics are susceptible to showing this increase were the ones responsible for the 80 percent increase. In that case, this protocol would work for only one cycle, after which the only cells present would be those not susceptible to this increase. However, since normal cells also show this 80 percent increase, then the increase can't be due to different responses due to different genetic makeups. It must be due to random chance, which means that every time you do this treatment, you would expect to see 80 percent of cells with lots more iAR, even those cells that showed no increase in iAR the previous time they were treated (Hsieh et al. 2011).

36. It is possible that men with a varicocele may benefit more by not using external testosterone. For these men, if the testosterone produced by the testicles enters the prostate at levels around a hundred times higher than what is in the blood serum, then external testosterone should be avoided, since it shuts down the production of testosterone by the testicles.

37. Friedman 2012. Three months would allow for the destruction of those prostate cancer cells that didn't divide without staying longer than needed in either of these two treatments. When the cells divide, iAR won't necessarily be divided equally, and the buildup of pro-apoptotic proteins will be diluted. Essentially, after a cell divides, you have to start all over on the process of killing it. You could think about it like a bathtub overflowing. Imagine a bathtub filling up with pro-apoptotic proteins, and once it overflows you've killed the cell. In this analogy, cell division would be like pulling the plug in the bathtub and letting half the liquid drain. If no plug is pulled, you would get the overflow and kill the cell, but once the plug is pulled, you would have to start up again, although not from scratch, since you're still halfway there. From our discussion in chapter 4, we know that low Gleason (the Gleason scale is a measure of the aggressiveness of prostate cancer, with higher numbers representing more aggression) prostate cancer cells die on average every seventy days, and high Gleason PCa cells die on average every seventy-six days. However, there's a substantial standard deviation, so by going ninety days, we're more likely to kill all the cells that didn't divide and in this way reduce the size of the prostate tumor.

38. Nanda et al. 2009.

39. Cells that will die more rapidly in the presence of estradiol (cells with lots of ER-beta) should already be dead, and cells that survived (which have lots of ER-alpha) would be expected to thrive in the presence of estradiol; and an AI reduces estradiol, thus reducing the risk of cancer.

40. Because of the potential harm that high local levels of estradiol can cause, it makes sense to totally block aromatase activity. However, the problem with doing this is that having too little estradiol can cause other health problems. One solution would be to totally block aromatase activity and then add enough *estriol* to maintain overall health. Since estriol preferentially binds to ER-beta (which is known to reduce inflammation, downregulate Bcl-2 production, and help prevent Alzheimer's), this should result in other health benefits as well as helping fight prostate cancer. Unfortunately, the ideal serum level of estriol (if used in place of estradiol) has not yet been determined.

41. Gandy et al. 2001.

42. For any men considering androgen deprivation, there is one other important consideration to keep in mind. Researchers who uncovered the fact that defects in internal spermatic veins raise the local level of testosterone in the prostate stated that if a man does have such a defect (usually a varicocele) and undergoes androgen deprivation, typically the testosterone level in his prostate will be roughly the same as that of a man without the defect who does not undergo androgen deprivation (Gat, Joshua, and Gornish 2009). There is no telling how many men have undergone androgen deprivation and suffered through its side effects without realizing that, since they did not undergo the surgery necessary to correct the defect in their internal spermatic vein, they did not even lower the testosterone level in their prostate to below what it normally is for most men.

43. Webb and Collins 2010.

44. Laaksonen et al. 2004.

45. Morsink et al. 2007.

46. Moffat et al. 2004.

47. Morgentaler and Rhoden 2006.

48. One recent study found that less than one-fourth of the men had any problem with increased red blood count in seventy-two men followed for two years (Hajjar, Kaiser, and Morley 1997).

49. Dr. John Crisler, a leader in the use of testosterone replacement therapy (TRT), favors the use of transdermal gels (Crisler 2009; Crisler 2004). Both documents are widely available online, and both are an excellent summary of how to do blood tests before and after TRT, how to use TRT for best effect, and how to use human chorionic gonadotropin (HCG) as an adjunct to TRT. Also of note is that while most doctors are familiar with only intramuscular testosterone injections, new research indicates that subcutaneous injections (through an insulin needle) are equally effective—and much less painful.

50. Canonico et al. 2007.

51. Unfortunately, there are no clinical studies yet using my treatment protocol because it is too new for any clinical studies to have been done.

52. Since prostate cancer typically grows so slowly, a fifteen-year study (and more patients) is needed in order to definitively find out how well any protocol, including my Systemic Treatment Protocol, is working. Ideally, this book will result in more researchers exploring these treatment options.

53. Isaacs et al. 2012.

54. Iverson, Madsen, and Corle 1995.

55. Shores et al. 2006.

56. Kjellman et al. 2008.

57. Wang et al. 2008.

58. Both high testosterone alone and high testosterone plus finasteride lead to a better quality of life.

59. Lu-Yao and Yao 1997.

60. You'll have to put up with a lot of pressure from your urologist if you have a high PSA and refuse a biopsy. But in my opinion, you *should* refuse the biopsy, since the procedure risks spreading bacteria, no matter how much you doctor claims that the needle is too thin to cause bacteria to escape into the bloodstream. A small number of men are dying from biopsies due to infection by antibiotic-resistant bacteria. While the percentage is very small, if you're the one who dies, you won't care what the percentage was, especially since the percentage is zero if you don't undergo a biopsy. A recent study indicated that biopsies increased the percentage of men who required hospitalization within thirty days of the procedure by 4.2 percent (Loeb et al. 2011). There's also a small but real possibility that a needle biopsy might spread prostate cancer. See, e.g., Bastacky et al. 1991. In all fairness, there may not be a large risk since prostate cancer cells that are in the bloodstream may not easily be able to metastasize to other parts of the body.

CHAPTER 13. THE STANDARD TREATMENT FOR BREAST CANCER

1. Treating breast cancer presents more of a challenge than treating prostate cancer. PSA is a fairly reliable marker for monitoring prostate cancer progression, although some rare, extremely aggressive prostate cancers do not produce PSA. However, there is no such reliable marker for monitoring breast cancer progression, although some markers are known to be produced by a significant proportion of breast cancers.

2. There are a number of different classifications of breast cancer, and doctors try to tailor their treatment protocols to optimize their success rate for the type of cancer they're treating. For simplicity's sake, we'll address the standard therapeutic protocols usually followed.

3. "Breast Cancer," Mayo Clinic, http://www.mayoclinic.org/breast-cancer/treatment.html (accessed November 3, 2012).

4. Presumably, estrogen receptor–positive cells contain mostly estrogen receptor-alpha. However, to be scientifically accurate, doctors should determine how much estrogen receptor-alpha and how much estrogen receptor-beta is present. Premenopausal estrogen receptor–negative women actually benefit from tamoxifen if they have estrogen receptor-beta (Gruvberger-Sahl et al. 2007).

5. Right now, systemic treatment of breast cancer is pretty much limited to attacking the production of protection by ER-alpha. Since ER-alpha increases Bcl-2, attacking this receptor decreases Bcl-2 and therefore increases the rate of cell death. The drug tamoxifen works by blocking ER-alpha (and ER-beta as well) directly. Aromatase inhibitors work by reducing the amount of estradiol converted from testosterone. The fact that these drugs are so effective highlights the importance of attacking protection. However, if attacking protection is the goal, then the most effective way to accomplish this is by using androgens to bind to the androgen receptors.

6. In addition, a drug should be used that blocks ER-alpha but not ER-beta. Currently, there is such a drug called toremifene, which can be added to treatment. In low dosages, the side effects of toremifene are minimal. However, if too much toremifene is given, it blocks ER-beta too. It's not clear exactly what dosage needs to be given to each individual woman to block only ER-alpha. (I would be more willing to recommend a drug if it blocked only ER-alpha at all dosages, but no such drug is currently FDA-approved.) Once ER-alpha is blocked, adding estriol may further decrease protection by binding to ER-beta. There are no known adverse side effects from adding estriol. Finally, it would be useful to block the membrane estrogen receptor, but no drug is yet available to do that. This combination should first be used in animal studies to see if in fact it can totally eliminate early-stage breast cancer.

7. Desta et al. 2004.

8. Early Breast Cancer Trialists' Collaborative Group 2011.

9. Mundhenke, Schem, and Jonat 2008.

10. Arimidex, Tamoxifen, Alone or in Combination (ATAC) Trialists' Group 2008.

11. Smith and Dowsett 2003.

12. Tai et al. 2004.

13. "Large Review Study Confirms Herceptin's Benefits," BREASTCANCER.ORG, http://www.breastcancer.org/treatment/targeted_therapies/new_research/20120420.jsp (accessed November 3, 2012).

14. Slamon et al. 2001.

15. Cutler and Schlemenson 1948.

16. Glaser 2010.

17. Tieszen et al. 2011.

18. One other important thing that finasteride does is to prevent the formation of "bad progesterone." This increases the odds that the breast cancer treatment I discussed may actually be curative. It also improves the effectiveness of the finasteride arm in prostate cancer when you alternate between finasteride and high testosterone.

19. Fjelldal et al. 2010.

20. It is known that some breast cancers are lacking intracellular androgen receptors. To maximize survival, breast cancer should eventually eliminate membrane androgen receptor as well. However, if membrane androgen receptors were to be eliminated before intracellular androgen receptors, then breast cancer would no longer be able to proliferate. It is not known if there are any cases of both intracellular and membrane androgen receptors being eliminated, largely because breast cancer researchers have almost totally ignored the membrane androgen receptor.

21. Alevizopoulos et al. 2008.

22. This protocol is expected to be effective against human breast cancer since it has already been shown to be effective for a combination of testosterone conjugated with beef serum albumin (Kampa et al. 2005).

23. There is one type of drug that has not yet been discovered, but it may well be able to cure both breast cancer and prostate cancer. If any drug company were to develop a drug that safely and effectively blocks membrane androgen receptor, then this drug, along with sex-appropriate teenage levels of testosterone plus an aromatase inhibitor, should stop any breast cancer or prostate cancer cell that has functional intracellular androgen receptor from being able to proliferate. This is because the only thing stopping the intracellular androgen receptor from producing enough AS3 to stop the cancer from being able to proliferate is the action of the membrane androgen receptor opposing this.

From the point of view of a drug company, attempting to develop such a drug is a win-win financial investment. If the company succeeds in developing a drug that blocks (acts as an antagonist) only the membrane androgen receptor, then breast and prostate cancer patients from around the world would want this drug. On the other hand, if the company fails, and the best it can do is to develop a drug that stimulates (acts as an agonist) only the membrane androgen receptor, then breast and prostate cancer patients would still want this drug to help slow down the growth rate of their cancers. If the drug company ends up developing both types of drugs, then most patients would choose the drug that blocks the membrane receptor, but patients whose cancer lacks intracellular androgen receptors would use the drug that stimulates membrane androgen receptor.

24. Gordon et al. 2006.

25. According to Ray Kurzweil and Terry Grossman, nanotechnology is one of the more promising new health technologies that will revolutionize anti-aging medicine in our lifetime (Kurzweil and Grossman 2004:193–94).

26. Zahl, Getzsche, and Maehlen 2011.

27. There actually are two ways that testosterone (T) can promote the growth of breast cancer (BCa)—either through its conversion to estradiol or its conversion to 3-beta Adiol. Dr. Glaser's protocol stops the first possibility but does nothing to stop the second. However, I'm a strong believer in the adage "If it ain't broke, don't fix it," and Dr. Glaser is 100 percent successful so far. However, if some patient should have their BCa progress even with Dr. Glaser's protocol, then one improvement would be to add finasteride to prevent T from being converted to DHT and thereby preventing any 3-beta Adiol from being made. The downside of this is that DHT binds to iAR around five times more strongly than T does, so you would probably have to up the T level five times in order to compensate. Since nobody has given five times normal T to women before, this is something that should first be done in animal studies to verify that there are no adverse side effects. However, the principle is that for any woman with BCa that progresses under Dr. Glaser's protocol, there are improvements that may be possible. Of course, five times the ordinary amount of T with no DHT present would also increase the amount of pro-apoptotic proteins produced by mAR, so this might be a major improvement—possibly even curative, especially if combined with RU-486 plus progesterone.

28. Choudhuri et al. 2002.

29. Kim et al. 2002.

30. Scarlatti et al. 2003.

31. Arunasree 2010.

32. Rahman et al. 2000.

33. Hong et al. 2002.

34. Vucenik et al. 2005.

35. Li, Ya. et al. 2010.

36. Yu et al. 1999.

37. Kurzweil and Grossman do an excellent job of spelling out the optimal dosage for many supplements, including curcumin and green tea extract (Kurzweil and Grossman 2004:178, 217, 220, 334).

38. Kim Carollo, "Survival at a Cost: Common Cancer Treatment Carries Huge Risks," ABC News, March 7, 2012, http://abcnews.go.com/Health/radiation-therapy-linked-development-secondary-cancers-heart-disease/story?id=15864706#.UET9YKDi58E (accessed November 11, 2012).

39. The normal maximum is 1.9 ng/dL, so I would aim for a free testosterone level of 9.5 ng/dL.

40. If you're treating breast cancer (BCa) with five times the teenage levels of testosterone (T), finasteride, vitamin D3, and aromatase inhibitors, you can also add turkey tail mushroom extract (turkey tail mushrooms themselves are inedible). This will minimize Bcl-2 production (high T), increase pro-apoptotic proteins (high mAR/iAR ratio due to high T/DHT ratio), help kill BCa with vitamin D, and help kill BCa with turkey tail mushrooms. Turkey tail mushrooms are very effective against prostate cancer and should be effective against BCa too. Their only downside is that they block the conversion of T to DHT, but that's already being done by finasteride. The icing on the cake would be to add RU-486 plus progesterone, but the FDA has made it illegal to treat cancer patients with RU-486; it can only be used to induce abortions.

41. An intriguing new aromatase reducer, Myomin®, appears to have therapeutic value in reducing estradiol and estrone and increasing the most benign estrogen—estriol—providing a more favorable estrogen balance. It achieves this balance by blocking aromatase's conversion of testosterone to estradiol and blocking aromatase's conversion of androstenedione to estrone but leaving untouched estrone's conversion to estriol and DHEA's conversion to estriol (Chi 2012). Myomin can also be used by men to achieve a better estrogen balance and improve prostate health.

42. In theory, RU-486 could legally be used if permission is granted by an Institutional Review Board (IRB). However, in practice this is extremely unlikely to happen because IRBs are reluctant to approve any multipronged approach such as is detailed here.

43. Of course, once Rexin-G becomes FDA-approved in this country, there is no reason to go to another country for it.

CHAPTER 14. A NEW PROTOCOL FOR CURING EARLY-STAGE ALZHEIMER'S

1. Papasozomenos and Shanavas 2002.

2. No research has yet been published for patients with Alzheimer's disease being treated with the protocols I advocate in chapter 6. However, rumor has it that men who have initially been diagnosed with Alzheimer's and who have received testosterone at levels much greater than the low levels used in the 2005 study mentioned later in this chapter have seen their symptoms disappear.

3. I was unable to locate any studies at all involving estriol and the enzymes that produce or break down beta amyloid. However, I did find one researcher who pointed out that estrogen receptor-beta is an important target for the treatment of neurodegenerative diseases (Smith 2000).

4. As one expert points out, "Estriol binds to a different estrogen receptor (estrogen receptor-beta) that actually inhibits some of the undesirable effects of estradiol" (Clarke n.d.).

5. As one frustrated science writer put it, contemporary physicians aren't educated by medical schools, they're educated by pharmaceutical companies. "Clever marketing by drug companies creates thousands of confused doctors who, to this day, do not understand the difference between progestins and progesterone. It's right there in their medical school texts, but textbooks do not educate our doctors, drug companies educate our doctors" (Hopkins n.d.b).

6. Gouras et al. 2000.

7. Lu et al. 2006.

8. Shumaker et al. 2004.

9. Stomati et al. 2002.

10. "Investigating the Role of Testosterone in Alzheimer's Disease," McCusker Alzheimer's Research Foundation, http://www.alzheimers.com.au/research/testosterone.php (accessed November 1, 2012).

11. Rusanen et al. 2011.

12. Rossor 2003:85.

13. Rossor 2003:85.

14. "Interpretive Handbook," Mayo Clinic, http://www.mayomedicallaboratories.com/interpretive-guide/index.html?alpha=P&unit_code=8141 (accessed November 1, 2012).

15. Green et al. 2008.

16. Lim et al. 2001.

17. Perry et al. 2003; Akhondzadeh et al. 2003.

18. Pengelly et al. 2012.

19. Ryan Jaslow, "Three Cups of Coffee per Day Might Prevent Alzheimer's in Older Adults," CBS News, June 5, 2012, http://www.cbsnews.com/8301-504763_162-57447490-10391704/three-cups-of-coffee-per-day-might-prevent-alzheimers-in-older-adults/ (accessed November 1, 2012).

20. Van der Auwera et al. 2005.

21. Maalouf, Rho, and Mattson 2009.

22. Reger et al. 2004.

23. You can also cook with coconut oil. In addition, coconut butter has a similar composition to coconut oil. There is intriguing evidence that medium-chain triglycerides can help with weight reduction (St-Onge and Bosarge 2008; see also St-Onge et al. 2008, and Han et al. 2007).

24. "Alternative Treatments," alz.org, http://www.alz.org/alzheimers_disease_alternative_treatments.asp#Caprylic_Acid (accessed November 1, 2012).

CHAPTER 15. QUESTIONS AND ANSWERS

1. Oncolink 2012.
2. "Vitamin D Supplementation Viable for Reducing Pain during Breast Cancer Therapy," ASCO Daily News, http://chicago2012.asco.org/ASCODailyNews/Abstract 9000.aspx (accessed November 1, 2012).
3. Gallicchio et al. 2011.
4. Many anti-aging practitioners follow the adage "Start low and go slow."
5. Pijpe et al. 2012. Thermography may be a superior diagnostic tool for the detection of breast cancer because it can find tumors earlier and is a passive technique that involves no radiation or potentially harmful compression of breast tissue (Saputo 2010). Especially for younger women, the carcinogenic radiation risk of mammography may outweigh its value as a diagnostic tool (Nekolla, Griebel, and Brix 2008).
6. Shrivastava et al. 2006.
7. Stefanick et al. 2006.
8. Million Women Study Collaborators 2003.
9. Berges et al. 1995.
10. Moyer 2012.
11. Loeb et al. 2011.
12. In addition to vitamin D, sunlight's UVB rays produce "feel-good" endorphins and antimicrobial peptides that kill bacteria and viruses (Holick 2010; Zaslof 2005; Dorschner et al. 2001).
13. A significant amount of misinformation about sunlight is propagated by pharmaceutical companies that profit from sunscreen products.
14. Melanoma is more likely to result from severe sunburns, non-melanoma from non-burning sun exposure (Holick 2010).
15. Holick 2009. In a curious irony, Dr. Holick was fired from the dermatology department by a rather shortsighted chair after he recommended sun exposure in his book *The UV Advantage* (2004). Turns out Holick was right after all. He continues to receive prestigious awards for his vitamin D research (including the Merit Award from the National Institutes of Health), he's still a professor of medicine at Boston University Medical Center, and the dermatology department has embarrassed itself by sounding paranoid about reasonable sun exposure. Says Holick, "They continue to have blinders on" (Holick 2009). See also Wright 2011.
16. Tuohimaa et al. 2007.

17. Mercola 2013.
18. Morgentaler 2006:936.
19. Morgentaler and Traish 2009.
20. Morgentaler et al. 2011.
21. Umekita et al. 1996.
22. Hatzoglou et al. 2005.
23. Friedman 2011.
24. Roddam et al. 2008.
25. Daniels et al. 2010.
26. Aromatase works directly by converting androstenedione to estrone or indirectly by converting testosterone to estradiol, which can then be converted to estrone by oxidation.
27. Theoret et al. 2011.
28. Imamov, Lopatkin, and Gustafsson 2004.
29. "Dr. Bob's Recommended Vitamin List," CompassionateOncology.org, http://www.compassionateoncology.org/pdfs/RECOMMENDEDVITAMINLIST.050305.pdf (accessed November 2, 2012).
30. Mirkovic et al. 1997.
31. Phytoestrogens will increase Bcl-2 only if there is a lot of ER-beta present and high local levels of estradiol. If there is little or no estradiol present, then phytoestrogens should decrease Bcl-2 levels.
32. Johnson et al. 1997.
33. Jorm, Korten, and Henderson 1987.
34. Koudinov and Berezov 2004.
35. Jon Hamilton, "Gene Mutation Offers Clue for Drugs to Stave Off Alzheimer's," NPR, July 11, 2012, http://www.npr.org/blogs/health/2012/07/11/156616799/gene-mutation-offers-clue-for-drugs-to-stave-off-alzheimers (accessed November 2, 2012).

CHAPTER 16. A BETTER TOMORROW

1. Gary Taubes had a similar reaction to the power of the Internet in facilitating research. Regarding his magnum opus *Good Calories, Bad Calories,* he said, "Just ten years ago, the research for this book would have taken the better part of a lifetime" (Taubes 2007:453).
2. Fjelldal et al. 2010.
3. Asher Mullard, "What Is the Link between Autism and Testosterone?" *Nature,* http://www.nature.com/news/2009/090113/full/news.2009.21.html (accessed November 2, 2012).
4. Walsh et al. 2001.
5. Folch et al. 1998.

6. Singh and Hanson 2006.

7. "Causes. Etiology and Biochemical Abnormalities of Autism," Springboard, http://www.springboard4health.com/notebook/health_autism2.html (accessed November 2, 2012).

8. Sparks et al. 2002.

9. Acid production continues to decline with age (Wright and Lenard 2001:20).

10. Wright and Lenard 2001.

11. If you still aren't convinced that *low* stomach acid is the cause of GERD, think about the logic of why it's not a good idea to eat three hours before bedtime. If you have excess stomach acid, the food would be digested quickly. It's only because there's *too little* stomach acid that it takes so long to be fully digested.

12. Whenever you want to discontinue a prescription medication, it's a good idea to speak with your doctor about it first.

13. While it is not known exactly why bitters increase stomach acid production, one possibility is that as the human race evolved, at one point wild-growing berries were a food staple. Some poisonous berries are very bitter in taste. There would be a survival advantage to maximizing stomach acid production after ingesting poisonous berries in order to break down toxins before they could enter the bloodstream.

14. I'm not sure whether temperature sensitivity is widespread or just peculiar to John. One possible explanation for why it might be widespread is that higher temperatures relax muscles. You don't want your lower esophageal sphincter muscle to be relaxed.

15. Dr. Wright has noted that his patients with low stomach acid tend to be depressed. He attributes this to low stomach acid not being able to totally break down proteins into amino acids. Amino acids are the building blocks for the neurotransmitters inside the brain. Antidepressants work by raising the effective level of neurotransmitters.

16. Underscoring the long-recognized human need for antioxidants, new research also implicates oxidation, along with estradiol-caused proliferation, as part of the genesis of cancer (Bhat et al. 2003).

BIBLIOGRAPHY

Abate-Shen, Cory, and Michael M. Shen

2000. Molecular genetics of prostate cancer. *Genes & Development* 14(19):2410–34.

Aikey, Jeremy L., John G. Nyby, David M. Anmuth, and Peter J. James

2002. Testosterone rapidly reduces anxiety in male house mice (Mus musculus). *Hormones and Behavior* 42(4):448–60.

Akhondazdeh, S., M. Noroozian, M. Mohammadi, S. Ohadinia, A. H. Jamshidi, and M. Khani

2003. *Salvia officinalis* extract in the treatment of patients with mild to moderate Alzheimer's Disease: A double blind, randomized and placebo-controlled trial. *Journal of Clinical Pharmacy and Therapeutics* 28(1):53–59.

Al-Sader, Hassan, Hani Abdul-Jabar, Zahra Allawi, and Yasser Haba

2009. Alcohol and breast cancer: The mechanisms explained. *Journal of Clinical Medicine Research* 1(3):125–31.

Alevizopolous, K., N. Bacapoulos, N. Papadopoulou, K. Dambaki, and C. Stoumaras

2008. Preclinical studies of MDX-12C, a selective membrane androgen receptor ligand with activity in prostate cancer. *American Association of Clinical Oncology*, Annual Meeting, Abstract No. 14549.

Alzheimer's Association

N.d. Medications for memory loss. Web.

Ambady, Nalini, Mark Hallahan, and Robert Rosenthal

1995. On judging and being judged accurately in zero-acquaintance situations. *Journal of Personality and Social Psychology* 69(2):518–29.

Amtul, Z., L. Wang, D. Westaway, and R. F. Rozmahel

2010. Neuroprotective mechanism conferred by 17beta estradiol on the biochemical basis of Alzheimer's Disease. *Neurodegeneraiton, Neuroprotection, and Disease-Oriented Neuroscience* 169(2):781–86.

Anderson, Carl W., and Ettore Appella

2005. Posttranslational modifications of p53: Upstream signalling pathways. In *The p53 Tumor Suppressor Pathway and Cancer*. Edited by Gerard P. Zambetti. New York: Springer Science + Business Media Inc.

Araujo, Andre B., Gretchen R. Esche, Varant Kupelian, et al.

2007. Prevalence of symptomatic androgen deficiency in men. *Journal of Clinical Endocrinology & Metabolism* 92(11):4241–47.

ARIMIDEX, TAMOXIFEN, ALONE OR IN COMBINATION (ATAC) TRIALISTS' GROUP 2008

2008. Effect of anastrozole and tamoxifen as adjuvant treatment for early-stage breast cancer: 100-month analysis of the ATAC trial. *Lancet Oncology* 9(1):45–53.

ARUNASREE, K. M.

2010. Anti-proliferative effects of carvacrol on a human metastatic breast cancer cell line, MDA-MB 231. *Phytomedicine* 17(8–9):581–88.

AXELL, ANNA-MAREE, HELEN E. MACLEAN, DAVID R. PLANT, ET AL.

2006. Continuous testosterone administration prevents skeletal muscle atrophy and enhances resistance to fatigue in orchidectomized male mice. *American Journal of Physiology–Endocrinology and Metabolism* 291(3):E506–16.

BACHMANN, GLORIA, JOHN BANCROFT, GLENN BRAUNSTEIN, ET AL.

2002. Female androgen insufficiency: The Princeton consensus statement on definition, classification, and assessment. *Fertility and Sterility* 77(4):660–65.

BACHMEIER, CORBIN, DANIEL PARIS, DAVID BEAULIEU-ABDELAHAD, BENOIT MOUZON, MICHAEL MULLON, AND FIONA CRAWFORD

2013. A multifaceted role for ApoE in the clearance of beta-amyloid across the blood-brain barrier. *Neurodegenerative Diseases* 11(1):13–21.

BACHNER-MELMAN, R., I. GRITSENKO, L. NEMANOV, A. H. ZOHAR, C. DINA, AND R. P. EBSTEIN

2005. Dopaminergic polymorphisms associated with self-report measures of human altruism: A fresh phenotype for the dopamine D4 receptor. *Molecular Psychiatry* 10(4): 333–35.

BAI, V. UMA, EUGENIA CIFUENTES, MANI MENON, EVELYN R. BARRACK, AND G. PREM-VEER REDDY

2005. Androgen receptor regulates Cdc6 in synchronized LNCaP cells progressing from G1 to S phase. *Journal of Cellular Physiology* 204(2):381–87.

BALUNAS, MARCY J., BIN SU, ROBERT W. BRUEGGEMEIER, AND A. DOUGLAS KINGHORN

2008. Natural products as aromatase inhibitors. *Anti-Cancer Agents in Medicinal Chemistry* 8(6):646–82.

BARRETT-CONNOR, ELIZABETH, DENISE G. VON MÜHLEN, AND DONNA KRITZ-SILVERSTEIN

1999. Bioavailable testosterone and depressed mood in older men: The Rancho Bernardo Study. *Journal of Clinical Endocrinology & Metabolism* 84(2):573–77.

BASARIA, SHEHZAD, ANDREA D. COVIELLO, THOMAS G. TRAVISON, ET AL.

2010. Adverse events associated with testosterone administration. *NEJM* 363(2):109–22.

BASARIA, SHEHZAD, MAITHILI N. DAVDA, THOMAS G. TRAVISON, JAGADISH ULLOOR, RAVINDER SINGH, AND SHALENDER BHASIN

2013. Risk factors associated with cardiovascular events during testosterone administration in older men with limited mobility. *Journals of Gerontology. Series A: Biological Sciences and Medical Science* 68(2):153–60.

BASINA, MARINA, HAU LIU, ANDREW R. HOFFMAN, AND DAVID FELDMAN

2012. Successful long-term treatment of Cushings Disease with mifepristone (RU486). *Endocrine Practice* 18(5):e114–20.

BASTACKY, S. S., P. C. WALSH, AND J. I. EPSTEIN

1991. Needle biopsy associated tumor tracking of adenocarcinoma of the prostate. *Journal of Urology* 145(5):1003–1007.

BECK, MELINDA

2012. Hormone use benefits may trump risks; age matters. *Wall Street Journal.* Web.

BERGES, RICHARD R., JASMINKA VUKANOVIC, JONATHAN I. EPSTEIN, ET AL.

1995. Implication of cell kinetic changes during the progression of human prostatic cancer. *Clinical Cancer Research* 1(5):473–80.

BETTUZZI, SAVERIO, MAURIZIO BRAUSI, FEDERICA RIZZI, GIOVANNI CASTAGNATTI, GIANCARLO PERACCHIA, AND ARNALDO CORTI

2006. Chemoprevention of human prostate cancer by oral administration of green tea catechins in volunteers with high-grade prostate intraepithelial neoplasia: A preliminary report from a one-year proof-of-principle study. *Cancer Research* 66(2):1234–40.

BHASIN, SHALENDER, ROBERT A. PARKER, FRED SATTLER, ET AL.

2007. Effects of testosterone supplementation on whole body and regional fat mass and distribution in human immunodeficiency virus-infected men with abdominal obesity. *Journal of Clinical Endocrinology & Metabolism* 92(3):1049–57.

BHAT, HARI K., GLORIA CALAF, TOM K. HEI, THERESA LOYA, AND JAYDUTT V. VADGAMA

2003. Critical role of oxidative stress in estrogen-induced carcinogenesis. *PNAS* 100(7):3913–18.

BILL-AXELSON, ANNA, LARS HOLMBERG, MIRJA RUUTU, ET AL.

2005. Radical prostatectomy versus watchful waiting in early prostate cancer. *NEJM* 352(19):1977–84.

BIRRELL, STEPHEN N., LISA M. BUTLER, JONATHAN M. HARRIS, GRANT BUCHANAN, AND WAYNE D. TILLEY

2007. Disruption of androgen receptor signaling by synthetic progestins may increase risk of developing breast cancer. *FASEB Journal* 21(10):2285–93.

BIXLER, EDWARD O., ALEXANDROS N. VGONTZAS, HUNG-MO LIN, ET AL.

2001. Prevalence of sleep-disordered breathing in women: Effects of gender. *American Journal of Respiratory and Critical Care Medicine* 163(3):608–13.

BONKHOFF, HELMUT, THOMAS FIXEMER, ISABEL HUNSICKER, AND KLAUS REMBERGER

1999. Estrogen receptor expression in prostate cancer and premalignant prostatic lesions. *American Journal of Pathology* 155(2):641–47.

BONKHOFF, HELMUT, AND RICHARD BERGES

2009. The evolving role of oestrogens and their receptors in the development and progression of prostate cancer. *European Urology* 55(3):533–42.

BOORJIAN, STEPHEN A., R. HOUSTON THOMPSON, MATTHEW K. TOLLEFSON, ET AL.

2011. Long-term risk of clinical progression after biochemical recurrence following radical prostatectomy: The impact of time from surgery to recurrence. *European Urology* 59(6):893–99.

BOSETTI, C., M. FILOMENO, P. RISO, ET AL.

2012. Cruciferous vegetables and cancer risk in a network of case-control studies. *Annals of Oncology* 23(8):2198–2203.

BOSLAND, MAARTEN C., HELEN FORD, AND LORI HORTON

1995. Induction at high incidence of ductal prostate adenocarcinoma in NBL/Cr and Sprague-Dawley Hsd:SD rats treated with a combination of testosterone and estradiol-17β or diethylstilbestrol. *Carcinogenesis* 16(6):1311–17.

BOUKER, KERRIE B., AND LEENA HILAKIVI-CLARKE

2000. Genistein: Does it prevent or promote breast cancer? *Environmental Health Perspective* 108(8):701–708.

BRAWLEY, OTIS W.

2012. Prostate cancer epidemiology in the United States. *World Journal of Urology* 30(2):195–200.

BRINTON, L. A., R. HOOVER, AND J. F. FRAUMENI JR.

1983. Reproductive factors in the aetiology of breast cancer. *British Journal of Cancer* 47(6):757–62.

BURGER, HENRY, JEAN HAILES, JOY NELSON, AND MARGARET MENELAUS

1987. Effect of combined implants of oestradiol and testosterone on libido in post-menopausal women. *BMJ* 294(6577): 936–37.

CALDERÓN-GARCIDUEÑAS, LILIAN, WILLIAM REED, ROBERT R. MARONPOT, ET AL.

2004. Brain inflammation and Alzheimer's-like pathology in individuals exposed to severe air pollution. *Toxicologic Pathology* 32(6):650–58.

CANONICO MARIANNE, EMMANUEL OGER, GENEVIÈVE PLU-BUREAU, ET AL.

2007. Hormone therapy and venous thromboembolism among postmenopausal women: Impact of the route of the estrogen administration: The ESTHER Study. *Circulation* 115(7):840–45.

CAO, CHUANHAI, DAVID A. LOEWENSTEIN, XIAOYANG LIN, ET AL.

2012. High blood caffeine levels in MCI linked to lack of progression to dementia. *Journal of Alzheimer's Disease* 30(3):550–72.

CARROLL, JENNA C., EMILY R. ROSARIO, ANGELA VILLAMAGNA, AND CHRISTIAN J. PIKE

2010. Continuous and cyclic progesterone differentially interact with estradiol in the regulation of Alzheimer-like pathology in female 3xtransgenic-Alzheimer's Disease mice. *Endocrinology* 151(6):2713–22.

CASTAGNETTA, LUIGI A., M. DORA MICELI, CARMELA M. G. SORCI, ET AL.

1995. Growth of LNCaP human prostate cancer cells is stimulated by estradiol via its own receptor. *Endocrinology* 136:2309–19.

CAVALLINI, G., S. CARACCIOLO, G. VITALI, F. MODENINI, AND G. BIAGIOTTI

2004. Carnitine versus androgen administration in the treatment of sexual dysfunction, depressed mood, and fatigue associated with male aging. *Urology* 63(4):641–46.

CHAM, BILL ELLIOT, AND TANIA ROBYN CHASE

2012. Solasodine rhamnosyl glycosides cause apoptosis in cancer cells. Do they also prime the immune system resulting in long-term protection against cancer? *Planta Medica* 78(4):349–53.

CHAU, MY N., LARA H. EL TOUNY, SHANKAR JAGADEESH, AND PARTHA P. BANERJEE

2007. Physiologically achievable concentrations of genistein enhance telomerase activity in prostate cancer cells via the activation of STAT3. *Carcinogenesis* 28(11):2282–90.

CHEN, S., S. PHUNG, S. KWOK, ET AL.

2005. Chemopreventative properties of mushrooms against breast cancer and prostate cancer. *International Journal of Medicinal Mushrooms* 7(3):342–43.

CHEN, SHIUAN, SEI-RYANG OH, SHERYL PHUNG, ET AL.

2006. Anti-aromatase activity of phytochemicals in white button mushrooms (Agaricus bisporus). *Cancer Research* 66(24):12026–34.

CHEN, ZHONG, IVAN S. YUHANNA, ZOYA GALCHEVA-GARGOVA, RICHARD H. KARAS, MICHAEL E. MENDELSOHN, AND PHILIP W. SHAUL

1999. Estrogen receptor α mediates the nongenomic activation of endothelial nitric oxide synthase by estrogen. *Journal of Clinical Investigation* 103(3):401–406.

CHERRIER, M. M., S. PLYMATE, S. MOHAN, ET AL.

2004. Relationship between testosterone supplementation and insulin-like growth factor-I levels and cognition in healthy older men. *Psychoneuroendocrinology* 29(1):65–82.

CHI, TSU-TSAIR

2012. Achieve a healthy estrogen quotient with myomin. *JANMA* 15(4):10–15.

CHIEFFI, P., A. KISSLINGER, A. A. SINISI, C. ABBONDONZA, AND D. TRAMONTANO

2003. 17β-estradiol-induced activation of ERK1/2 through endogenous androgen receptor α-src complex in human prostate cells. *International Journal of Oncology* 23(3):797–801.

CHLEBOWSKI ROWAN T., SUSAN L. HENDRIX, ROBERT D. LANGER, ET AL.

2003. Influence of estrogen and progestin on breast cancer and mammography in healthy postmenopausal women: The women's health initiative randomized trial. *JAMA* 289:3243–53.

CHOUDHURI, TATHAGATA, SUMAN PAL, MUNNA L. AGARWAL, TANYA DAS, AND GAURISANKAR SA

2002. Curcumin induces apoptosis in human breast cancer cells through p53-dependent Bax induction. *FEBS Letters* 512(1-3):334–40.

CLARKE, LEWIS K.

N.d. Truth about estriol: A laughing matter. Web .

COCCARO, EMIL F., RICHARD J. KAVOUSSI, RICHARD L. HAUGER, THOMAS B. COOPER, AND CRAIG F. FERRIS

1998. Cerebrospinal fluid vasopressin levels. Correlates with aggression and serotonin function in personality-disordered subjects. *Archives of General Psychiatry* 55(8):708–14.

COFFEY, J. C., J. H. WANG, M. J. F. SMITH, D. BOUCHIER-HAYES, T. G. KOTTER, AND H. P. REDMOND

2003. Excisional surgery for cancer cure: Therapy at a cost. *Lancet Oncology* 4(12):760–68.

COHEN, P. G.

1999. The hypogonadal-obesity cycle: Role of aromatase in modulating the testosterone-estradiol shunt—A major factor in the genesis of morbid obesity. *Medical Hypotheses* 52(1):49–51.

COLE, SARAH L., AND ROBERT VASSAR

2007. The Alzheimer's Disease β-secretase enzyme, BACE1. *Molecular Neurodegeneration* 2:22.

CRISLER, JOHN

2004. An update to the Crisler HCG protocol. Web.

2009. My current best thoughts on how to administer TRT for men: A recipe for success. Second edition. Web.

CUTLER, MAX, AND MELVIN SCHLEMENSON

1948. Treatment of advanced mammary cancer with testosterone. *JAMA* 138(3):187–90.

CUTTS, J. HARRY, AND R. L. NOBLE

1964. Estrone-induced mammary tumors in the rat. *Cancer Research* 24:1116–23.

DAMBAKI, CONSTANTINA, CHRISTINA KOGIA, MARLENA KAMPA, ET AL.

2005. Membrane testosterone binding sites in prostate carcinoma as a potential new marker and therapeutic target: Study in paraffin tissue sections. *BMC Cancer* 5:148.

DANIELS, NICHOLAS A., CARRIE M. NIELSON, ANDREW R. HOFFMAN, AND DOUGLAS C. BAUER

2010. Sex hormones and the risk of incident prostate cancer. *Urology* 76(5):1034–40.

DAVIS, PAUL A., VIHAS T. VASU, KISHORCHANDRA GOHIL, ET AL.

2012. A high-fat diet containing whole walnuts (Juglans regia) reduces tumour size and growth along with plasma insulin-like growth factor 1 in the transgenic adenocarcinoma of the mouse prostate model. *British Journal of Nutrition* 108(10):1764–72.

DAVIS, SUSAN R., AND JANE TRAN

2001. Testosterone influences libido and well being in women. *Trends in Endocrinology & Metabolism* 12(1):33–37.

DAVIS SUSAN R., M. MOREAU, R. KROLL, ET AL.

2008. Testosterone for low libido in postmenopausal women not taking estrogen. *NEJM* 359(19):2005–17.

DAVIS, SUSAN R.

2009. Testosterone for low libido in postmenopausal women not using systemic oestrogen therapy. *Medical Journal of Australia* 191(3):134–35.

DAVIS, WILLIAM

2011. *Wheat Belly: Lose the Wheat, Lose the Weight, and Find Your Path Back to Health.* New York: Rodale.

DAVISON, S. L., R. BELL, S. DONATH, J. G. MONTALTO, AND S. R. DAVIS

2005. Androgen levels in adult females: Changes with age, menopause, and oopherectomy. *Journal of Endocrinology & Metabolism* 90(7):3847–53.

DAVISON, SONIA L., ROBIN J. BELL, MARIA GAVRILESCU, ET AL.

2011. Testosterone improves verbal learning and memory in postmenopausal women: Results from a pilot study. *Maturitas* 70(3):307–11.

DELVILLE, YVON, KARIM M. MANSOUR, AND CRAIG F. FERRIS

1996. Testosterone facilitates aggression by modulating vasopressin receptors in the hypothalamus. *Physiology & Behavior* 60(1):25–29.

DEMICHELIS, F., K. FALL, S. PERNER, ET AL.

2007. *TMPRSS2:ERG* gene fusion associated with lethal prostate cancer in a watchful waiting cohort. *Oncogene* 26:4596–99.

DESTA, ZERUESENAY, BRYAN A. WARD, NADIA V. SOUKHOVA, AND DAVID A. FLOCKHART

2004. Comprehensive evaluation of tamoxifen sequential transformation by the human cytochrome P450 system in vitro: Prominent roles for CYP3A and CYP2D6. *Journal of Pharmacology and Experimental Therapeutics* 310(3):1062–75.

DIMITRAKAKIS, CONSTANTINE, JIAN ZHOU, JIE WANG, ET AL.

2003. A physiologic role for testosterone in limiting estrogenic stimulation of the breast. *Menopause* 10(4):292–98.

DIMITRAKAKIS, CONSTANTINE, ROBERT A. JONES, AIYI LIU, CAROLYN A. BONDY

2004. Breast cancer incidence in postmenopausal women using testosterone in addition to usual hormone therapy. *Menopause* 11(5):531–35.

DIMITRAKAKIS, CONSTANTINE, AND CAROLYN BONDY

2009. Androgens and the breast. *Breast Cancer Research* 11:212.

DIMITRAKAKIS, CONSTANTINE, DAVID ZAVA, SPYROS MARINOPOULOS, ALEXANDRA TSIGGINOU, ARIS ANTSAKLIS, AND REBECCA GLASER

2010. Low salivary testosterone levels in patients with breast cancer. *BMC Cancer* 10:547.

DORSCHNER, ROBERT A., VASUMATI K. PESTONJAMASP, SEEMA TAMAKUWALA, ET AL.

2001. Cutaneous injury induces the release of cathelicidin anti-microbial peptides active against Group A *Streptococcus. Journal of Investigative Dermatology* 117(1):91–97.

DRISCOLL, IRA, AND SUSAN M. RESNICK

2007. Testosterone and cognition in normal aging and Alzheimer's Disease: An update. *Current Alzheimer Research* 4(1):33–45.

EARLY BREAST CANCER TRIALISTS' COLLABORATIVE GROUP

2011. Relevance of breast cancer hormone receptors and other factors to the efficacy of adjuvant tamoxifen: Patient-level meta-analysis of randomised trials. *Lancet* 378(9793):771–84.

EBINGER, M., C. SIEVERS, D. IVAN, H. J. SCHNEIDER, AND G. K. STALLA

2009. Is there a neuroendocrinological rationale for testosterone as a therapeutic option in depression? *Journal of Psychopharmacology* 23(7):841–53.

ELLEM, S. J., AND G. P. RISBRIDGER

2006. Aromatase and prostate cancer. *Minerva Endocrinologica* 31(1):1–12.

FALOON, WILLIAM

2008. The FDA indicts itself. *Life Extension Magazine*, July. Web.

2012a. As we see it: The testosterone controversy. *Life Extension Magazine*, June. Web.

2012b. New study warns against excessive vitamin D intake. *Life Extension Magazine*, May. Web.

FARNSWORTH, WELLS E.

1996. Roles of estrogen and SHBG in prostate physiology. *Prostate* 28(1):17–23.

FDA

2008. Transcript of FDA press conference on FDA actions on bio-identical hormones. Moderator: Susan Cruzan. January 9:13. Web.

FEIGELSON, HEATHER SPENCER, AND BRIAN E. HENDERSON

1996. Estrogens and breast cancer. *Carcinogenesis* 17:2279–84.

FERNÖ, M., Å. BORG, U. JOHANSSON, ET AL.

1990. Estrogen and progesterone receptor analyses in more than 4,000 breast cancer samples: A study with special reference to age at diagnosis and stability of analyses. *Acta Oncologica* 29(2):129–35.

FJELLDAL, RENATHE, BJØRN T. MOE, ANNE ØRBO, AND GEORG SAGER

2010. MCF-7 cell apoptosis and cell cycle arrest: Non-genomic effects of progesterone and mifepristone (RU-486). *Anticancer Research* 30(12):4835–40.

FOLCH, JAUME, ARTURO ORTEGA, MARIA CABRÉ, AND JOSÉ L. PATERNÁIN

1998. Urinary levels of metallothioneins and metals in subjects from a semiindustrialized area in Tarragona Province of Spain. *Biological Trace Element Research* 63(2):113–21.

FOLLINGSTAD, ALVIN H.

1978. Estriol, the forgotten estrogen? *JAMA* 239:29–30.

FOURNIER, AGNÈS, FRANCO BERRINO, AND FRANÇOIS CLAVEL-CHAPELON

2008. Unequal risks for breast cancer associated with different hormone replacement therapies: Results from the E3N Cohort Study. *British Cancer Research and Treatment* 107(1):103–11.

FOWLER, JACKSON E. JR., AND WILLET F. WHITMORE JR.

1981. The response of metastatic adenocarcinoma of the prostate to exogenous testosterone. *Journal of Urology* 126(3):372–75.

FRIEDMAN, A. EDWARD

2005. The estradiol-dihydrotestosterone model of prostate cancer. *Theoretical Biology and Medical Modelling* 2:10.

2007. Can a single model explain both breast cancer and prostate cancer? *Theoretical Biology and Medical Modelling* 4:28.

2011. Re: testosterone therapy in men with untreated prostate cancer: A. Morgentaler, L. I. Lipshultz, R. Bennett, M. Sweeney, D. Avila, Jr., and M. Khera. *J Urol 2011; 185: 1256–1261. Journal of Urology* 186(4):1559–60.

2012. Comment on "Finasteride upregulates expression of androgen receptor in hyperplastic prostate and LNCaP cells: Implications for chemoprevention of prostate cancer." By Hsieh et al. *Prostate* 72(7):703–704.

GALLACCHIO, LISA, RYAN MACDONALD, BETHANY WOOD, ERROL RUSHOVICH, AND KATHY J. HELZLSOUER

2011. Androgens and musculoskeletal symptoms among breast cancer patients on aromatase inhibitor therapy. *Breast Cancer Research and Treatment* 130(2):569–77.

GANDY, SAM, OSVALDO P. ALMEIDA, JUSTIN FONTE, ET AL.

2001. Chemical andropause and amyloid-β peptide. *JAMA* 285(17):2195–96.

GARBER, KEN

2010. A tale of two cells: Discovering the origin of prostate cancer. *Journal of the National Cancer Institute* 102:1528–35.

GAT, Y., S. JOSHUA, AND M. G. GORNISH

2009. Prostate cancer: A newly discovered route for testosterone to reach the prostate. *Andrologia* 41(5):305–15.

GECK, PETER, MARICEL V. MAFFINI, JOZSEF SZELEI, CARLOS SONNENSCHEIN, AND ANA M. SOTO

2000. Androgen-induced proliferative quiescence in prostate cancer cells: The role of AS3 as its mediator. *PNAS* 97:10185–90.

GIOVANNUCCI, EDWARD, MEIR J. STAMPFER, KRISHNA KRITHIVAS, ET AL.

1997. The CAG repeat within the androgen receptor gene and its relationship to prostate cancer. *PNAS* 94(7):3320–23.

GLASER, R. L.

2010. Subcutaneous testosterone-anastrozole implant therapy in breast cancer survivors. *American Society of Clinical Oncology* Breast Cancer Symposium, Abstract No. 221.

GLASER, REBECCA, ANNE E. YORK, AND CONSTANTINE DIMITRAKAKIS

2011. Beneficial effects of testosterone therapy in women measured by the validated menopause rating scale (MRS). *Maturitas* 68(4):355–61.

GONG, CHEN-XIN, FEI LIU, INGE GRUNDKE-IQBAL, AND KHALID IQBAL

2006. Impaired brain glucose metabolism leads to Alzheimer neurofibrillary degeneration through a decrease in tau O-GlcNAcylation. *Journal of Alzheimer's Disease* 9(1):1–12.

GONZALEZ, LUIS O., MARIA D. CORTE, JULIO VAZQUEZ, ET AL.

2008. Androgen receptor expression in breast cancer: Relationship with clinicopathological characteristics of the tumors, prognosis, and expression of metalloproteases and their inhibitors. *BMC Cancer* 8:149.

GORDON, ERLINDA M., FRANCISCO F. LOPEZ, GERARDO H. CORNELIO, ET AL.

2006. Pathotropic nanoparticles for cancer gene therapy Rexin-G™ IV: Three-year clinical experience. *International Journal of Oncology* 29(5):1053–64.

GORLOV, IVAN P., JINYOUNG BYUN, OLGA Y. GORLOVA, ANA M. APARICIO, ELENI EFSTATHIOU, AND CHRISTOPHER J. LOGOTHETIS

2009. Candidate pathways and genes for prostate cancer: A meta-analysis of gene expression data. *BMC Medical Genomics* 2:48.

GOSS, PAUL E., JAMES N. INGLE, JOSÉ E. ALÉS-MARTINEZ, ET AL.

2011. Exemestane for breast-cancer prevention in postmenopausal women. *NEJM* 364(25):2381–91.

GOUDSMIT, ELMER, ERIC FLIERS, AND DICK F. SWAAB

1988. Testosterone supplementation restores vasopressin innervation in the senescent rat brain. *Brain Research* 473(2):306–13.

GOUDSMIT, ELMER, ERIC FLIERS, AND DICK F. SWAAB

1989. Changes in vasopressin neurons and fibers in aging and Alzheimer's Disease: Reversibility in the rat. *Progress in Clinical and Biological Research* 317:1193–1208.

GOURAS, GUNNAR K., HUAXI XU, RACHEL S. GROSS, ET AL.

2000. Testosterone reduces neuronal secretion of Alzheimer's β-amyloid peptides. *PNAS* 97(3):1202–1205.

GOURLAY, CAMPBELL W., AND KATHRYN R. AYSCOUGH

2005. The actin cytoskeleton: A key regulator of apoptosis and ageing? *Nature Reviews Molecular Cell Biology* 6(7):583–89.

GRANN, VICTOR R., KATHERINE S. PANAGEAS, WILLIAM WHANG, KAREN H. ANTMAN, AND ALFRED I NEUGUT

1998. Decision analysis of prophylactic mastectomy and oophorectomy in *BRCA1*-positive or *BRCA2*-positive patients. *Journal of Clinical Oncology* 16:979–85.

GRAY, ANNA, HENRY A. FELDMAN, JOHN B. MCKINLAY, AND CHRISTOPHER LONGCOPE

1991. Age, disease, and changing sex hormone levels in middle-aged men: Results of the Massachusetts Male Aging Study. *Journal of Clinical Endocrinology and Metabolism* 73(5):1016–25.

GREEN, KIM N., JOAN S. STEFFAN, HILDA MARTINEZ-CORIA, ET AL.

2008. Nicotanimide restores cognition in Alzheimer's Disease transgenic mice via a mechanism involving sirtuin inhibition and selective reduction of Thr231-phosphotau. *Journal of Neuroscience* 28(45):11500–510.

GREENWELL, IVY

2002. Grumpy no more: Testosterone deficiency & depression. *Life Extension Magazine*, August. Web.

GRUVBERGER-SAAL, SOFIA K., PÄR-OLA BENDAHL, LAO H. SAAL, ET AL.

2007. Estrogen receptor β expression is associated with tamoxifen response in ERα-negative breast carcinoma. *Clinical Cancer Research* 13(7):1987–94.

GU, SHUCHEN, NATALIA PAPADOPOULOU, EVA-MARIA GEHRING, ET AL.

2009. Functional membrane androgen receptors in colon tumors trigger pro-apoptotic responses *in vitro* and reduce drastically tumor incidence *in vivo*. *Molecular Cancer* 8:114.

GU, SHUCHEN, NATALIA PAPADOPOULOU, OMAIMA NASIR, ET AL.

2011. Activation of membrane androgen receptors in colon cancer inhibits the prosurvival signals Akt/Bad in vitro and in vivo and blocks migration via vinculin/actin signaling. *Molecular Medicine* 17(1–2):48–58.

GUAY, A. T., AND JERILYNN JACOBSON

2002. Decreased free testosterone and dehydroepiandrosterone-sulfate (DHEA-S) levels in women with decreased libido. *Journal of Sex & Marital Therapy* 28(suppl 1):129–42.

GULLINO, PIETRO M.

1977. Natural history of breast cancer progression from hyperplasia to neoplasia as predicted by angiogenesis. *Cancer* 39(6):2697–2703.

GUZEY, MERAL, SHINICHI KITADA, AND JOHN C. REED

2002. Apoptosis induction by 1α,25-dihydroxyvitamin D_3 in prostate cancer. *Molecular Cancer Therapeutics* 1(9):667–77.

HAJJAR, RAMZI R., FRAN E. KAISER, AND JOHN E. MORLEY

1997. Outcomes of long-term testosterone replacement in older hypogonadal males: A retrospective analysis. *Journal of Clinical Endocrinology & Metabolism* 82(11):3793–96.

HALL, J. A.

1979. Gender, gender roles, and nonverbal skills. In *Skill in Nonverbal Communication: Individual Differences* (pp. 32–67). Edited by R. Rosenthal. Cambridge, MA: Oelgeschlager, Gunn, & Hain.

1984. *Nonverbal Sex Differences: Communication Accuracy and Expressive Styles.* Baltimore: Johns Hopkins University Press.

HAN, JIAN RONG, BIN DENG, JING SUN, ET AL.

2007. Effects of dietary medium-chain triglyceride on weight loss and insulin sensitivity in a group of moderately overweight free-living type 2 diabetic Chinese subjects. *Metabolism* 56(7):985–91.

HATZOGLOU, ANASTASSIA, MARILENA KAMPA, CHRISTINA KOGIA, ET AL.

2005. Membrane androgen receptor activation induces apoptotic regression of human prostate cancer cells *in vitro* and *in vivo. Journal of Clinical Endocrinology & Metabolism* 90(2):893–903.

HERMANS, ERNO J., PETER PUTMAN, JOHANNA M. BAAS, HANS P. KOPPESCHAAR, AND JACK VAN HONK

2006. A single administration of testosterone reduces fear potentiated startle in humans. *Biological Psychiatry* 59(9):872–74.

HERMANS, ERNO J., NICK F. RAMSEY, AND JACK VAN HONK

2008. Exogenous testosterone enhances responsiveness to social threat in the neural circuitry of social aggression in humans. *Biological Psychiatry* 63(3):263–70.

HERNSMEYER, R. KENT, THERESA L. THOMPSON, GERALD M. POHOST, AND JUAN CARLOS KASKI

2008. Cardiovascular effects of medroxyprogesterone acetate and progesterone: A case of mistaken identity? *Nature Clinical Practice Cardiovascular Medicine* 5(7):387–95.

HERTOGHE, THIERRY WITH JULES-JACQUES NABET

2002. *The Hormone Solution: Stay Younger Longer with Natural Hormone and Nutrition Therapies.* New York: Harmony Books.

2010. Medical Consultation by Dr Thierry Hertoghe.wmv. Web.

HILL, MARTIN, DUŠAN LUKÁC, OLDRRICH LAPCÍK, ET AL.

2005. Age relationships and sex differences in serum levels of pregnenolone and 17-hydroxypregnenolone in normal subjects. *Clinical Chemistry and Laboratory Medicine* 37(4):439–47.

HOLICK, MICHAEL

2009. Quoted in *Scientific American.* Five years after being fired from one post, sun exposure proponent keeps up the fight, by Coco Ballantyne. Web.

HOLICK, MICHAEL F.

2010. *The Vitamin D Solution: A 3-Step Strategy to Cure Our Most Common Health Problems.* New York: Hudson Street Press.

HOLT, RICHARD I. G., AND NEIL A. HANLEY

2012. *Essential Endocrinology and Diabetes.* 6th edition. Chichester, West Sussex: Wiley-Blackwell.

HOLTORF, KENT

2009. The bioidentical hormone debate: Are bioidentical hormones (estradiol, estriol, and progesterone) safer or more efficacious than commonly used synthetic versions in hormone replacement therapy? *Postgraduate Medicine* 121(1):73–85.

HONG, CHIBO, HYEON-A. KIM, GARY L. FIRESTONE, AND LEONARD F. BJELDANES

2002. 3,3'-diindolylmethane (DIM) induces a G_1 cell cycle arrest in human breast cancer cells that is accompanied by Sp1-mediated activation of $p21^{WAF1/CIP1}$ expression. *Carcinogenesis* 23(8):1297–1305.

HOPKINS, VIRGINIA

N.d.a Estriol, the safest hormone. Web.

N.d.b Hysterectomy and bioidentical (natural) hormones. Web.

HOYOS, CAMILLA M., ROO KILLICK, BRENDON J. YEE, RONALD R. GRUNSTEIN, AND PETER Y. LIU

2012. Effects of testosterone therapy on sleep and breathing in obese men with severe obstructive sleep apnea: A randomized placebo-controlled trial. *Clinical Endocrinology* 77(4):599–607.

HSIEH, JU-TON, SHYH-CHYAN CHEN, HONG-JENG YU, AND HONG-CHIANG CHANG

2011. Finasteride upregulates expression of androgen receptor in hyperplastic prostate and LNCaP Cells: Implications for chemoprevention of prostate cancer. *Prostate* 71(10):1115–21.

HU, WEN-YANG, GUANG-BIN SHI, HUNG-MING LAM, ET AL.

2011. Estrogen-initiated transformation of prostate epithelium derived from normal human prostate stem-progenitor cells. *Endocrinology* 152(6):2150–63.

HUGGINS, CHARLES, R. E. STEVENS JR., AND CLARENCE V. HODGES

1941. The effect of castration on advanced carcinoma of the prostate gland. *Archives of Surgery* 43(2):209–23.

HYDE, ZOË, PAUL E. NORMAN, LEON FLICKER, ET AL.

2012. Low free testosterone predicts mortality from cardiovascular disease but not other causes: The Health in Men Study. *Journal of Clinical Endocrinology & Metabolism* 97:179–89.

IMAMOV, OTABEK, NIKOLAY A. LOPATKIN, AND JAN-AKE GUSTAFSSON

2004. Estrogen receptor β in prostate cancer. *NEJM* 351(26):2773–74.

ISAACS, JOHN T., JASON M. D'ANTONIO, SHUANGLING CHEN, ET AL.

2012. Adaptive auto-regulation of androgen receptor provides a paradigm shifting rationale for bipolar androgen therapy (BAT) for castrate resistant human prostate cancer. *Prostate* 72(14):1491–1505.

ISBARN, HENDRIK, JEHONATHAN H. PINTHUS, LEONARD S. MARKS, ET AL.

2009. Testosterone and prostate cancer: Revisiting old paradigms. *European Urology* 56(1):48–56.

ISIDORI, ANDREA M., ELISA GIANNETTA, EMANUELA A. GRECO, ET AL.

2005. Effects of testosterone on body composition, bone metabolism and serum lipid profile in middle-aged men: A meta-analysis. *Clinical Endocrinology* 63(3):280–93.

ITO, SHINGO, SUMIO OHTSUKI, YASUKO NEZU, YUSUKE KOITABASHI, SHO MURATO, AND TETSUYA TERASAKI.

2011. 1α,25-dihydroxyvitamin D_3 enhances cerebral clearance of human amyloid-β peptide(1-40) from mouse brain across the blood-brain barrier. *Fluids and Barriers of the CNS* 8:20.

IVERSEN, P., P. O. MADSEN, AND D. K. CORLE

1995. Radical prostatectomy versus expectant treatment for early carcinoma of the prostate. Twenty-three year follow-up of a prospective randomized study. *Scandinavian Journal of Urology and Nephrology. Supplementum* 172:65–72.

JAMINET, PAUL, AND SOU-CHING JAMINET

2010. *Perfect Health Diet: Four Steps to Renewed Health, Youthful Vitality, and Long Life.* Cambridge, MA: YinYang Press.

JANKOWSKA, EWA A., PIOTR ROZENTRYT, BEATA PONIKOWSKA, ET AL.

2009. Circulating estradiol and mortality in men with systolic chronic heart failure. *JAMA* 301(18):1892–1901.

JANOWSKY, JERI S., SHELIA K. OVIATT, AND ERIC S. ORWOLL

1994. Testosterone influences spatial cognition in older men. *Behavioral Neuroscience* 108(2):325–32.

JOHNSON, C. C., B. A. RYBICKI, G. BROWN, ET AL.

1997. Cognitive impairment in the Amish: A four county survey. *International Journal of Epidemiology* 26(2):387–94.

JONSSON, THORLAKUR, JASVINDER K. ATWAL, STACY STEINBERG, ET AL.

2012. A mutation in *APP* protects against Alzheimer's Disease and age-related cognitive decline. *Nature* 488(7409):96–99.

JORM, A. F., A. E. KORTEN, AND A. E. HENDERSON

1987. The prevalence of dementia: A quantitative integration of the literature. *Acta Psychiatrica Scandinavica* 76(5):465–79.

JOYAL, STEVEN

2010. Mainstream doctors' ineptitude put on display in the New England Journal of Medicine. *Life Extension Magazine*, November. Web.

KAMPA, MARILENA, ARTEMISSIA-PHOEBE NIFLI, IOANNIS CHARALAMPOPOULOS, ET AL.

2005. Opposing effects of estradiol- and testosterone-membrane binding sites on T74D breast cancer cell apoptosis. *Experimental Cell Research* 307(1):41–51.

KAMPA MARILENA, CHRISTINA KOGIA, PANAYIOTIS A. THEODOROPOULOS, ET AL.

2006. Activation of membrane androgen receptors potentiates the antiproliferative effects of paclitaxel on human prostate cancer cells. *Molecular Cancer Therapeutics* 5(5):1342–51.

KAMRADT, JOERN, CARSTEN DROSSE, SASCHA KALKBRENNER, ET AL.

2003. Telomerase activity and telomerase subunit gene expression levels are not related in prostate cancer: A real-time quantification and *in situ* hybridization study. *Laboratory Investigation* 83(5):623–33.

KAPOOR D., E. GOODWIN, K. S. CHANNER, AND T. H. JONES
2006. Testosterone replacement therapy improves insulin resistance, glycaemic control, visceral adiposity and hypercholesterolaemia in hypogonadal men with type 2 diabetes. *European Journal of Endocrinology* 154(6):899–906.

KARAKIEWICZ, PIERRE I., MICHEL BAZINET, ARMEN G. APRIKIAN, SIMON TANGUAY, AND MOSTAFA M. ELHILALI
1998. Thirty-day mortality rates and cumulative survival after radical retropubic prostatectomy. *Urology* 52(6):1041–46.

KELLY, L., S. ROEDDE, S. HARRIS, ET AL.
2001. Evidence-based practical management of type 2 diabetes. Type 2 diabetes flow chart-2001. Society of Rural Physicians of Canada. Web.

KEY, T., P. APPLEBY, I. BARNES, G. REEVES, AND ENDOGENOUS HORMONES AND BREAST CANCER COLLABORATIVE GROUP
2002. Endogenous sex hormones and breast cancer in postmenopausal women: Reanalysis of nine prospective studies. *Journal of the National Cancer Institute* 94(8):606–16.

KHALIL, R. A.
2005. Sex hormones as potential modulators of vascular function in hypertension. *Hypertension* 46(2):249–54.

KIM, JEONG-MI, EUN-MI NOH, KANG-BEAM KWON, ET AL.
2012. Curcumin suppresses the TPA-induced invasion through inhibition of PKCa-dependent MMP-expression in MCF-7 human breast cancer cells. *Phytomedicine* 19(12):1085–92.

KIM, NAM DEUK, RAJENDRA MEHTA, WEIPING YU, ET AL.
2002. Chemopreventative and adjuvant therapy potential of pomegranate (*Punica granatum*) for human breast cancer. *Breast Cancer Research and Treatment* 71(3):203–17.

KJELLMAN, ANDERS, OLOF AKRE, ULF NORMING, MAGNUS TÖRNBLUM, AND OVE GUSTAFSSON
2008. Dihydrotestosterone levels and survival in screening-detected prostate cancer: A 15-yr follow-up study. *European Urology* 53(1):106–11.

KLEIN, GEORGE
2007. P53 as seen by an outsider. In *25 Years of p53 Research.* Edited by Pierre Hainaut and Klas G. Wiman. Dordrecht, The Netherlands: Springer.

KORACH, KENNETH
1994. Estrogen receptor knockout yields insights in clinical and basic research areas. *NIH Catalyst,* Web.

KOUDINOV, ALEXEI R., AND TEMIRBOLAT T. BEREZOV
2004. Alzheimer's amyloid-beta (Aβ) is an essential synaptic protein, not neurotoxic junk. *Acta Neurobiologiae Experimentalis* 64(1):71–79.

KRIEG, MICHAEL, RALF NASS, AND SABINE TUNN

1993. Effect of aging on endogenous level of 5α-dihydrotestosterone, testosterone, estradiol, and estrone in epithelium and stroma of normal and hyperplastic human prostate. *Journal of Clinical Endocrinology and Metabolism* 77(2):375–81.

KRISHNAN, A. V., S. SWAMI, AND D. FELDMAN

2012. The potential therapeutic benefits of vitamin D in the treatment of estrogen receptor positive breast cancer. *Steroids* 77(11):1107–12.

KRISTAL, ALAN R., AND JOHANNE W. LAMPE

2002. Brassica vegetables and prostate cancer risk: A review of the epidemiological evidence. *Nutrition and Cancer* 42(1):1–9.

KRYGER, ABRAHAM HARVEY

2007. *A Woman's Guide to Men's Health.* Berkeley, CA: RDR Books.

KUIPER, GEORGE G. J. M., CARLSSON B., GRANDIEN K., ET AL.

1997. Comparison of the ligand binding specificity and transcript tissue distribution of estrogen receptors α and β. *Endocrinology* 138:863–70.

KUMLE, MERETHE, ELISABETE WIDERPASS, TONJE BRAATEN, INGEMAR PERSSON, HANS-OLOV ADAMI, AND EILIV LUND

2002. Use of oral contraceptives and breast cancer risk: The Norwegian-Swedish women's lifestyle and health cohort study. *Cancer Epidemiology, Biomarkers & Prevention* 11(11):1375–81.

KURZWEIL, RAY, AND TERRY GROSSMAN

2004. *Fantastic Voyage: Live Long Enough to Live Forever.* New York: Rodale.

LAAKSONEN, DAVID E., LEO NISKANEN, KARI PUNNONEN, ET AL.

2004. Testosterone and sex hormone-binding globulin predict the metabolic syndrome in middle-aged men. *Diabetes Care* 27(5):1036–41.

LACHMAN, MARGIE E., AND KIMBERLY M. PRENDA FIRTH

2004. The adaptive value of feeling in control during midlife. In *How Healthy Are We? A National Study of Well-Being at Midlife,* edited by Orville Gilbert Brim, Carol D. Ryff, and Ronald C. Kessler, pp. 320–349. Chicago: University of Chicago Press.

LAKSHMAN, MINALINI, LI XU, VIJAYALAKSHMI ANANTHANARAYANAN, ET AL.

2008. Dietary genistein inhibits metastasis of human prostate cancer in mice. *Cancer Research* 68(6):2024–32.

LANDAU, SUSAN M., SHAWN M. MARKS, ELIZABETH C. MORMINO, ET AL.

2012. Association of lifetime cognitive engagement and low β-amyloid deposition. *Archives of Neurology* 69(5):623–29.

LANNERT, H., P. WIRTZ, V. SCHUHMANN, AND R. GALMBACHER

1998. Effects of estradiol (-17β) on learning, memory, and cerebral energy metabolism in male rats after intracerebroventricular administration of streptozotocin. *Journal of Neural Transmission* 105(8–9):1045–63.

LAYDE, PETER M., LINDA A. WEBSTER, ANDREW L. BAUGHMAN, PHYLLIS A. WINGO, GEORGE L. RUBIN, AND HOWARD W. ORY

1989. The independent associations of parity, age at first full term pregnancy, and duration of breastfeeding with the risk of breast cancer. *Journal of Clinical Epidemiology* 42(10):963–73.

LEE, J. H., J. S.CHAE, S. J. KOH, S. M. KANG, D. H. CHOI, AND Y. S. JANG

2003. Caloric restriction vs testosterone treatment; the effect on body fat distribution and serum lipid levels in overweight male patients with coronary artery disease. *Korean Journal of Nutrition* 36(9):924–32.

LEE, JOHN R., DAVID ZAVA, AND VIRGINIA HOPKINS

2002. *What Your Doctor May Not Tell You about Breast Cancer: How Hormone Balance Can Help Save Your Life.* New York: Warner Books.

LEIBOWITZ, ROBERT L., TANYA B. DORFF, STEVEN TUCKER, JAMES SYMANOWSKI, AND NICHOLAS J. VOGELZANG

2010. Testosterone replacement in prostate cancer survivors with hypogonadal symptoms. *BJU International* 105(10):1397–1401.

LEITZMANN, MICHAEL F., ELIZABETH A. PLATZ, MEIR J. STAMPFER, WALTER C. WILLETT, AND EDWARD GIOVANNUCCI

2004. Ejaculation frequency and subsequent risk of prostate cancer. *JAMA* 291(13):1578–86.

LI, CHAOYANG, EARL S. FORD, BENYI LI, WAYNE H. GILES, AND SIMIN LIU

2010. Association of testosterone and sex hormone–binding globulin with metabolic syndrome and insulin resistance in men. *Diabetes Care* 33(7):1618–24.

LI, YANYAN, TAO ZHANG, HASAN KORKAYA, ET AL.

2010. Sulforaphane, a dietary component of broccoli/broccoli sprouts, inhibits breast cancer stem cells. *Clinical Cancer Research* 16(9):2580–90.

LI, YUANYUAN, YIH-YING YUAN, SYED M. MEERAN, AND TRYGVE O.TOLLEFSBOL

2010. Synergistic epigenetic reactivation of estrogen receptor-α (ER-α) by combined green tea polyphenol and histone deacetylase inhibitor in ERα-negative breast cancer cells. *Molecular Cancer* 9:274.

LIANG, KAIWEI, LIUQING YANG, CHEN YIN, ET AL.

2010. Estrogen stimulates degradation of β-amyloid peptide by up-regulating neprilysin. *Journal of Biological Chemistry* 285(2):935–42.

LIEDE, ALEXANDER, BETH Y. KARLAN, AND STEVEN A. NAROD

2004. Cancer risks for male carriers of germline mutations in *BRCA1* or *BRCA2*: A review of the literature. *Journal of Clinical Oncology* 22:735–42.

LIEHR, JOACHIM G.

2000. Is estradiol a genotoxic mutagenic carcinogen? *Endocrine Reviews* 21:40–54.

LIENING, SCOTT H., AND ROBERT A. JOSEPHS

2010. It is not just about testosterone: Physiological mediators and moderators of testosterone's behavioral effects. *Social and Personality Psychology Compass* 4(11):982–94.

LIM, GISELLE P., TERESA CHU, FUSHENG YANG, WALTER BEECH, SALLY A. FRAUTSCHY, AND GREG M. COLE

2001. The curry spice curcumin reduces oxidative damage and amyloid pathology in an Alzheimer transgenic mouse. *Journal of Neuroscience* 21(21):8370–77.

LIPPMAN, MARC, MARIE E. MONACO, AND GAIL BOLAN

1977. Effects of estrone, estradiol, and estriol on hormone-responsive human breast cancer in long-term tissue culture. *Cancer Research* 37(6):1901–1907.

LITVINOV, IVAN V., ANGELO M. DE MARZO, AND JOHN T. ISAACS

2003. Is the Achilles' heel for prostate cancer therapy a gain in androgen receptor signaling? *Journal of Clinical Endocrinology & Metabolism* 88:2972–82.

LIU, P. Y., A. K. DEATH , AND DAVID J. HANDELSMAN

2003. Androgens and cardiovascular disease. *Endocrine Reviews* 24:313–40.

LOEB, STACY, H. BALLENTINE CARTER, SONJA I. BERNDT, WINNIE RICKER, AND EDWARD M. SCHAEFFER

2011. Complications after prostate biopsy: Data from SEER-Medicare. *Journal of Urology* 186(5):1830–34.

LÖFGREN, L., L. SAHLIN, B. VON SCHOULTZ, R. FERNSTAD, L. SKOOG, AND E. VON SCHOULTZ

2006. Expression of sex steroid receptor subtypes in normal and malignant breast tissue—A pilot study in menopausal women. *Acta Oncologica* 45(1):54–60.

LÓPEZ-OTÍN, CARLOS, AND ELEFTHERIOS P. DIAMANDIS

1998. Breast and prostate cancer: An analysis of common epidemiological, genetic, and biochemical features. *Endocrine Reviews* 19:365–96.

LU, PO H., DONNA A. MASTERMAN, RUTH MULNARD, ET AL.

2006. Effects of testosterone on cognition and mood in male patients with mild Alzheimer Disease and healthy men. *Archives of Neurology* 63(2):177–85.

LU-YAO, GRACE L., AND SIU-LONG YAO

1997. Population-based study of long-term survival in patients with clinically localised prostate cancer. *Lancet* 349(9056):906–10.

LUK, SZE UE, WEI NEY YAP, YUNG-TUEN CHIU, ET AL.

2010. Gamma-tocotrienol as an effective agent in targeting prostate cancer stem cell-like population. *International Journal of Cancer* 128(9):2182–91.

LUK, SZE-UE, TERENCE KIN-WAH LEE, JI LIU, ET AL.

2011. Chemopreventative effect of PSP through targeting of prostate cancer stem cell-like population. *PLoS ONE* 6(5):e19804.

MA, YONGXIAN, PRAGATI KATIYAR, LAUNDETTE P. JONES, ET AL.

2006. The breast cancer susceptibility gene BRCA1 regulates progesterone receptor signaling in mammary epithelial cells. *Molecular Endocrinology* 20:14–34.

MAALOUF, MARWAN, JONG M. RHO, AND MARK P. MATTSON

2009. The neuroprotective properties of calorie restriction, the ketogenic diet, and ketone bodies. *Brain Research Reviews* 59(2):293–315.

MALET, CATHERINE, ANNE GOMPEL, POLI SPRITZER, ET AL.

1988. Tamoxifen and hydroxytamoxifen isomers versus estradiol effects on normal human breast cells in culture. *Cancer Research* 48(24 Pt 1):7193–99.

MALKIN C. J., P. J. PUGH, R. D. JONES, T. H. JONES, AND K. S. CHANNER

2003. Testosterone as a protective factor against atherosclerosis—Immunomodulation and influence upon plaque development and stability. *Journal of Endocrinology* 178(3):373–80.

MARTIKAINEN, PAULA AND JOHN ISAACS

1990. Role of calcium in the programmed cell death of rat prostatic glandular cells. *Prostate* 17(3):175–87.

MATTHEWS, JASON, AND JAN-ÅKE GUSTAFSSON

2003. Estrogen signaling: A subtle balance between ERα and ERβ *Molecular Interventions* 3(5):281–92.

MAYO CLINIC; MAYO MEDICAL LABORATORIES

N.d. Test ID: TTFB. testosterone, total, bioavailable, and free, serum. Web.

MCALLISTER, CARRIE, JIANGANG LONG, ADRIENNE BOWERS, ET AL.

2010. Genetic targeting aromatase in male amyloid precursor protein transgenic mice down-regulates β-secretase (BACE1) and prevents Alzheimer-like pathology and cognitive impairment. *Journal of Neuroscience* 30(21):7326–34.

MENDELSOHN, MICHAEL E., AND GIUSEPPE M. C. ROSANO

2003. Hormonal regulation of normal vascular tone in males. *Circulation Research* 93(12):1142–45.

MERCOLA, JOSEPH

2009a. Avoid routine mammograms if you are under 50. Web.

2009b. Little-known secrets about optimal iron levels. Web.

2010. Feeling fatigued or irritable? There's a 1 in 4 chance you suffer from this disease. September 02. Web.

2012. Little sunshine mistakes that can give you cancer instead of vitamin D. Web.

2013. How vitamin D performance testing can help you optimize your health, and aid the health freedom movement. Web.

MICHAELSON, JAMES S., ELKAN HALPERN, AND DANIEL B. KOPANS

1999. Breast cancer: Computer simulation method for estimating optimal intervals for screening, *Radiology* 212:551–60.

MILLION WOMEN STUDY COLLABORATORS

2003. Breast cancer and hormone-replacement therapy in the Million Women Study. *Lancet* 362(9382):419–27.

MINERS, JAMES SCOTT, ZOË VAN HELMOND, KATY CHALMERS, GORDON WILCOCK, SETH LOVE, AND PATRICK GAVIN KEHOE

2006. Decreased expression and activity of neprilysin in Alzheimer Disease are associated with cerebral amyloid angiopathy. *Journal of Neuropathology* 65(10):1012–21.

MIRKOVIC, NENA, DAVID W. VOEHRINGER, MICHAEL D. STORY, DAVID J. MCCONKEY, TIMOTHY J. MCDONNELL, AND RAYMOND E. MEYN

1997. Resistance to radiation-induced apoptosis in Bcl-2 expressing cells is reversed by depleting cellular thiols. *Oncogene* 15(12):1461–70.

MOFFAT, S. D., A. B. ZONDERMAN, E. J. METTER, ET AL.

2004. Free testosterone and risk for Alzheimer Disease in older men. *Neurology* 62(2):188–93.

MORGENTALER, ABRAHAM

2006. Testosterone and prostate cancer: An historical perspective on a modern myth. *European Urology* 50(5):935–39.

2008. *Testosterone for Life*. New York: McGraw-Hill.

MORGENTALER, ABRAHAM, AND EMANI LUIS RHODEN

2006. Prevalance of prostate cancer among hypogonadal men with prostate-specific antigen levels of 4.0 ng/mL or less. *Urology* 68(6):1263–67.

MORGENTALER, ABRAHAM, AND ABDULMAGED M. TRAISH

2009. Shifting the paradigm of testosterone and prostate cancer: The saturation model and the limits of androgen-dependent growth. *European Urology* 55(2):310–21.

MORGENTALER, ABRAHAM, LARRY I. LIPSHULTZ, RICHARD BENNETT, MICHAEL SWEENEY, DESIDERIO AVILA JR., AND MOHIT KHERA

2011. Testosterone therapy in men with untreated prostate cancer. *Journal of Urology* 185(4):1256–61.

MORINAGA, AKIYOSHI, MIE HIROHATA, KENJIRO ONO, AND MASAHITO YAMADA

2007. Estrogen has anti-amyloidogenic effects on Alzheimer's β-amyloid fibrils in vitro. *Biochemical and Biophysical Research Communications* 359(3):697–702.

MORRIS, MICHAEL J., DAISY HUANG, WILLIAM K. KELLY, ET AL.

2009. Phase 1 trial of high-dose exogenous testosterone in patients with castrate-resistant metastatic prostate cancer. *European Urology* 56(2):237–44.

MORSINK, LISETTE F., NICOLE VOGELSANGS, BARBARA J. NICKLAS, ET AL.

2007. Associations between sex steroid hormone levels and depressive symptoms in elderly men and women: Results from the health ABC study. *Psychoneuroendocrinology* 32(8–10):874–83.

MOSKOWITZ, DEBORAH

2006. A comprehensive review of the safety and efficacy of bioidentical hormones for the management of menopause and related health risks. *Alternative Medicine Review* 11(3):208–23.

MOSS, DAVID K., VIRGINIE M. BETIN, SOAZIG D. MALESINSKI, AND JON D. LANE
2006. A novel role for microtubules in apoptotic chromatin dynamics and cellular fragmentation. *Journal of Cell Science* 119(pt 11):2362–74.

MOTE, PATRICIA A., JENNIFER A. LEARY, KELLY A. AVERY, ET AL.
2004. Germ-line mutations in *BRCA1* or *BRCA2* in the normal breast are associated with altered expression of estrogen-responsive proteins and the predominance of progesterone receptor A. *Genes, Chromosomes & Cancer* 39:236–48.

MOYER, VIRGINIA A. AND ON BEHALF OF THE U.S. PREVENTIVE SERVICES TASK FORCE
2012. Screening for prostate cancer: U.S. Preventive Services Task Force Recommendation Statement. *Annals of Internal Medicine* 157(2):120–34.

MULLER, ROBERTO L., LEAH GERBER, DANIEL M. MOREIRA, GERALD ANDRIOLE, RAMIRO CASTRO-SANTAMARIA, AND STEPHEN J. FREEDLAND
2012. Serum testosterone and dihydrotestosterone and prostate cancer risk in the placebo arm of the reduction by dutasteride of Prostate Cancer Events Trial. *European Urology* 62(5):e83–e94.

MUNDHENKE, CRISTOPH, CHRISTIAN SCHEM, AND WALTER JONAT
2008. Adjuvant endocrine therapy in early postmenopausal breast cancer. *Breast Care* 3(5):317–24.

NAKAI, YASUTOMO, AND NORIO NONOMURA
2013. Inflammation and prostate carcinogenesis. *International Journal of Urology* 20(2):150–60.

NANDA, AKASH, MING-HUI CHEN, MICHELLE H. BRACCIOFORTE, BRIAN J. MORAN, AND ANTHONY V. D'AMICO
2009. Hormonal therapy use for prostate cancer and mortality in men with coronary heart failure or myocardial infarction. *JAMA* 302(8):866–73.

NANNI, SIMONA, MICHELA NARDUCCI, LINDA DELLA PIETRA, ET AL.
2002. Signaling through estrogen receptors modulates telomerase activity in human prostate cancer. *Journal of Clinical Investigation* 110(2):219–27.

NARVAEZ, CARMEN J., AND JOELLEN WELSH
2001. Role of mitochondria and caspases in vitamin D-mediated apoptosis of MCF-7 breast cancer cells. *Journal of Biological Chemistry* 276(12):9101–9107.

NATHAN, D. G., G. F. CAHILL JR., AND F. H. GARDNER
1963. The effect of large doses of testosterone on the body fat of elderly men. *Metabolism* 12:850–62.

NATHANSON, KATHERINE N.
2001. Breast cancer genetics: What we know and what we need. *Nature Medicine* 7:552–56.

NATIONAL CANCER INSTITUTE
N.d. BRCA1 and BRCA2: Cancer risk and genetic testing. Web.

NEKOLLA, E. A., J. GRIEBEL, AND G. BRIX

2008. [Radiation risk associated with mammography screening examinations for women younger than 50 years of age]. *Zeitschrift fürMedizinische Physik* 18(3):170–79.

NEYCHEV, V. K., AND V. I. MITEV

2005. The aphrodisiac herb Tribulus terrestris does not influence the androgen production in young men. *Journal of Ethnopharmacology* 101(1–3):319–23.

NIELSEN, JOHANNES, BJARNE PELSEN, AND KURT SØRENSEN

1988. Follow-up of 30 Klinefelter males treated with testosterone. *Clinical Genetics* 33(4):262–69.

NIESCHLAG, EBERHARD

1998. If testosterone, which testosterone? Which androgen regimen should be used for supplementation in older men? Formulation, dosing, and monitoring issues. *Journal of Clinical Endocrinology and Metabolism* 83:3443–45.

NIXON, RALPH A.

2000. A protease activation cascade in the pathogenesis of Alzheimer's Disease. *Annals of the New York Academy of Sciences* 924:117–31.

NOBLE, ROBERT L.

1977. The development of prostatic adenocarcinoma in Nb rats following prolonged sex hormone administration. *Cancer Research* 37(6):1929–33.

ONCOLINK.COM

2012. Aromatase inhibitor-related joint pain. Web.

ORSHAL, JULIA M., AND RAOUF A. KHALIL

2004. Gender, sex hormones, and vascular tone. *American Journal of Physiology–Regulatory, Integrative and Comparative Physiology* 286(2):R233–49.

PALACIOS, NATALIA, XIANG GAO, MARJORIE L. MCCULLOUGH, ET AL.

2012. Caffeine and risk of Parkinson's Disease in a large cohort of men and women. *Movement Disorders* 27(10):1276–82.

PANJARI, MARY, ROBIN J. BELL, FIONA JANE, JENNY ADAMS, CORALLEE MORROW, AND SUSAN R. DAVIS

2009. The safety of 52 weeks of oral DHEA therapy for postmenopausal women. *Maturitas* 63(3):240–45.

PAOLETTI, A. M., S. CONGIA, S. LELLO, ET AL.

2004. Low androgenization index in elderly women and men with Alzheimer's Disease. *Neurology* 62(2):301–303.

PAPADOPOULOU, NATALIA, IOANNIS CHARALAMPOPOULOS, VASILEIA ANAGNOSTOPOULOU, ET AL.

2008. Membrane androgen receptor activation triggers down-regulation of PI-3K/Akt/NF-kappaB activity and induces apoptotic responses via Bad, FasL and caspase-3 in DU145 prostate cancer cells. *Molecular Cancer* 7:88.

PAPADOPOULOU, NATALIA, EVANGELIA A. PAPAKONSTANTI, GALATEA KALLERGI, KONSTANTINOS ALEVIZOPOULOS, AND CHRISTOS STOURNARAS

2009. Membrane androgen receptor activation in prostate and breast tumor cells: Molecular signaling and clinical impact. *IUBMB Life* 61(1):56–61.

PAPASOZOMENOS, SOZOS CH., AND ALIKUNJU SHANAVAS

2002. Testosterone prevents the heat shock-induced overactivation of glycogen synthase kinase-3β but not of cyclin-dependent kinase 5 and c-Jun NH_2-terminal kinase and concomitantly abolishes hyperphosphorylation of τ: implications for Alzheimer's Disease. *PNAS* 99(3):1140–45.

PARKER-POPE, TARA

2011. *The Women's Health Initiative and the Body Politic.* Web.

PARSONS, J. KELLOGG, H. BALLENTINE CARTER, ELIZABETH A. PLATZ, E. JAMES WRIGHT, PATRICIA LANDIS, AND E. JEFFREY METTER

2005. Serum testosterone and the risk of prostate cancer: Potential implications for testosterone therapy. *Cancer Epidemiology, Biomarkers & Prevention* 14:2257–60.

PENGELLY, ANDREW, JAMES SNOW, SIMON Y. MILLS, ANDREW SCHOLEY, KEITH WESNES, AND LEAH REEVES BUTLER

2012. Short-term study on the effects of rosemary on cognitive function in elderly population. *Journal of Medicinal Food* 15(1):10–17.

PERMAN, CINDY

2012. Wall Street's secret weapon for getting an edge. Web.

PERRY, NICOLETTE S. L., CHLOE BOLLEN, ELAINE K. PERRY, AND CLIVE BALLARD

2003. Salvia for dementia therapy: Review of pharmacological activity and pilot tolerability clinical trial. *Pharmacology Biochemistry and Behavior* 75(3):651–59.

PETROVA, ROUMYANA D., SOLOMON P. WASSER, JAMAL A. MAHAJNA, CVETOMIR M. DENCHEV, AND EVIATAR NEVO

2005. Potential role of medicinal mushrooms in breast cancer treatment: Current knowledge and future perspectives. *International Journal of Medicinal Mushrooms* 7(1–2):141–56.

PHILLIPS, GERALD B., WILLIAM P. CASTELLI, ROBERT D. ABBOTT, AND PATRICIA M. MCNAMARA

1983. Association of hyperestrogenemia and coronary heart disease in men in the Framingham Cohort. *American Journal of Medicine* 74:863–69.

PICH, A., E. MARGARIA, L. CHIUSA, G. CANDELARESI, AND O. DAL CANTON

1999. Androgen receptor expression in male breast carcinoma: Lack of clinicopathological association. *British Journal of Cancer* 79:959–64.

PIJPE, ANOUK, NADINE ANDRIEU, DOUGLAS F. EASTON, ET AL.

2012. Exposure to diagnostic radiation and risk of breast cancer among carriers of BRCA1/2 mutations: Retrospective cohort study (GENE-RAD-RISK). *BMJ* 345:e5660.

PIRSKANEN, MIA, MIKKO HILTUNEN, ARTO MANNERMAA, ET AL.

2005. Estrogen receptor beta gene variants are associated with increased risk of Alzheimer's Disease in women. *European Journal of Human Genetics* 13(9):1000–1006.

PIZZORNO, LARA

2012. Progestin drugs: More side effects & risks. Web.

POOLE, ALEKSANDRA JOVANOVIC, YING LI, YOON KIM, SUH-CHIN J. LIN, WEN-HWA LEE, AND EVA Y.-H. P. LEE

2006. Prevention of *BRCA1*-mediated mammary tumorigenesis in mice by a progesterone antagonist. *Science* 314(5804):1467–70.

POPE, HARRISON G. JR., ELENA M. KOURI, AND JAMES I. HUDSON

2000. Effects of supraphysiologic doses of testosterone on mood and aggression in normal men: A randomized controlled trial. *Archives of General Psychiatry* 57(2):133–40.

POTOSKY, ARNOLD L., WILLIAM W. DAVIS, RICHARD M. HOFFMAN, ET AL.

2004. Five-year outcomes after prostatectomy or radiotherapy for prostate cancer: The prostate cancer outcomes study. *Journal of the National Cancer Institute* 96(18):1358–67.

POWERS, M. LINDA, AND JAMES R. FLORINI

1975. A direct effect of testosterone on muscle cells in tissue culture. *Endocrinology* 97(4):1043–47.

PRICE, DAVID, BARRY STEIN, PAUL SIEBER, ET AL.

2006. Toremifene for the prevention of prostate cancer in men with high grade intraepithelial neoplasia: Results of a double-blind placebo controlled, phase IIB clinical trial. *Journal of Urology* 176(3):965–71.

PRYSTUPA, ANDRZEJ, MONIKA WÓJTOWICZ, AGNIESZKA STYGAR, WOJCIECH GÓRSKI, PATRYCJA LACHOWSKA-KOTOWSKA, AND JERZY MOSIEWICZ.

2012. NSAID-induced acute liver failure—A case report. *Baltic Journal of Comparative & Clinical Systems Biology* 1:31–37.

RABKIN, JUDITH G., GLENN J. WAGNER, AND RICHARD RABKIN

1999. Testosterone therapy for human immunodeficiency virus-positive men with and without hypogonadism. *Journal of Clinical Psychopharmacology* 19(1):19–27.

RAFFO, ANTHONY J., HARRIS PERLMAN, MIN-WEI CHEN, MARK L. DAY, JACK S. STREITMAN, AND RALPH BUTTYAN

1995. Overexpression of Bcl-2 protects prostate cancer cells from apoptosis *in vitro* and confers resistance to androgen depletion *in vivo*. *Cancer Research* 55:4438–45.

RAHMAN, K. M. WAHIDUR, OLIVIA ARANHA, ALEXEY GLAZYRIN, SREENIVASA R. CHINNI, AND FAZLUL H. SARKAR

2000. Translocation of Bax to mitochondria induces apoptotic cell death in indole-3-carbinol (I3C) treated breast cancer cells. *Oncogene* 19(50):5764–71.

RAKHA, EMAD A., JORGE S. REIS-FILHO, AND IAN O. ELLIS

2008. Basal-like breast cancer: A critical review. *Journal of Clinical Oncology* 26(15):2568–81.

RAZANDI, MAHNAZ, ALI PEDRAM, ISTVAN MERCHENTHALER, GEOFFREY L. GREENE, AND ELLIS R. LEVIN

2004. Plasma membrane estrogen receptors exist and functions as dimers. *Molecular Endocrinology* 18:2854–65.

READY, R. E., J. FRIEDMAN, J. GRACE, AND H. FERNANDEZ

2004. Testosterone deficiency and apathy in Parkinson's Disease: A pilot study. *Journal of Neurology, Neurosurgery & Psychiatry* 75(9):1323–26.

REGER, MARK A., SAMUEL T. HENDERSON, CATHY HALE, ET AL.

2004. Effects of β-hydroxybutarate on cognition in memory-impaired adults. *Neurobiology of Aging* 25(3):311–14.

RICE, DONNA, ROBERT E. BRANNIGAN, R. KEITH CAMPBELL, ET AL.

2008. Men's health, low testosterone, and diabetes: Individualized treatment and a multidisciplinary approach. *Diabetes Educator* 34(suppl 5):97S–112S.

RICKE, WILLIAM A., STEPHEN J. MCPHERSON, JOSEPH J. BIANCO, GERALD R. CUNHA, YUZHUO WANG, AND GAIL P. RISBRIDGER

2008. Prostatic hormonal carcinogenesis is mediated by *in situ* estrogen production and estrogen receptor alpha signaling. *FASEB Journal* 22(5):1512–20.

RISBRIDGER, G. P., J. J. BIANCO, S. J. ELLEM, AND S. J. MCPHERSON

2003. Oestrogens and prostate cancer. *Endocrine-Related Cancer* 10(2):187–91.

RISBRIDGER, GAIL P., STUART J. ELLEM, AND STEPHEN J. MCPERSON

2007. Estrogen action on the prostate gland: A critical mix of endocrine and paracrine signaling. *Journal of Molecular Endocrinology* 39(3):183–88.

RODDAM, A. W., N. E. ALLEN, P. APPLEBY, AND T. J. KEY

2008. Endogenous sex hormones and prostate cancer: A collaborative analysis of 18 prospective studies. *Journal of the National Cancer Institute* 100(3):170–83.

ROGERS, GARY S., ROBERT L. VAN DE CASTLE, WILLIAM S. EVANS, AND JOSEPH W. CRITELLI

1985. Vaginal pulse amplitude response patterns during erotic conditions and sleep. *Archives of Sexual Behavior* 14(4):327–42.

ROLF, C., S. VON ECKARDSTEIN, U. KOKEN, AND E. NIESCHLAG

2002. Testosterone substitution of hypogonadal men prevents the age-dependent increases in body mass index, body fat and leptin seen in healthy ageing men: Results of a cross-sectional study. *European Journal of Endocrinology* 146(4):505–11.

ROSANO, GIUSEPPE M. C., FILIPPO LEONARDO, PAOLO PAGNOTTA, ET AL.

1999. Acute anti-ischemic effect of testosterone in men with coronary artery disease. *Circulation* 99(13):1666–70.

ROSENBERG, LENA U., CECILIA MAGNUSSON, EMMA LINDSTRÖM, SARA WEDRÉN, PER HALL, AND PAUL W. DICKMAN

2006. Menopausal hormone therapy and other breast cancer risk factors in relation to the risk of differential histological subtypes of breast cancer: A case-control study. *Breast Cancer Research* 8(1):R11.

ROSSOR, MARTIN NEIL

2003. How to write a case report. In *How to Write a Paper*, pp. 85–91. 3rd edition. Edited by George M. Hall. London: BMJ Books.

ROSSOUW, J. E., G. L. ANDERSON, R. L. PRENTICE, ET AL.

2002. Risks and benefits of estrogen plus progestin in healthy postmenopausal women: Principal results from the Women's Health Initiative Randomized Controlled Trial. *JAMA* 288(3):321–33.

ROUNDY, J. N., J. S. TURNER, AND R. L. LEIBOWITZ

2011. Primary triple androgen blockade (TAB) followed by finasteride maintenance (FM) for clinically localized prostate cancer (CL-PC): Ten year follow-up. *Journal of Clinical Oncology* 29(15_suppl):e15198.

RUSANEN, MINNA, MILO KIVIPELTO, CHARLES P. QUESENBERRY JR., JUFEN ZHOU, AND RACHEL A. WHITMER

2011. Heavy smoking in midlife and long-term risk of Alzheimer Disease and vascular dementia. *Archives of Internal Medicine* 171(4):333–39.

SAAD, FARID, AND LOUIS J. GOOREN

2011. The role of testosterone in the etiology and treatment of obesity, the metabolic syndrome, and diabetes mellitus type 2. *Journal of Obesity*, Article ID 471584, doi:10.1155/2011/471584.

SABOURIN, J. C., A. MARTIN, J. BARUCH, T. B. TRUC, A. GOMPEL, AND P. POITOUT

1994. Bcl-2 expression in normal breast tissue during the menstrual cycle. *International Journal of Cancer* 59:1–6.

SAHAY, R. K., A. G. UNNIKRISHNAN, S. K. BHADADA, AND J. K. AGRAWAL

2002. Hormone receptor disorders. *Journal, Indian Academy of Clinical Medicine* 3(1):65–80.

SAHELIAN, RAY

1997. *Pregnenolone: Nature's Feel Good Hormone.* Garden City Park, NY: Avery Publishing Group.

SAKR, W. A., G. P. HAAS, B. F. CASSIN, J. E. PONTES, AND J. D. CRISSMAN

1993. The frequency of carcinoma and intraepithelial neoplasia of the prostate in young male patients. *Journal of Urology* 150(2 pt 1):379–85.

SAKR, W. A., D. J. GRIGNON, J. D. CRISSMAN, ET AL.

1994. High grade prostatic intraepithelial neoplasia (HGPIN) and prostatic adenocarcinoma between the ages of 20–69: An autopsy study of 249 cases. *In Vivo* 8(3):439–43.

SALAM, RANABIR, ACHOUBA SINGH KSHETRIMAYUM, AND REETU KEISAM

2012. Testosterone and metabolic syndrome: The link. *Indian Journal of Endocrinology and Metabolism* 16(suppl 1):S12–S19.

SALOM, JUAN B., MARIA C. BURGUETE, FERNANDO J. PÉREZ-ASENSIO, GERMÁN TORREGROSA, AND ENRIQUE ALBORCH

2001. Relaxant effects of 17-β-estradiol in cerebral arteries through Ca^{2+} entry inhibition. *Journal of Cerebral Blood Flow & Metabolism* 21(4):422–29.

SANTEN, RICHARD J., WEI YUE, AND DANIEL F. HEITAN

2012. Modeling of the growth kinetics of occult breast tumors: Role in interpretation of studies of prevention and menopausal hormone therapy. *Cancer Epidemiology, Biomarkers & Prevention* 21(7):1038–48.

SAPUTO, LEN

2011. The FDA assaults breast thermography while protecting mammography industry. Web.

SARTORIUS, CAROL A., STEVE D. GROSHONG, LOUISE A. MILLER, ET AL.

1994. New T74D breast cancer cell lines for the independent study of progesterone receptor B- and A-receptors: Only antiprogestin-occupied B-receptors are switched to transcriptional agonists by cAMP. *Cancer Research* 54(14):3868–77.

SCARLATTI, FRANCESCA, GIUSY SALA, GIULIA SOMENZI, PAOLA SIGNORELLI, NICOLETTA SACCHI, AND RICCARDO GHIDONI

2003. Resveratrol induces growth inhibition and apoptosis in metastatic breast cancer cells via de novo ceramide signaling. *FASEB Journal* 17(15):2339–41.

SCHUTTER, DENNIS J. L. G., JISKA S. PEPER, HANS P. F. KOPPESCHAAR, RENÉ S. KAHN, AND JACK VAN HONK

2005. Administration of testosterone increases functional connectivity in a cortico-cortical depression circuit. *Journal of Neuropsychiatry and Clinical Neurosciences*17(3):372–77.

SCOTT, I. S., H. M. CHARLTON, B. S. COX, C. A. GROCOCK, J. W. SHEFFIELD, AND P. J. O'SHAUGHNESSY

1990. Effect of LH injections on testicular steroidogenesis, cholesterol side-chain cleavage P450 mRNA content and Leydig cell morphology in hypogonadal mice. *Journal of Endocrinology* 125(1):131–38.

SEIDMAN, STUART N., ANDRE B. ARAUJO, STEVEN P. ROOSE, AND JOHN B. MCKINLAY

2001. Testosterone level, androgen receptor polymorphism, and depressive symptoms in middle-aged men. *Biological Psychiatry* 50(5):371–76.

SEKINE, YOSHITAKA, KAZUTO ITO, TAKUMI YAMAMOTO, ET AL.

2007. Pretreatment total testosterone levels in patients with prostate cancer in the past two decades in Japan. *Cancer Detection and Prevention* 31:149–53.

SHAABAN, ABEER M., PENNY A. O'NEILL, MICHAEL P. A. DAVIES, ET AL.
2003. Declining estrogen receptor-[beta] expression defines malignant progression of human breast neoplasia. *American Journal of Surgical Pathology* 27(12):1502–12.

SHANKLE, WILLIAM RODMAN, AND DANIEL G. AMEN
2005. *Preventing Alzheimer's: Ways to Help Prevent, Delay, Detect, and Even Halt Alzheimer's Disease and Other Forms of Memory Loss.* NY: Perigee.

SHIBAYAMA, YUJIN, TATSUYA HIGASHI, KAZUTAKE SHIMADA, ET AL.
2009. Simultaneous determination of salivary testosterone dehydroepiandrosterone using LC-MS/MS method development and evaluation of applicability for diagnosis and medication for late-onset hypogonadism. *Journal of Chromatography B: Analytical Technologies in the Biomedical and Life Sciences* 877(25):2615–23.

SHOGO, ICHII, ENRICO FORCHIELLI, AND RALPH I. DORFMAN
1963. In vitro effect of gonadotropins on the soluble cholesterol side-chain cleaving enzyme system of bovine corpus luteum. *Steroids* 2(6):631–56.

SHORES, MOLLY M., ALVIN M. MATSUMOTO, KEVIN L. SLOAN, AND DANIEL R. KIVLAHAN
2006. Low serum testosterone and mortality in male veterans. *Archives of Internal Medicine* 166:1660–65.

SHRIVASTAVA, ASHUTOSH, MEENAKSHI TIWARI, ROHIT A. SINHA, ET AL.
2006. Molecular iodine induces caspase-independent apoptosis in human breast carcinoma cells involving the mitochondria-mediated pathway. *Journal of Biological Chemistry* 281(28):19762–771.

SHUMAKER, S. A., C. LEGAULT, S. R. RAPP, ET AL.
2003. Estrogen plus progestin and the incidence of dementia and mild cognitive impairment in postmenopausal women. *JAMA* 289:2651–62.

SHUMAKER, SALLY A., CLAUDINE LEGAULT, LEWIS KULLER, ET AL.
2004. Conjugated equine estrogens and incidence of probable dementia and mild cognitive impairment in postmenopausal women. *JAMA* 291(24):2947–58.

SIERI, SABINA, VITTORIO KROGH, GIANFRANCO BOLELLI, ET AL.
2009. Sex hormone levels, breast cancer risk, and cancer receptor status in postmenopausal women: The ORDET cohort. *Cancer Epidemiology, Biomarkers & Prevention* 18:169–76.

SIEVERS, CAROLINE, JENS KLOTSCHE, LARS PIEPER, ET AL.
2010. Low testosterone levels predict all-cause mortality and cardiovascular events in women: A prospective cohort study in German primary care patients. *European Journal of Endocrinology* 163(4):699–708.

SIMPSON, EVAN R., COLIN CLYNE, GARY RUBIN, ET AL.
2002. Aromatase—A brief overview. *Annual Review of Physiology* 64:93–127.

SIMPSON, KATHERINE
2001. The role of testosterone in aggression. *McGill Journal of Medicine* 6:32–40.

SINGH, P., A. UZGARE, I. LITVINOV, S. R. DENMEADE, AND J. T. ISAACS

2006. Combinatorial androgen receptor targeted therapy for prostate cancer. *Endocrine-Related Cancer* 13(3):653–66.

SINGH, VIJENDRA K., AND JEFF HANSON

2006. Assessment of metallothionein and antibodies to metallothionein in normal and autistic children having exposure to vaccine-derived thimerosal. *Pediatric Allergy and Immunology* 17(4):291–96.

SISSON, MARK

2012. *The Primal Blueprint.* 2nd edition. Malibu, CA: Primal Nutrition, Inc.

SLAMON, DENNIS J., BRIAN LEYLAND-JONES, STEVEN SHAK, ET AL.

2001. Use of chemotherapy plus a monoclonal antibody against HER2 for metastatic breast cancer that overexpresses HER2. *NEJM* 344(11):783–92.

SMITH, IAN E., AND MITCH DOWSETT

2003. Aromatase inhibitors in breast cancer. *NEJM* 348(24):2431–42.

SMITH, ROY G.

2000. The aging process: Where are the drug opportunities? *Current Opinion in Chemical Biology* 4(4):371–76.

SMITH-WARNER, STEPHANIE A., DONNA SPIEGELMAN, SHIAW-SHYUAN YAUN, ET AL.

1998. Alcohol and breast cancer in women: A pooled analysis of cohort studies. *JAMA* 279(7):535–40.

SOMERS, SUZANNE

2006. *Ageless: The Naked Truth about Bioidentical Hormones.* NY: Crown.

2009. *Knockout: Interviews with Doctors Who Are Curing Cancer—and How to Prevent Getting It in the First Place.* NY: Crown.

2012. *Bombshell: Explosive Medical Secrets That Will Redefine Aging.* NY: Crown.

SONG, LIANG-NIAN, MEGHAN COGHLAN, AND EDWARD P. GELMANN

2004. Antiandrogen effects of mifepristone on coactivator and corepressor interactions with the androgen receptor. *Molecular Endocrinology* 18(1):70–85.

SPARKS, B. F., S. D. FRIEDMAN, D. W. SHAW, ET AL.

2002. Brain structural abnormalities in young children with autism spectrum disorder. *Neurology* 59(2):184–92.

SPIES, P. E., D. SLATS, J. M. C. SJOGREN, ET AL.

2010. The cerebrospinal fluid amyloid β42/40 ratio in the differentiation of Alzheimer's Disease from non-Alzheimer's dementia. *Current Alzheimer Research* 7(5):470–76.

SPRATT, JOHN S. JR., MARY LOU KALTENBACH, AND JOHN A. SPRATT

1977. Cytokinetic definition of acute and chronic breast cancer, *Cancer Research* 37:226–30.

ST-ONGE, MARIE-PIERRE, AND AUBREY BOSARGE

2008. Weight-loss diet that includes consumption of medium-chain triacylglycerol oil leads to a greater rate of weight and fat mass loss than does olive oil. *American Journal of Clinical Nutrition* 87(3):621–26.

St-Onge, Marie-Pierre, Aubrey Bosarge, Laura Lee T. Goree, and Betty Darnell
2008. Medium chain triglyceride oil consumption as part of a weight loss diet does not lead to an adverse metabolic profile when compared to olive oil. *Journal of the American College of Nutrition* 27(5):547–52.

Stambolsky, Perry, Yuval Tabach, Giullia Fontemaggi, et al.
2010. Modulation of the vitamin D3 response by cancer-associated mutant p53. *Cancer Cell* 17(3):273–85.

Stathopoulos, Efstathios N., Constantina Dambaki, Marilena Kampa, et al.
2003. Membrane androgen binding sites are preferentially expressed in human prostate carcinoma cells. *BMC Clinical Pathology* 3:1.

Stefanick, Marcia L., Garnet L. Anderson, Karen L. Margolis, et al.
2006. Effects of conjugated equine estrogens on breast cancer and mammography screening in postmenopausal women with hysterectomy. *JAMA* 295(14):1647–57.

Stomati, Massimo, Francesca Bernardi, Stefano Luisi, et al.
2002. Conjugated equine estrogens, estrone sulfate and estradiol valerate oral administration in ovariectomized rats: Effects on central and peripheral allopregnanolone and β-endorphin. *Maturitas* 43(3):195–206.

Sun, Tong, Gwo-Shu Mary Lee, William K. Oh, et al.
2010. Single-nucleotide polymorphisms in p53 pathway and aggressiveness of prostate cancer in a Caucasian population. *Clinical Cancer Research* 16(21):5244–51.

Swerdloff, Ronald S., Christina Wang, Glenn Cunningham, et al.
2000. Long-term pharmacokinetics of transdermal gel in hypogonadal men. *Journal of Clinical Endocrinology & Metabolism* 85(12):4500–10.

Syed, G. M. S., S. Eagger, J. O'Brien, J. J. Barrett, and R. Levy
1992. Patterns of regional cerebral blood flow in Alzheimer's Disease. *Nuclear Medicine Communications* 13(9):656–63.

Szelei, Jozsef, Jesus Jimenez, Ana M. Soto, Maria F. Luizzi, and Carlos Sonnenschein
1997. Androgen-induced inhibition of proliferation in human breast cancer MCF7 cells transfected with androgen receptor. *Endocrinology* 38(4):1406–12.

Szmulewitz, Russell, Supriya Mohile, Edwin Posadas, et al.
2009. A randomized phase 1 study of testosterone replacement for patients with low-risk castration-resistant prostate cancer. *European Urology* 56(1):97–103.

Tai, Patricia, Edward Yu, Vincent Vinh-Hung, Gábor Cserni, and Georges Vlastos
2004. Survival of patients with metastatic breast cancer: Twenty-year data from two SEER registries. *BMC Cancer* 4:60.

Takahashi, Kentaro, Masako Okada, Tomoya Ozaki, et al.
2000. Safety and efficacy of oestriol for symptoms of natural or surgically induced menopause. *Human Reproduction* 15(5):1028–36.

TAKEDA, HIDEO, KOICHIRO AKAKURA, MOTOYUKI MASAI, SUSUMU AKIMOTO, RYUICHI YATANI, AND JUN SHIMAZAKI

1996. Androgen receptor content of prostate carcinoma cells estimated by immunohistochemistry is related to prognosis of patients with stage D2 prostate carcinoma. *Cancer* 77:934–40.

TAMBI, MOHD ISMAIL BIN MOHD, AND M. KAMARUL IMRAN

2010. *Eurycoma longifolia* Jack in managing idiopathic male infertility. *Asian Journal of Andrology* 12(3):376–80.

TAMIMI, R., L. A. MUCCI, E. SPANOS, A. LAGIOU, V. BENETOU, AND D. TRICHOPOULOS

2001. Testosterone and oestradiol in relation to tobacco smoking, body mass index, energy consumption and nutrient intake among adult men. *European Journal of Cancer Prevention* 10(3):275–80.

TAMIMI, RULLA M., SUSAN E. HANKINSON, WENDY Y. CHEN, BERNARD ROSNER, AND GRAHAM A. COLDITZ

2006. Combined estrogen and testosterone use and risk of breast cancer in postmenopausal women. *Archives of Internal Medicine* 166:1483–89.

TAUBES, GARY

2007. *Good Calories, Bad Calories: Challenging the Conventional Wisdom on Diet, Weight Control, and Disease.* NY: Knopf.

TAYLOR , RENEA A., ROXANNE TOLVANEN, AND GAIL P. RISBRIDGER

2010. Stem cells in prostate cancer: Treating the root of the problem. *Endocrine-Related Cancer* 17:R273–85.

TAYLOR , RENEA A., ROXANNE TOLVANEN, MARK FRYDENBERG, ET AL.

2012. Human epithelial basal cells are cells of origin of prostate cancer, independent of CD133 status. *Stem Cells* 30:1087–96.

TERBURG, DAVID, BARAK MORGAN, AND JACK VAN HONK

2009. The testosterone–cortisol ratio: A hormonal marker for proneness to social aggression. *International Journal of Law and Psychiatry* 32(4):216–23.

THEORET, MARC R., YANG-MIN NING, JENNY J. ZHANG, ROBERT JUSTICE, PATRICIA KEEGAN, AND RICHARD PAZDUR

2011. The risks and benefits of 5-α reductase inhibitors for prostate-cancer prevention. *NEJM* 365(2):97–99.

TIESZEN, CHELSEA R., ALICIA A. GOYENECHE, BREEANN N. BRANDHAGEN, CASEY T. ORTBAHN, AND CARLOS M. TELLERIA

2011. Antiprogestin mifepristone inhibits the growth of cancer cells of reproductive and non-reproductive origin regardless of progesterone receptor expression. *BMC Cancer* 11:207.

TORKLER, SARAH, HENRI WALLASCHOFSKI, SEBASTIAN E. BAUMEISTER, ET AL.

2011. Inverse association between total testosterone concentrations, incident hypertension and blood pressure. *Aging Male* 14(3):176–82.

TRAINOR, BRIAN C., KELLY M. GREIWE, AND RANDY J. NELSON

2006. Individual differences in estrogen receptor α in select brain nuclei are associated with individual differences in aggression. *Hormones and Behavior* 50(2):338–45.

TUOHIMAA, PENTTI, EERO PUKKALA, GHISLAINE SCÉLO, ET AL.

2007. Does solar exposure, as indicated by the non-melanoma skin cancers, protect from solid cancers: Vitamin D as a possible explanation. *European Journal of Cancer* 43(11):1701–12.

TURAN, V. K., R. I. SANCHEZ, J. J. LI, ET AL.

2004. The effects of steroidal estrogens in ACI rat mammary carcinogenesis: 17β-estradiol 2-hydroxyestradiol 4-hydroxyestradiol 16α-hydroxyestradiol, and 4-hydroxyestrone. *Journal of Endocrinology* 183:91–99.

TYLER, SUSAN J., DAVID DAWBARN, GORDON K. WILCOCK, AND SHELLEY J. ALLEN

2002. α- and β-secretase: Profound changes in Alzheimer's Disease. *Biochemical and Biophysical Research Communications* 299(3):373–76.

UMEKITA, YOSHIHISA, RICHARD A. HIIPAKKA, JOHN M. KOKONTIS, AND SHUTSUNG LIAO

1996. Human prostate tumor growth in athymic mice: Inhibition by androgens and stimulation by finasteride. *PNAS* 93(21):11802–11807.

URBAN, I. J. A., J. P. H. BURBACH, AND D. DE WIED (EDS.)

1998. *Advances in Brain Vasopressin.* Amsterdam and NY: Elsevier 1998.

VAN DER AUWERA, INGRID, STEFAAN WERA, FRED VAN LEUVEN, AND SAMUEL T. HENDERSON

2005. A ketogenic diet reduces amyloid beta 40 and 42 in a mouse model of Alzheimer's Disease. *Nutrition & Metabolism* 2:28.

VAN HONK, JACK, JISKA S. PEPER, AND DENNIS J. L. G. SCHUTTER

2005. Testosterone reduces unconscious fear but not consciously experienced anxiety: Implications for the disorders of fear and anxiety. *Biological Psychiatry* 58(3):218–25.

VAN LANDEGHEM, A. A. J., J. POORTMAN, M. NABUURS, AND J. H. H. THIJSSEN

1985. Endogenous concentration and subcellular distribution of estrogens in normal and malignant human breast tissue. *Cancer Research* 45(6): 2900–2906.

VAN WINGEN, GUIDO A., STAS A. ZYLICZ, SARA PIETERS, ET AL.

2009. Testosterone increases amygdala reactivity in middle-aged women to a young adulthood level. *Neuropsychopharmacology* 34(3):539–47.

VENKATESWARAN, VASUNDARA, AHMED Q. HADDAD, NEIL E. FLESHNER, ET AL.

2007. Association of diet-induced hyperinsulinemia with accelerated growth of prostate cancer (LNCaP) xenografts. *Journal of the National Cancer Institute* 99(23):1793–1800.

VERMEERSCH, HANS, GUY T'SJOEN, JEAN MARC KAUFMAN, JOHN VINCKE, AND MIEKE VAN HOUTTE

2010. Testosterone, androgen receptor gene CAG repeat length, mood and behaviour in adolescent males. *European Journal of Endocrinology* 163(2):319–28.

VERONESI, ANDREA, CLELIA DE GIACOMI, MARIA D. MAGRI, ET AL.

2005. Familial breast cancer: Characteristics and outcome of BRCA1-2 positive and negative cases. *BMC Cancer* 5:70.

VINCENT, BRUNO, AND PIYARAT GOVITRAPONG

2011. Activation of the α-secretase processing of AβPP as a therapeutic approach in Alzheimer's Disease. *Journal of Alzheimer's Disease* 24(S2):75–94.

VUCENIK, IVANA, AND ABULKALAM M. SHAMSUDDIN

2003. Cancer inhibition by inositol hexaphosphate (IP_6) and inositol: From laboratory to clinic. *Journal of Nutrition* 133(11):3778S–84S.

VUCENIK, IVANA, GAYATRI RAMAKRISHNA, KWANCHANIT TANTIVEJKUL, LUCY M. ANDERSON, AND DANICA RAMLJAK

2005. Inositol hexaphosphate (IP_6) blocks proliferation of human breast cancer cells through a PKCδ-dependent increase in p27 ^{Kip1} and decrease in retinoblastoma protein (pRb) phosphorylation. *Breast Cancer Research and Treatment* 91(1):35–45.

WAGNER, G. J., J. G. RABKIN, AND R. RABKIN

1998. Testosterone as a treatment for fatigue in HIV+ men. *General Hospital Psychiatry* 20(4):209–13.

WALKER, TAYLOR C.

1942. Use of testosterone propionate and estrogenic substance in treatment of essential hypertension, angina pectoris and peripheral vascular disease. *Journal of Clinical Endocrinology & Metabolism* 2(9):560–68.

WALSH, WILLIAM J., ANJUM USMAN, AND JEFFREY TARPEY

2001. Disordered metal metabolism in a large autism population. *Presented at the APA Annual Meeting, May 2001, New Orleans.* Web.

WANG, CHRISTINA, GERIANNE ALEXANDER, NANCY BERMAN, ET AL.

1996. Testosterone replacement therapy improves mood in hypogonadal men—A clinical research center study. *Journal of Clinical Endocrinology & Metabolism* 81(10): 3578–83.

WANG, CHRISTINA, RONALD S. SWERDLOFF, ALI IRANMANESH, ET AL.

2000. Transdermal testosterone gel improves sexual function, mood, muscle strength, and body composition parameters in hypogonadal men. *Journal of Clinical Endocrinology & Metabolism* 85(8):2839–53.

WANG, CHRISTINA, GLENN CUNNINGHAM, ADRIAN DOBS, ET AL.

2004. Long-term testosterone gel (AndroGel) treatment maintains beneficial effects on sexual function and mood, lean and fat mass, and bone mineral density in hypogonadal men. *Journal of Clinical Endocrinology & Metabolism* 89(5):2085–98.

WANG, THOMAS T. Y., TAMARO S. HUDSON, TIEN-CHUNG WANG, ET AL.

2008. Differential effects of resveratrol on androgen-responsive LNCaP human prostate cancer cells *in vitro* and *in vivo*. *Carcinogenesis* 29(10):2001–10.

WEBB, CARYOLYN M., AND PETER COLLINS

2010. Testosterone and coronary artery disease in men. *Maturitas* 67(1):15–19.

WEIHUA, ZHANG, MARGARET WARNER, AND JAN-ÅKE GUSTAFSSON

2002. Estrogen receptor beta in the prostate. *Molecular and Cellular Endocrinology* 193(1–2):1–5.

WHITE, RALPH W. DEVERE, ALEXANDER TSODIKOV, ESCHELLE C. STAPP, STEPHANIE E. SOARES, HAJIME FUJII, AND ROBERT M. HACKMAN

2010. Effects of a high dose, aglycone-rich soy extract on prostate specific antigen and serum isoflavone concentrations in men with localized prostate cancer. *Nutrition and Cancer* 62(8):1036–43.

WHITE, STEVEN R., PAULA WILLIAMS, KIMBERLY R. WOJCIK, ET AL.

2001. Initiation of apoptosis by actin cytoskeletal derangement in human airway epithelial cells. *American Journal of Respiratory Cell and Molecular Biology* 24(3):282–94.

WIEBE, JOHN P., DAVID MUZIA, JUNCAI HU, DAVID SZWAJCER, SCOTT A. HILL, AND JENNIFER L. SEACHRIST

2000. The 4-pregnene and 5α-pregnane progesterone metabolites formed in nontumorous and tumorous breast tissue have opposite effects on breast cell proliferation and adhesion. *Cancer Research* 60(4):936–43.

WIEBE, JOHN P.

2006. Progesterone metabolites in breast cancer. *Endocrine-Related Cancer* 13(3):717–38.

WILBERT, DIRK M., JAMES E. GRIFFIN, AND JEAN D. WILSON

1983. Characterization of the cytosol androgen receptor of the human prostate. *Journal of Clinical Endocrinology and Metabolism* 56:113–20.

WILLIAMS, MARO R. I., TYE DAWOOD, SHANHONG LING, ET AL.

2004. Dehydroepiandrosterone increases endothelial cell proliferation *in vitro* and improves endothelial function *in vivo* by mechanisms independent of androgen and estrogen receptors. *Journal of Clinical Endocrinology & Metabolism* 89(9):4708–15.

WINGFIELD, JOHN C., IGNACIO T. MOORE. WOLFGANG GOYMANN, DOUGLAS W. WACKER, & TODD SPERRY.

2006. Contexts and ethology of vertebrate aggression: Implications for the evolution of hormone-behavior interactions. In *Biology of Aggression,* edited by Randy Joe Nelson, pp. 179–210. Oxford and NY: Oxford University Press.

WORTHMAN, CAROL M., AND JOY F. STALLINGS

1997. Hormone measures in finger-prick blood spot samples: New field methods for reproductive endocrinology. *American Journal of Physical Anthropology* 104:1–21.

WRIGHT, JONATHAN V., AND LANE LENARD

2001. *Why Stomach Acid Is Good for You: Natural Relief from Heartburn, Indigestion, Reflux & GERD*. Lanham, MD: M. Evans.

WRIGHT, JONATHAN V.

2011. Skin cancer's top ally isn't what you think . . . Unlock the secret weapons in warding off even deadly melanoma. Web.

YANG, CHIH-MIN, YA-LING LU, HUEL-YAN CHEN, AND MIAO-LIN HU

2012. Lycopene and the LXRα agonist T0901317 synergistically inhibit the proliferation of androgen-independent prostate cancer cells via the PPARγ- LXRα-ABCA1 pathway. *Journal of Nutritional Biochemistry* 23(9):1155–62.

YEAP, B. B.

2009. Are declining testosterone levels a major risk factor for ill-health in aging men? *International Journal of Impotence Research* 21(1):24–36.

YOUNG, L. J., Z. WANG, T. T. COOPER, AND H. ELLIOTT ALBERS

2000. Vasopressin (V1a) receptor binding, mRNA expression and transcriptional regulation by androgen in the Syrian hamster brain. *Journal of Neuroendocrinology* 12(12):1179–85.

YU, SHAN, YAN ZHANG, MONG-TING YUEN, CHANG ZOU, DAVID DANIELPOUR, AND FRANKY L. CHAN

2011. 17-beta-estradiol induces neoplastic transformation in prostatic epithelial cells. *Cancer Letters* 304(1):8–20.

YU, WEIPING, MARIA SIMMONS-MENCHACA, ABDUL GAPOR, BOB G. SANDERS, AND KIMBERLY KLINE

1999. Induction of apoptosis in human breast cancer cells by tocopherols and tocotrienols. *Nutrition and Cancer* 33(1):26–32.

ZAHL, PER-HENRIK, PETER C. GETZSCHE, AND JAN MAEHLEN

2011. Natural history of breast cancers detected in the Swedish Mammography Screening Programme: A cohort study. *Lancet Oncology* 12(12):1118–1124.

ZAMOSKY, LISA

N.d. 7 Myths about Alzheimer's Disease. *WebMD*. Web.

ZASLOFF MICHAEL M.

2005. Sunlight, vitamin D, and the innate immune defenses of the human skin. *Journal of Investigative Dermatology* 125(5):xvi–xvii.

ZHANG, MIN, JIAN HUANG, XING XIE, AND C. D'ARCY J. HOLMAN

2009. Dietary intakes of mushrooms and green tea combine to reduce the risk of breast cancer in Chinese women. *International Journal of Cancer* 124(6):1404–1408.

ZHOU, JIANFENG, BILGIN GURATES, SIJUN YANG, SIBY SEBASTIAN, AND SERDAR E. BULUN

2001. Malignant breast epithelial cells stimulate aromatase expression via promoter II in human adipose fibroblasts: An epithelial-stromal interaction in breast tumors mediated by CCAAT/enhancer binding protein β. *Cancer Research* 61:2328–34.

ZHU, BAO TING, GUI-ZHEN HAN, JOONG-YOUN SHIM, YUJING WEN, AND XIANG-RONG JIANG

2006. Quantitative structure-activity relationship of various endogenous estrogen metabolites for human estrogen receptor α and β subtypes: Insights into the structural determinants favoring a differential subtype binding. *Endocrinology* 147(9):4132–50.

ZIETMAN, ANTHONY L.

1999. Consensus statements on radiation therapy of prostate cancer: Guidelines for radiation therapy with rising prostate-specific antigen levels after radical prostatectomy. *Journal of Clinical Oncology* 17(4):1155–63.

ZITMANN M., M. WECKESSER, O. SCHOBER, AND E. NIESCHLAG

2001. Changes in cerebral glucose metabolism and visuospatial capability in hypogonadal males under testosterone substitution therapy. *Experimental and Clinical Endocrinology & Diabetes* 109(5):302–304.

INDEX

Page numbers in *italic* refer to figures, charts, or captions; **bold** indicates important references.

ABBREVIATIONS USED IN THIS INDEX

BCa = breast cancer
PCa = prostate cancer
n = endnote
T = testosterone

ABOUT THE AUTHORS

Edward Friedman, PhD, is regarded as the world's foremost authority on models explaining how hormone receptors affect prostate cancer. Author of numerous articles about the relationship between hormones, hormone receptors, and disease, he earned his BA at Brown University and a PhD in biophysics and theoretical biology from the University of Chicago, where he currently works.

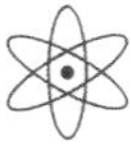

William Cane is the bestselling author of *Clubhouse Confidential* (with Luis Castillo), and *The Art of Kissing*. A former trial attorney, he taught English at Boston College and CUNY for two decades.